Self-Assessment Color Review

Canine Infectious Diseases

Self-Assessment Color Review

Canine Infectious Diseases

Katrin Hartmann
Professor Dr med vet, Dr habil
Diplomate ECVIM-CA (Internal Medicine)
Head of the Clinic of Small Animal Medicine
Centre for Clinical Veterinary Medicine
Ludwig Maximilian University Munich, Germany

Jane Sykes
BVSc, PhD
Diplomate ACVIM (Small Animal Internal Medicine)
Professor of Small Animal Internal Medicine
School of Veterinary Medicine
University of California-Davis, USA

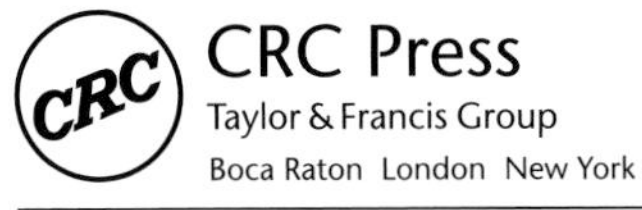

CRC Press
Taylor & Francis Group
Boca Raton London New York

CRC Press is an imprint of the
Taylor & Francis Group, an **informa** business

CRC Press
Taylor & Francis Group
6000 Broken Sound Parkway NW, Suite 300
Boca Raton, FL 33487-2742

Printed and bound in India by Replika Press Pvt. Ltd.

Printed on acid-free paper

International Standard Book Number-13: 978-1-4822-2515-0 (Paperback)

Visit the Taylor & Francis Web site at
http://www.taylorandfrancis.com

and the CRC Press Web site at
http://www.crcpress.com

Contents

Preface

Infectious diseases are very common in companion animals and the dog is at the forefront of emerging and newly discovered infections. Dogs also have been implicated in zoonoses and the spread of infections to and from wildlife.

In this book, we have provided an overview of canine infectious diseases in a case-based manner in the way clinicians encounter them in daily practice all over the globe. Because of the global nature of the case descriptions, several unique cases and images that have not been published elsewhere in the scientific literature can be found in this book. We hope this practice-oriented approach motivates the reader to contemplate the cases and to reflect on how they might have managed each case themselves.

The book was created for veterinary practitioners and veterinary students during their clinical rotations, to improve and practice their knowledge of infectious diseases. At the end of every case, questions for self-assessment by the reader are provided to test existing knowledge. The illustrations that accompany each case will help the reader to identify both classical and unique disease presentations.

We are very grateful for the expertise and hard work of all our co-authors. Further, we are extremely thankful to Monika Freisl for her hard work in providing the final editing of case descriptions and for acting as a point of liaison with co-authors. We would also like to thank the whole team at CRC Press for their patience and encouragement. Most of all we would like to thank our partners, families, friends, and colleagues in our teaching institutions for all their support and encouragement to turn this book into reality.

We invite the readers to approach this book in the way we approach each of our canine patients, as a series of mysteries awaiting our careful detective work in search of a happy outcome for our patients and the families that care for them. We hope that this book will inspire veterinarians to embrace the topic of canine infectious diseases and to contribute to the health and welfare of dogs everywhere.

Katrin Hartmann and Jane Sykes

Contributors

Ursula M. Dietrich
Professor Dr med vet, MRCVS
Diplomate ACVO
Diplomate ECVO
Royal Veterinary College
North Mymms, Hertfordshire, UK

Pedro Paulo Vissotto de Paiva Diniz
DVM, PhD
Associate Professor of Small Animal Internal Medicine
College of Veterinary Medicine
Western University of Health Sciences
Pomona, California, USA

René Dörfelt
Dr med vet
Diplomate ECVAA
Clinic of Small Animal Medicine
Centre for Clinical Veterinary Medicine
Ludwig Maximilian University Munich, Germany

Andrea Fischer
Professor Dr med vet, Dr habil
Diplomate ECVN
Diplomate ACVIM (Neurology)
Clinic of Small Animal Medicine
Centre for Clinical Veterinary Medicine
Ludwig Maximilian University Munich, Germany

Tadeusz Frymus
Professor Dr med vet
Head of the Division of Infectious Diseases
Department of Small Animal Diseases
Faculty of Veterinary Medicine
Warsaw University of Life Sciences (SGGW)
Warsaw, Poland

Daniel Guimarães Gerardi
DVM, MS, PhD
Departamento de Medicina Animal
Faculdade de Veterinária
Universidade Federal do Rio Grande do Sul (UFRGS)
Porto Alegre, Brazil

Bernhard Gerber
Priv-Doz, Dr med vet
Diplomate ACVIM
Diplomate ECVIM-CA (Internal Medicine)
Vetsuisse Faculty
University of Zurich
Zurich, Switzerland

Craig E. Greene
DVM, MS
Diplomate ACVIM (Internal Medicine and Neurology)
Emeritus Professor, Departments of Small Animal Medicine and Infectious Diseases
College of Veterinary Medicine
University of Georgia
Athens, Georgia, USA

Katrin Hartmann
Professor Dr med vet, Dr habil
Diplomate ECVIM-CA (Internal Medicine)
Clinic of Small Animal Medicine
Centre for Clinical Veterinary Medicine
Ludwig Maximilian University Munich, Germany

Lynelle Johnson
BA, DVM, MS, PhD
Diplomate ACVIM (Internal Medicine)
Professor, Medicine & Epidemiology
University of California-Davis
Davis, California, USA

Ralf S. Mueller
Professor Dr med vet, Dr habil
Diplomate ACVD
Diplomate ECVD
Clinic of Small Animal Medicine
Centre for Clinical Veterinary Medicine
Ludwig Maximilian University Munich, Germany

Maria Grazia Pennisi
DVM, PhD
Specialist in Applied Microbiology
Department of Veterinary Sciences
Polo Universitario dell'Annunziata
University of Messina
Messina, Italy

Bianka Schulz
Priv.-Doz., Dr med vet, Dr habil
Diplomate ECVIM-CA (Internal Medicine)
Clinic of Small Animal Medicine
Centre for Clinical Veterinary Medicine
Ludwig Maximilian University Munich, Germany

Jane E. Sykes
BVSc(Hons), PhD
Diplomate ACVIM
Professor of Small Animal Internal Medicine
School of Veterinary Medicine
University of California-Davis, USA

Stefan Unterer
Priv.-Doz., Dr med vet, Dr habil
Diplomate ECVIM-CA (Internal Medicine)
Clinic of Small Animal Medicine
Centre for Clinical Veterinary Medicine
Ludwig Maximilian University Munich, Germany

Gerhard Wess
Professor Dr med vet, Dr habil
Diplomate ACVIM (Cardiology)
Diplomate ECVIM-CA (Cardiology)
Diplomate ECVIM-CA (Internal Medicine)
Clinic of Small Animal Medicine
Centre for Clinical Veterinary Medicine
Ludwig Maximilian University Munich, Germany

Picture acknowledgments

4: courtesy of Craig Greene, © University of Georgia Research Foundation Inc.
5: courtesy of Craig Greene, © University of Georgia Research Foundation Inc.
10a, b: courtesy of Prof. Antonio Vicente Mundim
12: courtesy of the University of California-Davis, Veterinary Ophthalmology Service
13a, b: courtesy of the University of California-Davis, Veterinary Medical Teaching Hospital
16: courtesy of Dr. Suzane Beier
17a, 17b: courtesy of Dr. Cynthia Lucidi
23: courtesy of Chirurgische und Gynäkologische Kleintierklinik, LMU Munich
27: courtesy of the Clinical Laboratory, Vetsuisse Faculty, University of Zurich
28: courtesy of M. De Majo
29a, 29b: courtesy of G. Mazzullo
60a, 60b: courtesy of Dr. Gary Johnston
61a: courtesy of Dr. Gary Johnston
61b: courtesy of Kristin Nunez
74: courtesy of Prof. Dr. Tricia Maria Ferreira de Souza Oliveira
82: courtesy of Craig Greene, © University of Georgia Research Foundation Inc.
84: courtesy of Craig Greene, © University of Georgia Research Foundation Inc.
88: courtesy of Dr. Matt Eberts
92: courtesy of G. Lombardo
107: courtesy of the University of California-Davis, Veterinary Medical Teaching Hospital
113: courtesy of Teton New Media
114: courtesy of Craig Greene, © University of Georgia Research Foundation Inc.
115a, b: courtesy of Mark Kent, © University of Georgia Research Foundation Inc.
116: courtesy of Craig Greene, © University of Georgia Research Foundation Inc.
117a, 117b: courtesy of Dr. Matt Eberts
118: courtesy of Dr. Kristin Nunez
127a, 127b: courtesy of Craig Greene © University of Georgia Research Foundation Inc.
128: courtesy of the Department of Veterinary Pathology, UGA, © University of Georgia Research Foundation Inc.
133a, b: courtesy of Prof. Dr. Rafael Fighera
134: courtesy of Prof. Dr. Rafael A. Fighera
136: courtesy of the University of California-Davis, Veterinary Cardiology Service
139: courtesy of M. Masucci
140a, 140b: courtesy of M. De Majo
145: courtesy of Jacek Brzeski
146: courtesy of Jacek Brzeski
147: courtesy of the University of California-Davis, Veterinary Medical Teaching Hospital

154a, 154b: courtesy of Dr. Mitika Hagiwara
155a, 155b: courtesy of Flavio Paz
157: courtesy of the University of California-Davis Veterinary Medical Teaching Hospital
167: courtesy of Craig Greene, © University of Georgia Research Foundation Inc.
168: courtesy of the Department of Veterinary Pathology, UGA, © University of Georgia Research Foundation Inc.
172: courtesy of Dr. Matt Eberts
180a, 180b: courtesy of Chirurgische und Gynäkologische Kleintierklinik, LMU Munich
182a, 182b: courtesy of G. Malara
191: courtesy of Dr. Cynthia Lucidi
197: courtesy of the University of California-Davis, Veterinary Medical Teaching Hospital
199b: courtesy of Dr. José Luis Laus and Dr. Ivan Martinez

Abbreviations

ALP	alkaline phosphatase
ALT	alanine aminotransferase
aPTT	activated partial thromboplastin time
AST	aspartate aminotransferase
BAL	bronchoalveolar lavage
BCS	body condition score
bpm	beats per minute
BUN	blood urea nitrogen
CBC	complete blood count
CFU	colony-forming units
CNS	central nervous system
CRI	continuous rate infusion
CSF	cerebrospinal fluid
CT	computed tomography
DIC	disseminated intravascular coagulopathy
DNA	deoxyribonucleic acid
ECG	electrocardiography/electrocardiogram
ELISA	enzyme-linked immunosorbent assay
GABA	gamma-aminobutyric acid
hpf	high-power field
IFA	immunofluorescence assay
Ig	immunoglobulin
IRIS	International Renal Interest Society
IM	intramuscular(ly)
IMHA	immune-mediated hemolytic anemia
IV	intravenous(ly)
MCHC	mean cell hemoglobin content
MCV	mean cell volume
MRI	magnetic resonance imaging
OD	right eye (*oculus dextrus*)
OS	left eye (*oculus sinister*)
PCR	polymerase chain reaction
PO	orally (*per os*)
PT	prothrombin time
PU/PD	polyuria/polydipsia
RBC	red blood cell(s)
RI	reference interval
RNA	ribonucleic acid
SC	subcutaneous(ly)
T4	thyroxine
TSH	thyroid-stimulating hormone
UPCR	urine protein to creatinine ratio
UV	ultraviolet
WBC	white blood cell(s)

Broad classification of cases

Viral infections

CASE 1 An 8-year-old female intact Siberian Husky from Bern, Switzerland, was evaluated for acute onset of vomiting, lethargy, and increased thirst and urination. On physical examination, the dog was estimated to be 7–8% dehydrated and had a tense abdomen on palpation. The kidneys appeared to be slightly enlarged on palpation and a large bladder was noted. The BCS was 5/9 (**1**). A CBC, serum biochemistry panel, and urinalysis were performed:

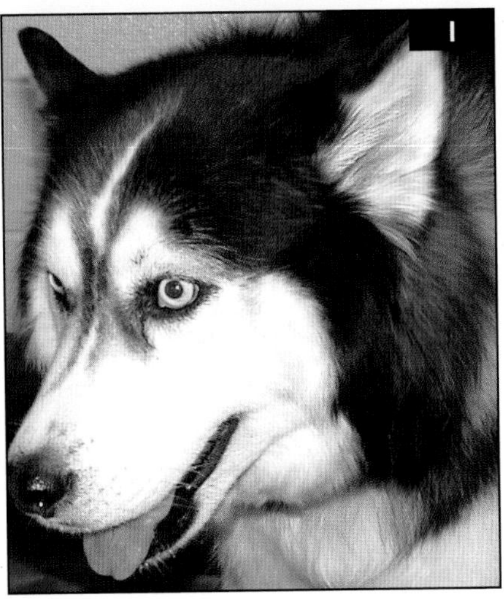

Complete blood count	Results	Reference interval
Hematocrit	0.32 l/l	0.42–0.55
Platelets	75×10^9/l	130–394
White blood cells	6.1×10^9/l	4.7–11.3

Biochemistry panel	Results	Reference interval
Creatinine	364 μmol/l	50–119
Urea	39 μmol/l	3.8–9.4
Glucose	4.8 mmol/l	4.1–5.9
Sodium	153 mmol/l	152–159
Potassium	4.5 mmol/l	4.3–5.3
Phosphorus	2.19 mmol/l	1–1.6

Urinalysis	Results
Collection method	Cystocentesis
Color, appearance	Yellow, clear
Specific gravity	1.022
pH	6.8
Protein	Negative
Glucose	++
Sediment	Inactive

1 How would you interpret the findings in this dog?
2 What are the differential diagnoses for this dog?

CASE 2 Case 2 is the same dog as case 1. On abdominal ultrasound, the kidneys were slightly enlarged and a small amount of perirenal fluid was visualized (2). Leptospirosis is suspected as the underlying disease.

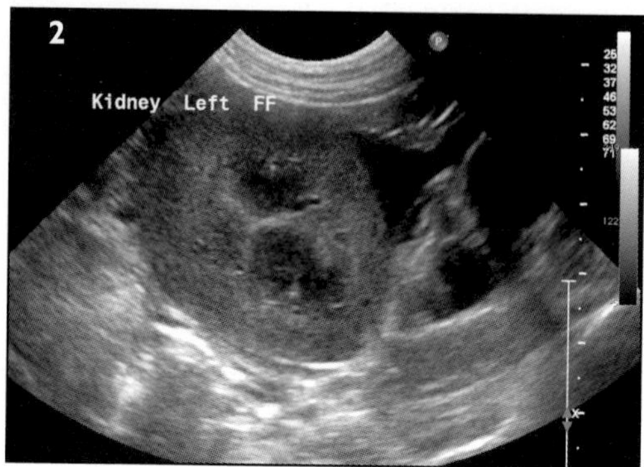

1 How would you make a specific diagnosis of leptospirosis?
2 How would you treat this dog?
3 Is there a risk of human infection when handling the dog?

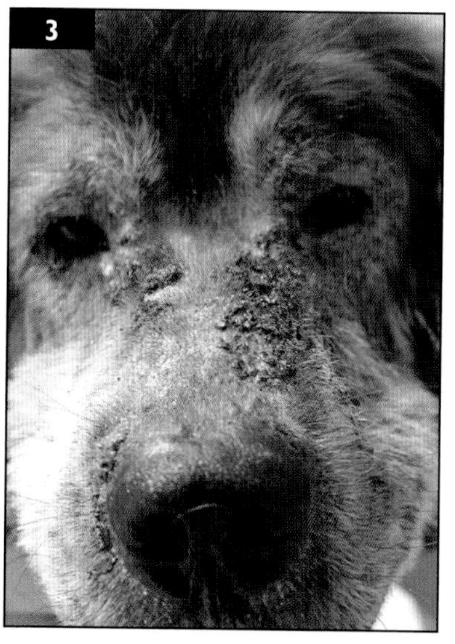

CASE 3 A 6-month-old intact male Labrador mix was evaluated for a 4-week history of facial skin disease (3). The dog was bright and alert, but showed prominent erythema, crusting, and alopecia periocularly as well as on the muzzle. The dog lived in Munich, Germany, had no travel history outside the country, was vaccinated with core vaccines and last treated with an endoparasiticide 6 weeks previously, and was fed a commercial puppy food. Besides the skin changes, the dog was unremarkable on physical examination.

1 What are the most likely differential diagnoses for this dog based on your assessment of the history and image provided?
2 What diagnostic tests should be done immediately?
3 Could this dog have a transmissible infectious disease?

CASE 4 A 3-year-old neutered male Border Collie was referred for skin lesions on his extremities that had been present for 4 months. Therapy with antibacterial drugs for the past month had not been effective. The dog appeared otherwise healthy. The owners owned farmland in Greensboro, Georgia, USA, and lived by a lake. The dog spent time inside and outside. There was no travel history. The dog had been regularly vaccinated and treated with parasiticides.

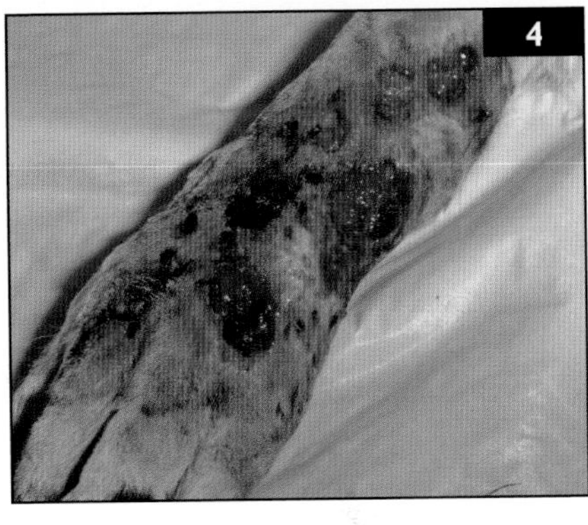

Physical examination, beside the skin lesions, was unremarkable. There were draining ulcerative skin lesions on the dog's extremities (**4**).

1 What are the differential diagnoses for draining skin lesions?
2 What diagnostic plan should be considered for the skin lesions?

CASE 5 Case 5 is the same dog as case 4. Serum biochemical abnormalities included increased serum globulin concentration and serum alkaline phosphatase activity. Cytologic findings were a predominance of neutrophils and a few macrophages. Poorly stained, slightly basophilic thin-walled, rarely septate hyphae were observed (**5**).

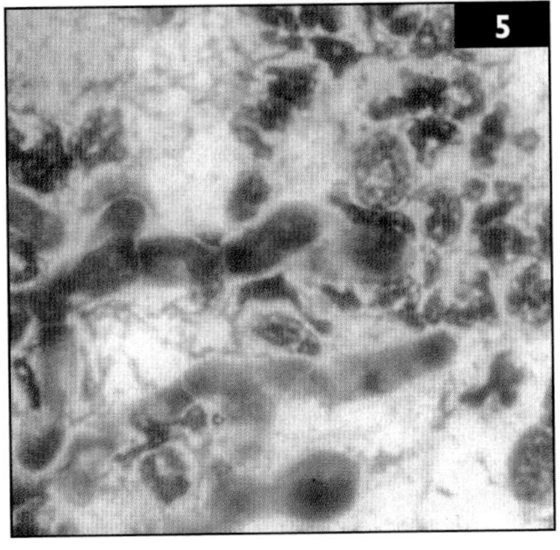

Hematoxylin and eosin-stained skin biopsy specimens showed diffuse infiltrates of lymphocytes, plasma cells, neutrophils, and macrophages, and a few giant cells. Necrotic cellular debris was interspersed with multifocal fibroplasia. Within the sections were thin-walled, rarely branching hyphae with occasional septa with bulbous enlargements. Gomori's methenamine silver stain highlighted the fungal hyphal elements within the lesions. Organisms grew on Sabouraud dextrose agar at 25°C. Colonies were smooth and yellow with radial folds. Smooth, thick-walled zygospores had copulatory beaks. The organisms were identified as *Basiobolus ranarum*. Fungal susceptibility testing suggested susceptibility to terbinafine, trimethoprim/sulfonamide, and amphotericin B.

1 What is the source of the organism isolated in this infection?
2 What treatment is indicated?

CASE 6 A 2-year-old intact male German Shepherd Dog mix was referred for a 4-day history of acute vomiting and anorexia. Two days before the dog was evaluated, the referring veterinarian reported icterus and had treated the dog with oral antibiotics (doxycycline) and a single injection of a short-acting glucocorticoid. Because the vomiting persisted, the owner did not administer the doxycycline. No previous health problems were known. The dog was up to date on vaccinations and regularly treated for endoparasites. He lived in a suburban area close to Munich, Germany, and had traveled to Southern Italy once, 10 months ago.

On presentation, the dog was lethargic, but still responsive and ambulatory. He was in a good body condition (BCS 4.5/9). Rectal body temperature was 39.8°C (103.6°F), pulse was 120 bpm, and respiratory rate was 32 breaths/min. Mucous membranes were icteric (**6**). On palpation, the abdomen was tense, but not painful. The remainder of the physical examination was unremarkable.

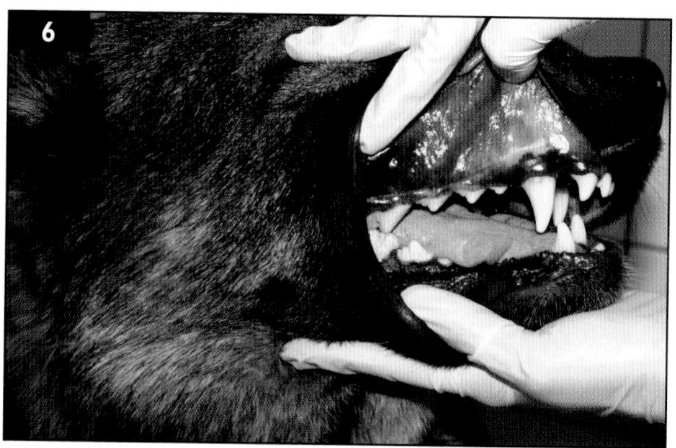

1 What is the differential diagnosis for icterus?
2 What non-invasive tests would you perform first to investigate this problem?

CASE 7 Case 7 is the same dog as case 6. A CBC revealed a hematocrit of 0.65 l/l (RI 0.35–0.58 l/l), a neutrophil count of 26.1 × 10^9/l (RI 5–16 × 10^9/l), and a band neutrophil count of 5.6 × 10^9/l (RI 0–0.5 × 10^9/l).

On abdominal ultrasound examination, the liver was of normal size and echogenicity. The gallbladder was not enlarged. No abnormal contents, such as stones, could be visualized in the gallbladder, and the wall was not thickened (**7a**). However, the common bile duct was distended and 1 cm in diameter (**7b**). Because of gas in the gastrointestinal tract, the enlarged bile duct could not be followed to its duodenal entrance.

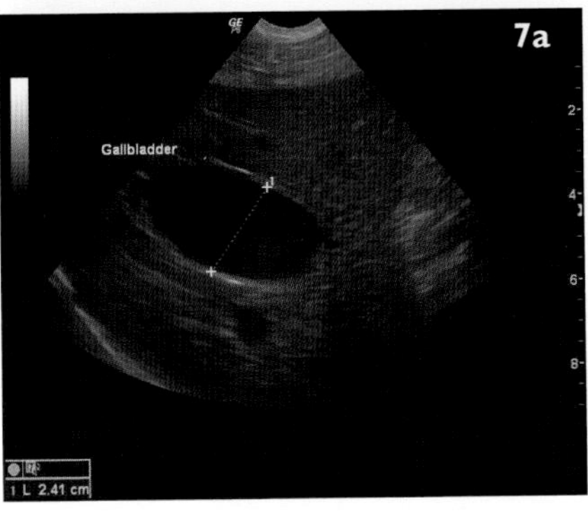

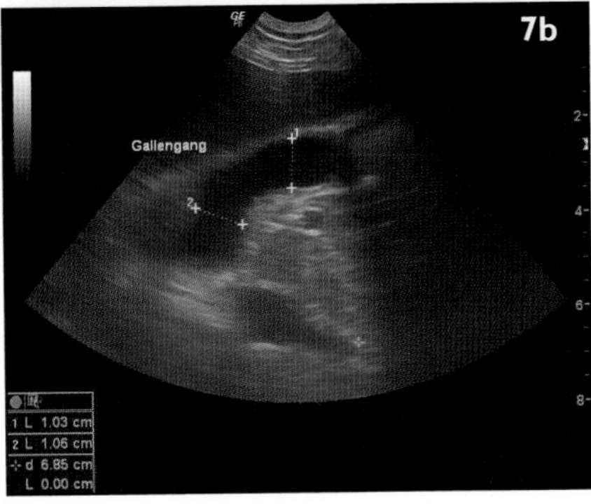

1 What form of icterus can be ruled out based on the results of the CBC?
2 What is your assessment of the neutrophilia observed in this dog?
3 What are reasons for distension of the common bile duct?
4 Which reason is more likely in this case, and what test would you perform to confirm your suspicion?

CASE 8 Case 8 is the same dog as cases 6 and 7. Cytologic examination of the aspirated bile showed neutrophilic inflammation and the presence of bacteria (**8a**). On bile culture, significant growth of *Escherichia coli* was noted.

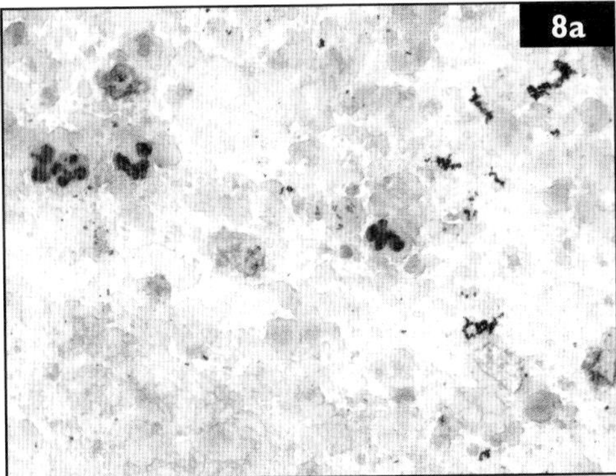

1 What are the most common bacterial species involved in bacterial cholangitis and, therefore, what antimicrobial would you choose empirically while the results of culture and susceptibility are pending?
2 Are bacterial infections of the hepatobiliary system common in dogs?
3 What predisposing factors contribute to ascending bacterial cholangitis?
4 For how long would you continue antimicrobial treatment?

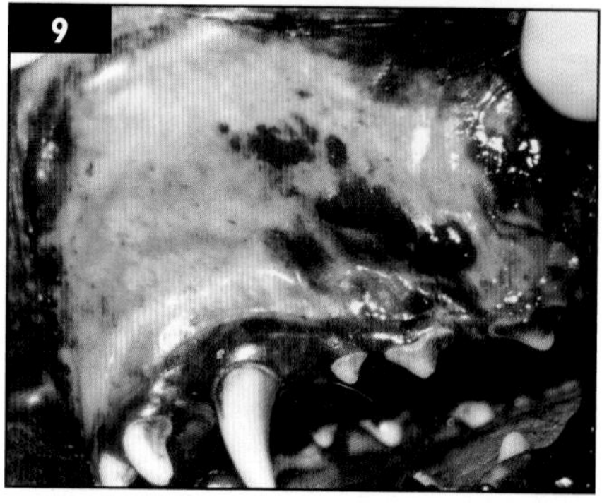

CASE 9 A 4-year-old intact female mixed-breed dog that lived in a rural community in the area of Porto Alegre, Brazil, was evaluated for anorexia, lethargy, and weight loss over the past 4 days. The dog had been properly vaccinated and recently treated for parasites. On physical examination, the dog had pale mucous membranes with ecchymosis (**9**), fever (39.7°C [103.5°F]), mild peripheral generalized lymphadenomegaly, and splenomegaly. Ticks found on the dog were identified as *Rhipicephalus sanguineus*. Significant findings on a CBC, serum biochemistry panel, and urinalysis are shown below. The anemia was normocytic and hypochromic.

Complete blood count	Results	Reference interval
Hematocrit	0.27 l/l	0.35–0.58
Reticulocytes	0 × 10^9/l	0–60
Platelets	3 × 10^9/l	150–500
White blood cells	108.7 × 10^9/l	5–16
Mature neutrophils	103.6 × 10^9/l	3–9

Biochemistry panel	Results	Reference interval
Total protein	84 g/l	56–78
Albumin	22 g/l	31–43
Globulins	62 g/l	24–35

1 Which infectious agents can be transmitted by *Rhipicephalus sanguineus*?
2 What are the two most striking abnormalities in the CBC, and which tick-borne diseases can cause these abnormalities?
3 What tests should be performed to diagnose these infections?

CASE 10 Case 10 is the same dog as case 9. A blood smear showed *Hepatozoon* organisms within neutrophils (**10a, 10b**). PCR confirmed infection with both *Hepatozoon canis* and *Ehrlichia canis*.

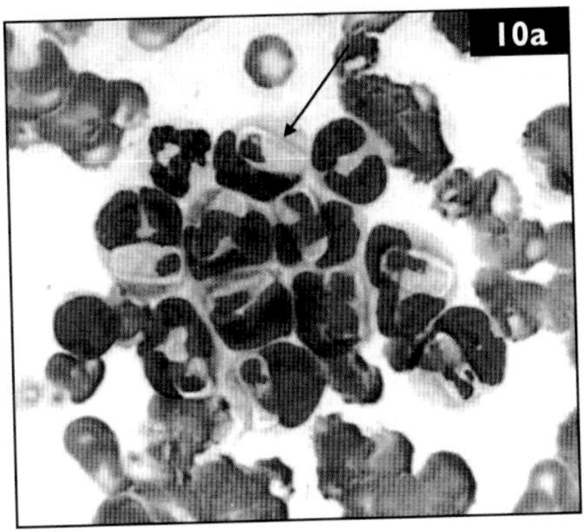

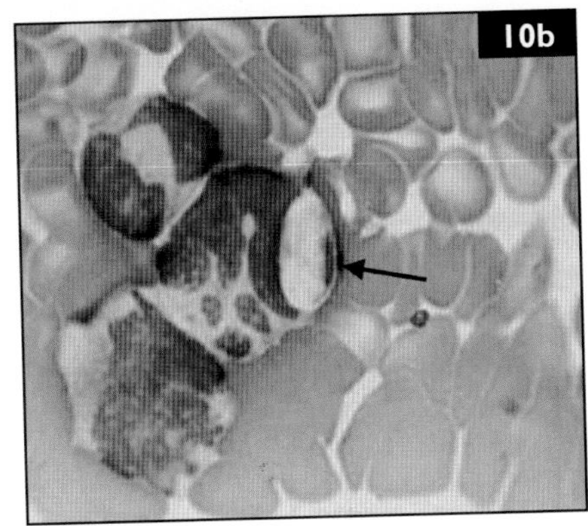

1 Which clinical signs and laboratory abnormalities in this dog are caused by *Hepatozoon canis* and which are more likely to be caused by *Ehrlichia canis*?
2 What are the differences between the mode of transmission of *Hepatozoon canis* and *Ehrlichia canis*?
3 What treatments are indicated for the two infections?

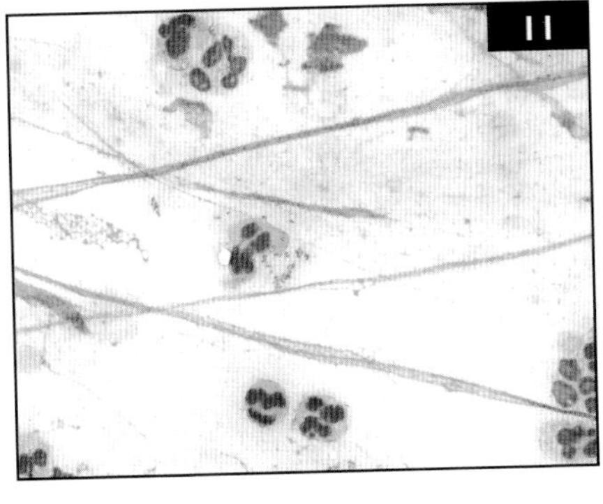

CASE 11 A 10-month-old neutered female Labrador Retriever living in a rural area in the region of Regensburg, Germany, was evaluated for a 7-day history of cough. For the 2 days before evaluation the dog was lethargic and anorexic. The dog had been vaccinated against distemper virus, adenovirus, parvovirus, *Leptospira* spp. infection, and rabies as a puppy and was treated every 3 months with a parasiticide. The owner reported that several dogs in a puppy class that the dog attended were also coughing. On physical examination pyrexia was noted (39.8°C [103.6°F]). A moist cough could be elicited on palpation of the trachea. Increased lung sounds were noted on auscultation. Thoracic radiographs revealed a mild bronchointerstitial lung pattern. A CBC showed a neutrophilia with a mild left shift. Bronchoalveolar lavage was performed, and the fluid was examined cytologically (**11**).

1 What is your assessment of this case, and how would you proceed?
2 How would you interpret the cytology of bronchoalveolar lavage fluid in this patient?
3 What treatment would you recommend?

CASE 12 A 3-year-old neutered female Labrador Retriever was evaluated for seizures. For the past week, she had shown signs of lethargy, trembling, and circling, and she had occasionally been found with her head pressed against the wall. She also had decreased appetite. On the day of evaluation, she had begun to show focal seizures that were described as side-to-side head movements. There had been no cough, sneezing, vomiting, or diarrhea. The dog lived in Shasta Lake, California, USA. There was no history of travel. Her owners had started digging up their garden 4 weeks ago. There had been no history of toxin exposure. The dog was treated regularly with flea and heartworm preventives and was up to date on vaccinations (distemper, canine infectious hepatitis, parvovirus infection, and leptospirosis). She was receiving no other medications.

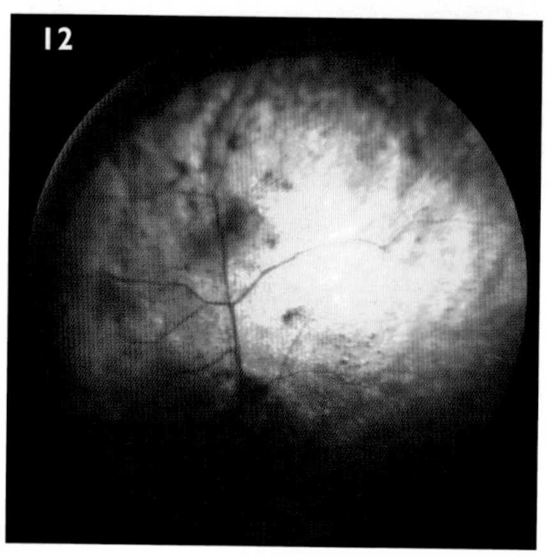

On physical examination, she was quiet, alert, responsive, and well hydrated. Body weight was 20 kg. The rectal body temperature was 38.8°C (101.8°F), pulse rate was 104 bpm, and she was panting. The remainder of the general physical examination was unremarkable. Neurologic examination showed mild obtundation, an absent menace response on the right side, and pain on lumbosacral palpation. Hopping was equivocally delayed in the pelvic and thoracic limbs. Funduscopic examination showed multifocal, indistinct gray opacities in the right eye (**12**).

1 What is the neuroanatomic localization of the problem?
2 What are your differential diagnoses for this dog's problem, and what infectious agents might be involved?
3 What is your plan for further work-up of this dog's problem?

CASE 13 Case 13 is the same dog as case 12. The CBC and urinalysis were normal. The biochemistry panel showed mild hyperglobulinemia (38 g/l, RI 17–35 g/l). Thoracic radiographs were normal, whereas lumbosacral spinal radiographs showed narrowing of the L4–L5 intervertebral disc space with a mineralized disc at the L1–L2 space. Abdominal ultrasound revealed enlarged mesenteric, ileocolic, hepatic, and pancreaticoduodenal lymph nodes, which were heterogeneous in echogenicity (**13a**). The surrounding mesentery

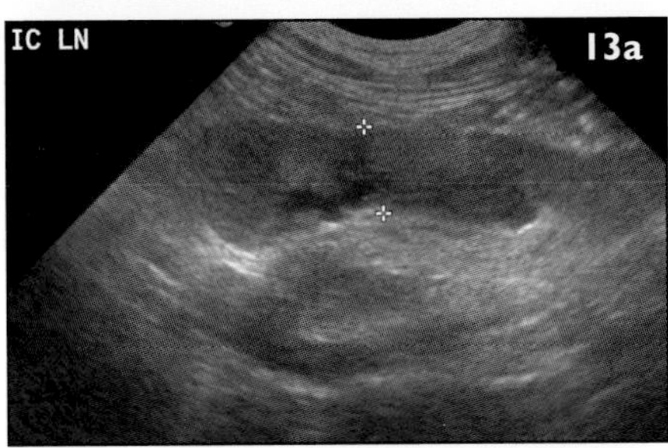

13a

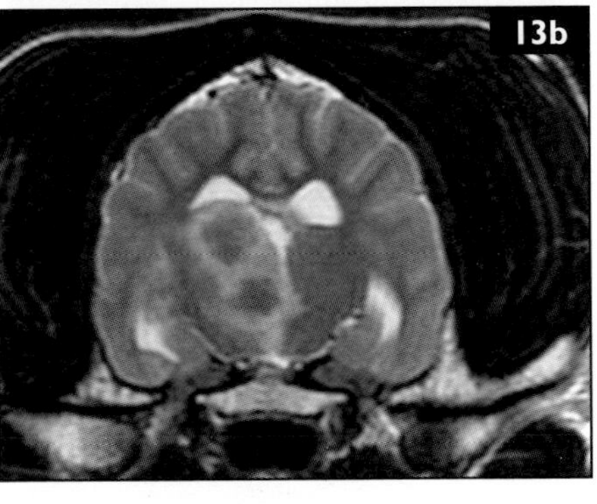
13b

was hyperechoic. There was segmental eccentric thickening of the muscularis throughout the jejunum. The wall layering in those regions was well defined.

Aspirates of multiple lymph nodes were obtained and revealed changes consistent with immune reactivity. MRI showed numerous, T1 hypointense, T2 hypo- to isointense, contrast-enhancing nodules distributed throughout the cerebral cortex, and within the thalamus and cerebellum. There was a lobular mass involving the olfactory bulbs bilaterally with regional meningeal enhancement. This lesion abutted the cribriform plate but no mass lesion was identified in the nasal cavity. There were numerous cerebral nodules throughout all lobes, the largest of which was in the left temporal region, measuring 1 cm. There were two large nodules in the left thalamic region, measuring 1.2 cm in diameter. These nodules resulted in mass effect with displacement of the interthalamic adhesion to the right (**13b**). There were multiple nodules in the cerebellum; the largest one was left sided and measured 0.6 cm. There was diffuse meningeal contrast enhancement including leptomeningeal enhancement. Moderate FLAIR hyperintensity was observed within the white matter around the described nodules and adjacent to the lateral ventricles and mesencephalic aqueduct.

Analysis of the CSF revealed a protein concentration of 1.07 g/l. There were 91 nucleated cells/μl, consisting of 37% neutrophils, 30% small mononuclear cells, and 33% large mononuclear cells. No infectious agents were seen, but culture of the CSF yielded *Cryptococcus neoformans*. A *Cryptococcus* antigen titer was 1:1024.

1 What species of *Cryptococcus* cause infections in dogs, and are there differences in their ecologic niches and clinical presentations?
2 What is the recommended treatment for this dog?
3 What are possible adverse effects of drug therapy and how should response to treatment be monitored?

CASE 14 An 8-month-old intact male Weimaraner (**14**) was evaluated for a 2-day history of oliguria and a 3-day history of vomiting and anorexia. The dog lived in a suburban area close to Munich, Germany, and had no travel history. He had been vaccinated against distemper virus, canine adenovirus, and parvovirus, and received parasite prevention once a month. On physical examination, the dog was lethargic, appeared overhydrated, and the kidneys were slightly painful on palpation. The remainder of the physical examination was unremarkable.

Initial laboratory examination revealed a severe neutrophilia (42×10^9 mature neutrophils/l, RI 3–115 $\times$ 10^9/l) with left shift (4.5×10^9 band neutrophils/l, RI 0–3 $\times$ 10^9/l), thrombocytopenia (65×10^9 platelets/l, RI 150–400 $\times$ 10^9/), increased serum urea concentration (48 mmol/l, RI 3.8–9.4 mmol/l), increased serum creatinine concentration (709 µmol/l , RI 45–125 µmol/l), and a urine specific gravity of 1.016.

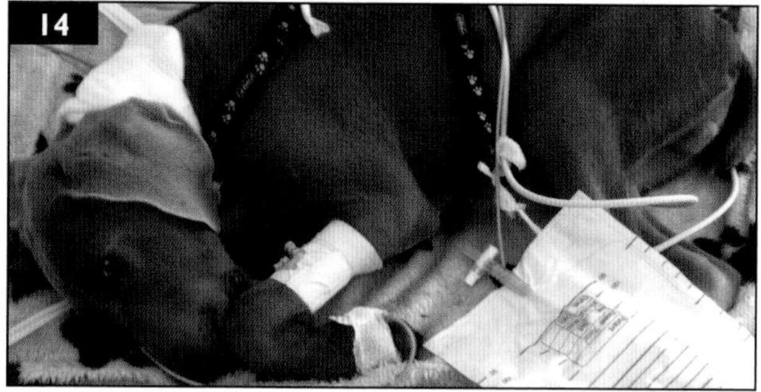

1 What is the primary problem in this dog and the most likely underlying disease?
2 What additional tests would you perform?
3 What treatment would you initiate?

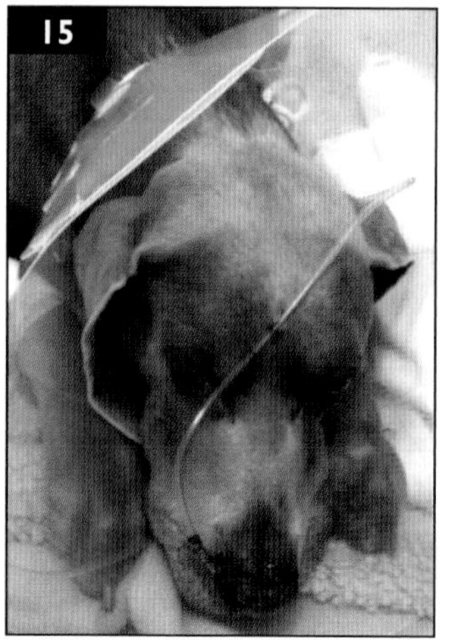

CASE 15 Case 15 is the same dog as case 14. The dog received aggressive supportive treatment and antimicrobials for possible leptospirosis (**15**). However, after 12 hours the dog became anuric with a heart rate of 60 bpm and a rectal body temperature of 37.1°C (98.8°F). After 24 hours the dog also developed respiratory distress with a respiratory rate of 64 breaths/min.

1 What should be the monitoring plan for this dog?
2 What are the next diagnostic and therapeutic considerations in regards to the respiratory distress?

CASE 16 A 5-year-old neutered female mixed-breed dog was brought to a veterinary clinic in San Diego, California, USA, for a routine dental cleaning procedure. The owner reported that the dog was healthy, but 2 weeks previously she had an episode of lethargy lasting 2–3 days, from which she recovered spontaneously. The owner believed that the incident was associated with travel that had occurred over that period, rather than illness. The dog had not traveled outside of California, was up to date on core vaccines, and had no history of ectoparasites, although preventives were not used.

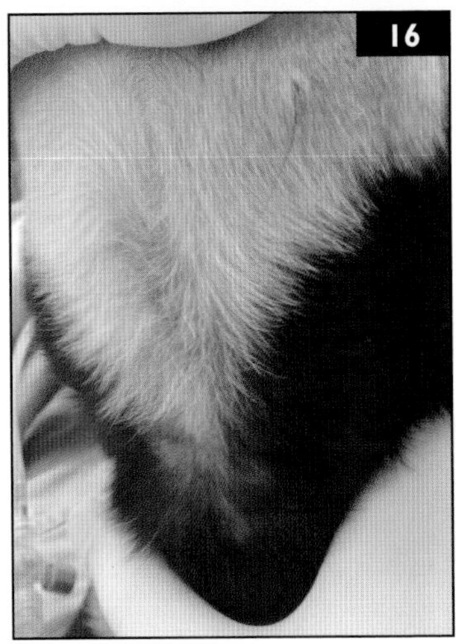

On physical examination, the dog was bright, alert, and responsive, and no abnormalities were detected. When blood was taken for routine pre-anesthetic bloodwork, prolonged bleeding at the site of venipuncture was noted, with subsequent development of a hematoma and ecchymoses (**16**). The CBC showed a low platelet count of 65×10^9 platelets/l. All other CBC results were within normal limits.

1 Would you proceed with the dental cleaning procedure?
2 What are the most likely differential diagnoses for the thrombocytopenia?

CASE 17 Case 17 is the same dog as case 16. Blood smears were obtained (**17a, 17b**).

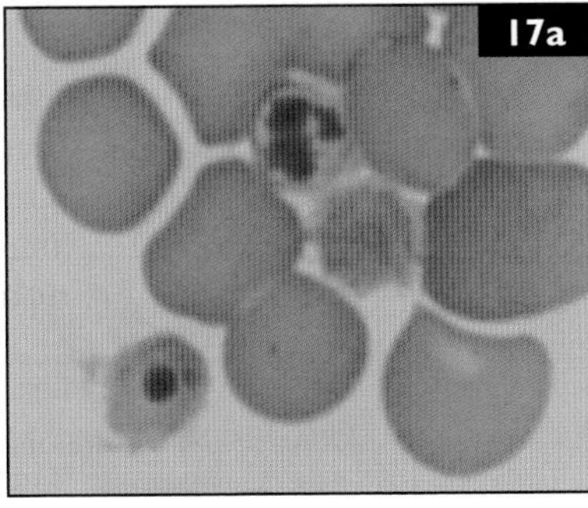

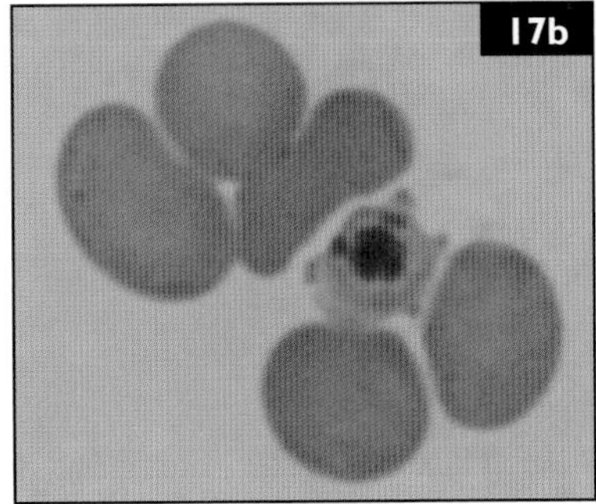

1 Describe the blood smear findings.
2 What tests could be performed to confirm the diagnosis?
3 Does this dog need specific therapy for this problem?

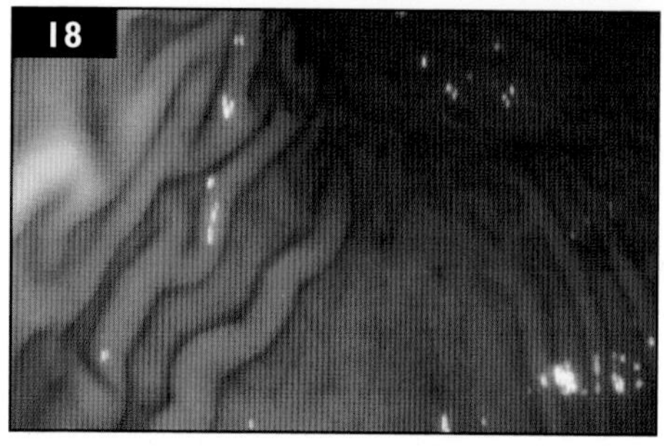

CASE 18 A 6-year-old intact male Labrador Retriever was evaluated for a 2-month history of vomiting. The vomiting occurred two to three times a week, contained bile or food, and was unrelated to food intake. There was no diarrhea. There had been no improvement following administration of a hypoallergenic diet for 4 weeks. The dog lived in Reggio Calabria, Italy, and had been regularly vaccinated and received prophylaxis for endoparasites and ectoparasites.

On physical examination, the dog had a thin body condition (BCS 3/9). Otherwise the physical examination was unremarkable. The results of a CBC, serum biochemistry panel, and urinalysis were all normal. Centrifugal zinc sulfate fecal flotation was negative. Abdominal imaging (radiographs and ultrasound) were unremarkable. Gastroduodenoscopy was performed. The duodenum and jejunum appeared grossly normal, while the stomach showed pathologic changes (**18**).

1 How would you interpret the gastroscopy picture?
2 What would be your diagnostic plan?

CASE 19 Case 19 is the same dog as case 18. Histopathology showed mucosal edema, lymphoplasmacytic infiltrates, and fibrosis (**19a**). Spiral-shaped organisms were also seen and stained positive with Warthin–Starry silver stain (**19b**).

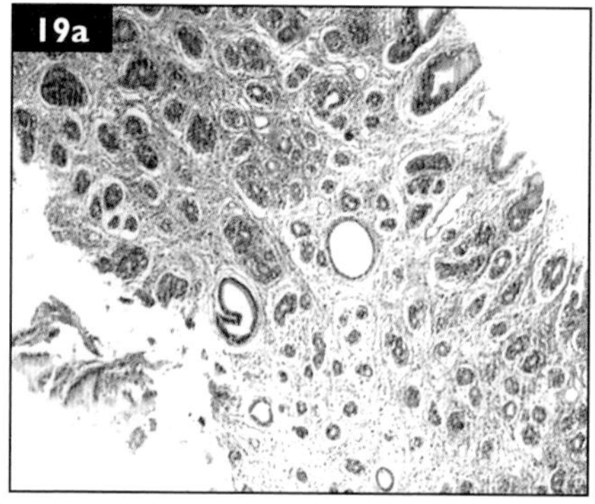

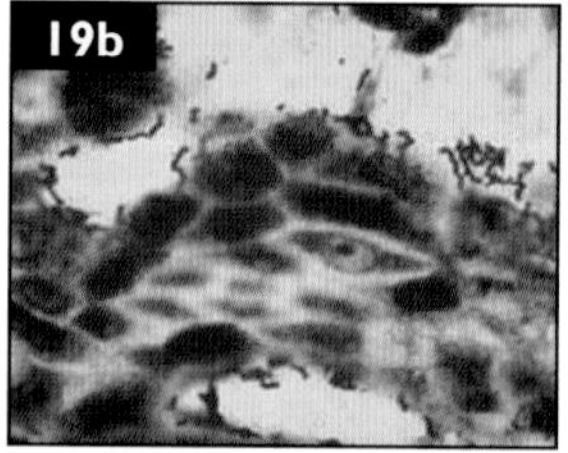

1 How would you interpret the results?
2 How should this dog be treated?

CASE 20 An 11-year-old neutered female Miniature Dachshund was evaluated for a 6-week history of pruritus and dermatitis. No other abnormalities were noted by the owner. The dog lived in Augsburg, Germany, and had occasionally traveled to northern Italy. It had received regular vaccinations (distemper virus, adenovirus, parvovirus, rabies, and *Leptospira* spp.) but had not received parasiticides for several years.

On physical examination, papules and pustules were found on the abdomen (**20**). Otherwise the physical examination was unremarkable.

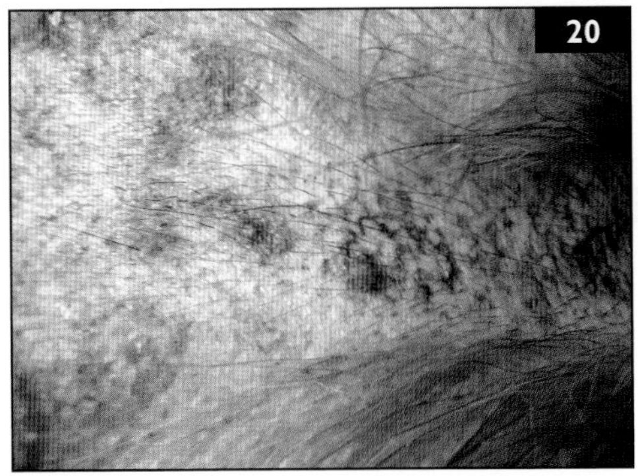

1 What are the most likely differential diagnoses for this dog?
2 What diagnostic tests should be done immediately?

CASE 21 Case 21 is the same dog as case 20. Skin scrapings were negative. An impression smear cytology was obtained (**21**).

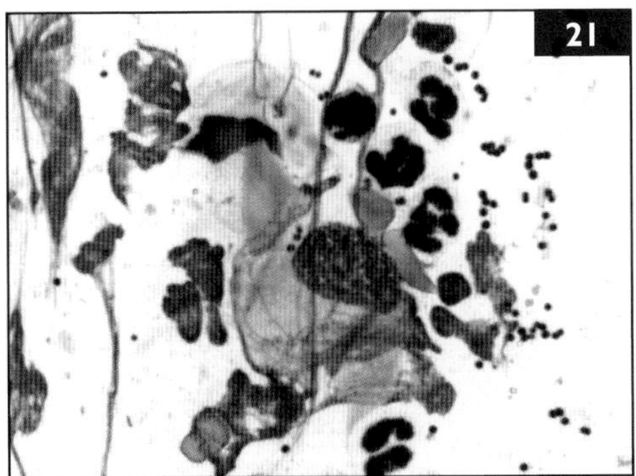

1 What questions should the owner be asked before performing further diagnostic tests?
2 How should you proceed based on the possible responses from the owner?

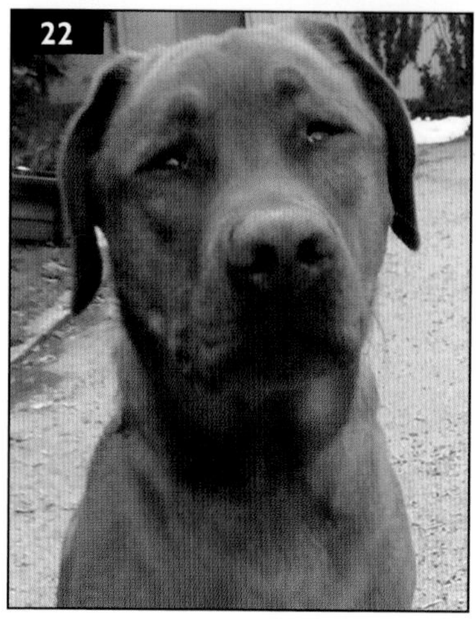

CASE 22 A 4-year-old intact male mixed-breed dog was referred for further assessment and treatment. The dog had a history of a split nail and swelling of the paw 2 weeks previously. Antibiotic treatment with amoxicillin–clavulanic acid was instituted and the swelling improved. On the morning of the referral, there was an onset of facial spasms and trismus (lockjaw) (**22**).

The dog came from Augsburg, Germany, and had never traveled outside the country. He had not been vaccinated since he was a puppy, and not received any parasiticides within the last year.

On neurologic examination, masticatory muscle atrophy and mild cervical pain were noted as additional findings. Besides the neurologic changes, physical examination was unremarkable.

1. What is the likely etiology of the clinical signs?
2. How would you describe the different clinical stages of this disease, and what is the prognosis?

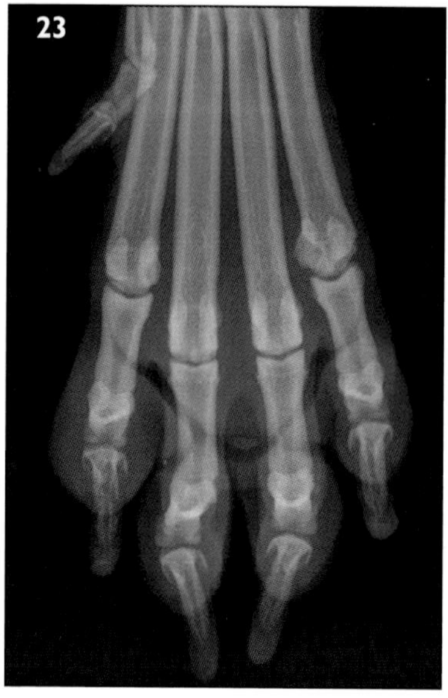

CASE 23 Case 23 is the same dog as case 22. Generalized tetanus was diagnosed on the basis of typical clinical signs. Close inspection of the paw with the split nail revealed that there was still some swelling evident. Therefore, a radiograph of the paw were taken (**23**). Prior to taking the radiograph, the dog was sedated in order to minimize exacerbation of tetanus by either excitement or pain from the procedure.

The dog was placed in a dark and noise-protected room with instructions for minimal handling, and ear plugs were applied. Initial management consisted of intravenous application of 100 units/kg of equine tetanus antitoxin (following a subcutaneous test dose) and intravenous application of diphenhydramine. Thereafter, treatment with metronidazole (10 mg/kg PO q8h) was instituted in order to control the anaerobic wound infection. Methocarbamol (10 mg/kg/h) was given as a central muscle relaxant. The dog also received intravenous fluids and hand-feeding. However, the dog's condition worsened during the following day and he developed generalized spasticity with intermittent recumbency and dysphagia.

1 How would you describe the radiographic findings?
2 What are your further treatment recommendations?

CASE 24 A 3-year-old intact female Miniature Schnauzer was evaluated for mild head tilt and ataxia (**24**). The owner reported an episode of conjunctivitis, coughing, and diarrhea 2 weeks ago and a generalized seizure 3 days ago. The dog lived in Munich, Germany, had never traveled outside the country, was current on vaccinations, and received regular parasiticide treatment.

A general physical examination revealed a rectal body temperature of 39.1°C (102.4°F) and mild conjunctivitis, but was otherwise unremarkable. Neurologic examination showed vestibular and proprioceptive ataxia, head tilt to the right, positional rotating nystagmus, no response to touch of the left nostril, and a loss of menace response of the left eye with normal pupillary light reflexes. Proprioceptive positioning and hopping of the left pelvic limb were delayed. There was no evidence of pain on spinal palpation.

Laboratory examination showed a mild neutrophilia (17.0×10^9/l). Serum chemistry and urinalysis were unremarkable.

Based on the neurologic examination, central vestibular disease was diagnosed. Neuroanatomic localization of lesions was multifocal brainstem and forebrain.

1 Why is the presence of CNS inflammation likely in this case?
2 What diagnostic tests should be performed?
3 What are the potential diagnostic pitfalls?
4 What treatment should be initiated?

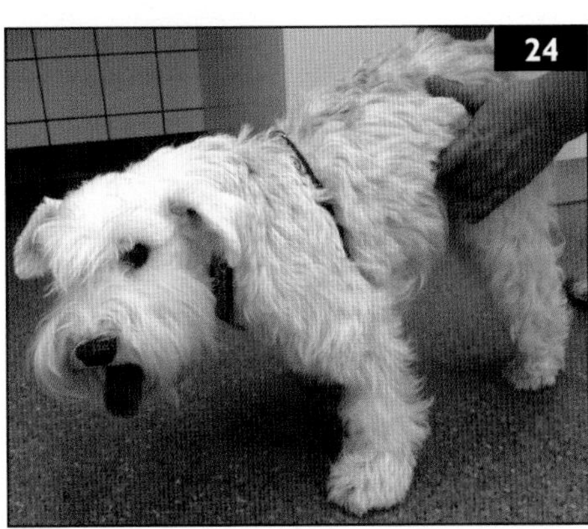
24

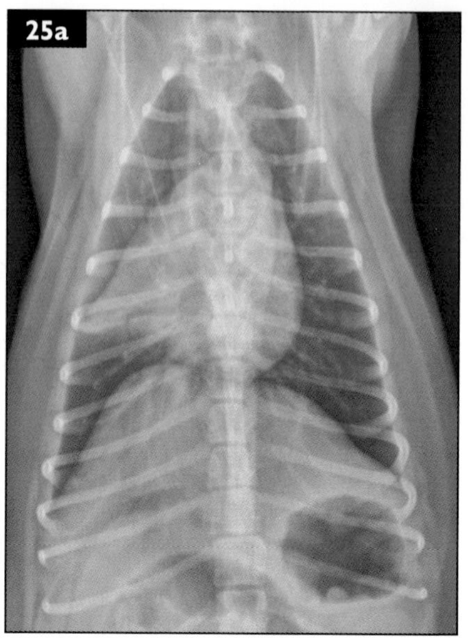

25a

CASE 25 A 4-year-old neutered female Maltese Terrier mix was evaluated for a 4-day history of cough and loss of appetite. The dog lived in the San Francisco Bay area, California, USA, and was up to date on vaccines, was on heartworm prophylaxis, and had no recent exposure to other dogs.

On physical examination, the dog was estimated to be 5% dehydrated, and had a pulse rate of 140 bpm and a respiratory rate of 44 breaths/min. Respiratory effort was mildly increased, and a cough was readily induced on tracheal palpation. Harsh bronchovesicular sounds were evident in all lung fields. The remainder of the physical examination was within normal limits. Thoracic radiographs were taken (**25a, 25b**).

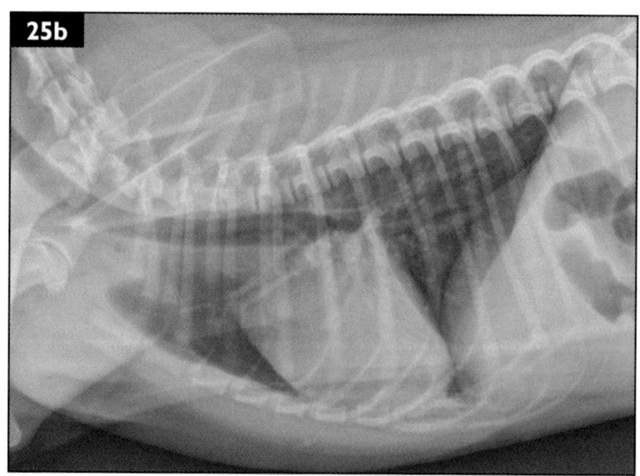

25b

1 What is your interpretation of the radiographs?
2 What differential diagnoses are most likely in this animal?
3 What additional tests should be performed?

CASE 26 Case 26 is the same dog as case 25. Bronchoscopy and bronchoalveolar lavage were performed (**26a, 26b**).

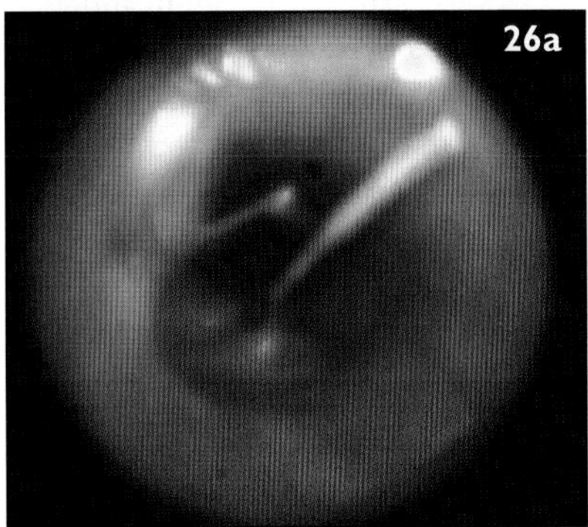
26a

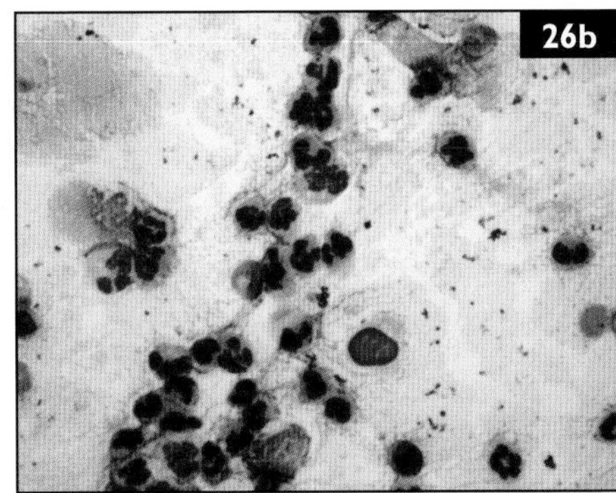
26b

1 What findings can be seen on bronchoscopy and on cytologic examination of the bronchoalveolar lavage fluid?
2 What additional tests should be submitted on the bronchoalveolar lavage fluid?

CASE 27 A 10-year-old neutered female Cocker Spaniel from Geneva, Switzerland, was evaluated for recurrent urinary tract infections, which were associated with lower urinary tract signs of hematuria, dysuria, and stranguria. These infections had been treated successfully with antimicrobial drugs in the past but, recently, treatment had not resulted in clinical improvement. The dog had a history of previous traumatic urethral injury that had been treated surgically. For further diagnostic work-up, urinalysis was performed with light microscopy of unstained urine sediment (**27**).

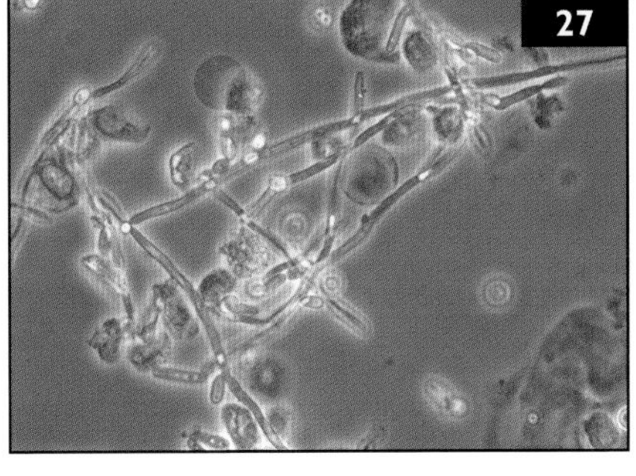
27

1 What can be seen in the urinary sediment?
2 How common are fungal urinary tract infections?
3 What are risk factors for this infection?
4 What treatment should be recommended?

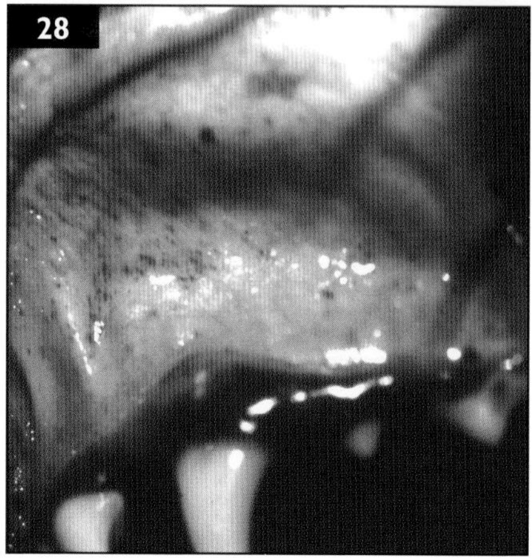

CASE 28 A 2-year-old intact male mixed-breed dog, living entirely outdoors in a rural area of Sicily, Italy, was evaluated because of a 2-day history of anorexia and lethargy. The dog had been vaccinated only for rabies and was only treated for internal parasites once as a puppy.

On physical examination, pyrexia (40.0°C [104.0°F]) and petechial lesions on the gingival mucosa were observed (**28**). There were no other abnormalities.

1 What are the differential diagnoses for the petechial lesions?
2 What useful information could be obtained from a CBC?
3 Antibody testing for which infectious diseases would be indicated, and what are the limitations of these assays for establishing a diagnosis?

CASE 29 Case 29 is the same dog as case 28. The CBC revealed a severe thrombocytopenia, mild non-regenerative anemia, and neutropenia. On the blood smear, morula-like cytoplasmic inclusion bodies were observed in a few mononuclear cells (**29a**) and in many platelets (**29b**).

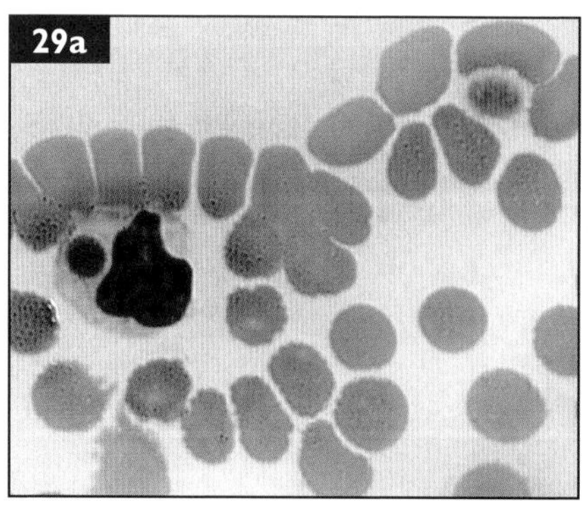

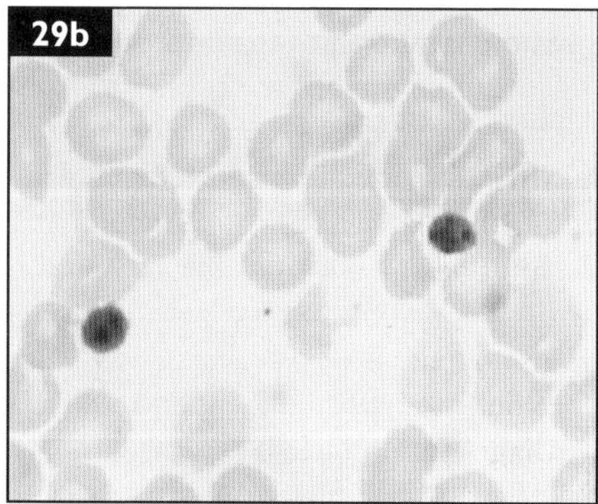

1 What is the diagnosis?
2 How should the dog be treated?

CASE 30 A 2-year-old neutered male American Pitbull Terrier (**30**) was evaluated for lethargy that had started 6 months previously but had become progressively worse over the last 2 months. The dog had been seen by a veterinarian 1 month previously; a mild anemia was diagnosed that was not further evaluated. The dog had been treated with doxycycline, but the clinical signs did not improve. The dog lived in Atlanta, Georgia, USA. He had been adopted by his owner about 1 year previously when the owner found the dog roaming around the streets of Atlanta. Within that year the dog had not traveled. The dog had been vaccinated at the time of adoption and now received monthly preventives for endo- and ectoparasites, including heartworm.

On physical examination, the dog was quiet, but responsive. Mucous membranes were slightly pale; capillary refill time was 2 seconds. Otherwise, the physical examination was unremarkable.

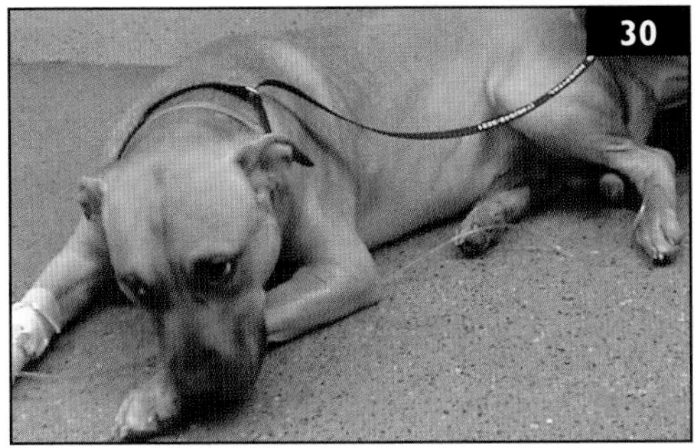
30

1 What would be the first step to work-up the problem of pale mucous membranes?
2 What infectious disease are American Pitbull Terriers predisposed to, and what is the likely reason for this breed predisposition?

CASE 31 Case 31 is the same dog as case 30. *Babesia gibsoni* was detected on a blood smear of the dog (**31**).

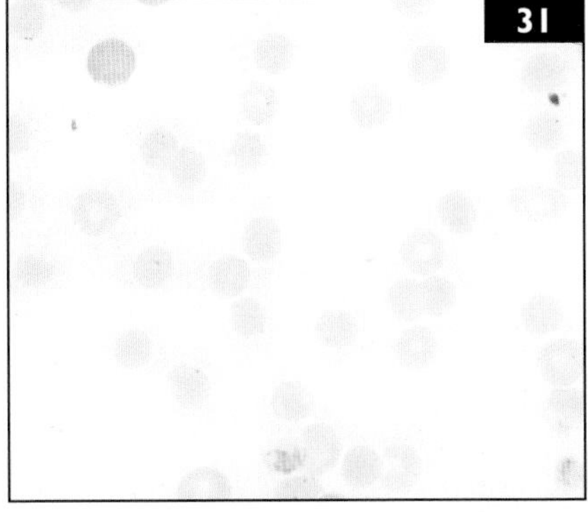
31

1 If no parasites can be found on a blood smear, what would be the diagnostic test of choice?
2 What is the recommended treatment?

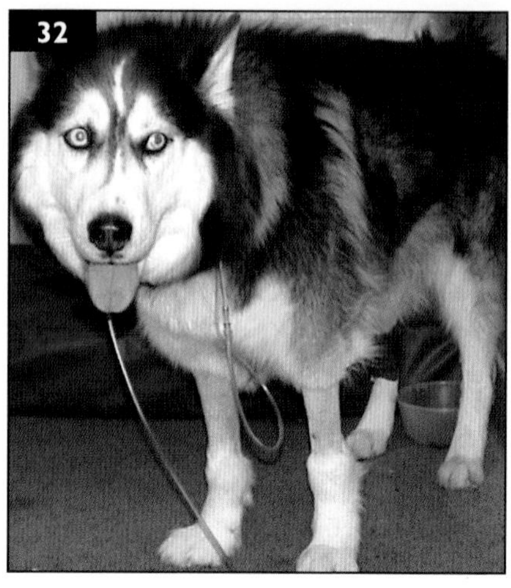

CASE 32 A 7-year-old neutered male Siberian Husky (**32**) was referred because of a 3-week history of exercise intolerance and dry cough. The dog lived in Munich, Germany, but had traveled in the past to several southern European countries. He had not received any ectoparasite control, nor was he ever treated for internal parasites. He had received only vaccinations against rabies. On physical examination, pulse quality was normal, no heart murmur was heard, and lung auscultation revealed harsh lung sounds during expiration. The dog had as slightly reduced BCS (3/9). Otherwise the physical examination was normal. According to the owner, bloodwork performed by the referring veterinarian had revealed moderate hypoalbuminaemia.

1 What is your initial assessment of this case, and what are your differential diagnoses for the dog's problems?
2 What diagnostic tests would you perform?

CASE 33 Case 33 is the same dog as case 32. Thoracic radiographs (**33a, 33b**), CBC, biochemistry panel, and urinalysis were performed. The most notable laboratory findings were a marked

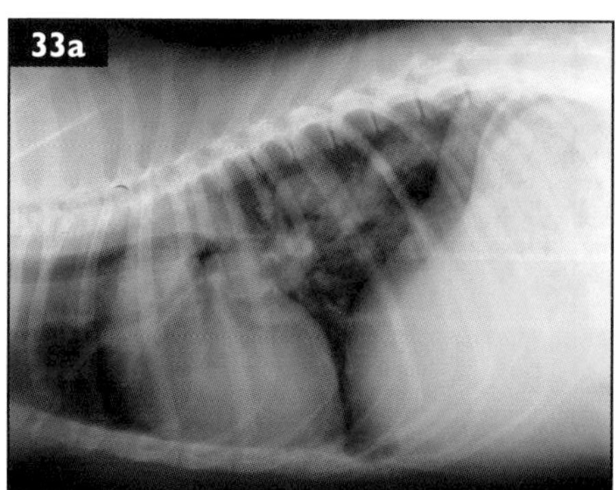

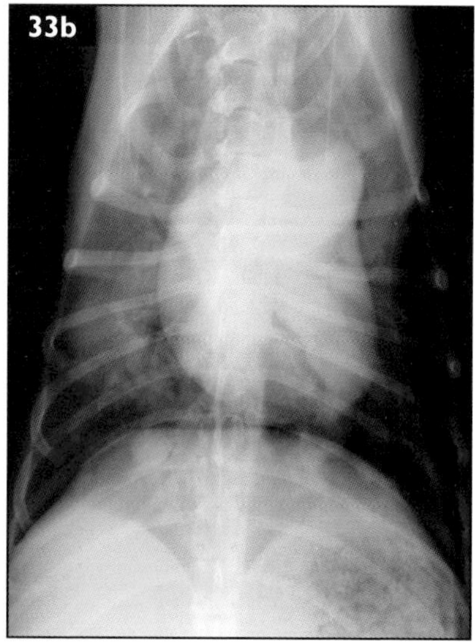

eosinophilia (2.946×10^9/l), hypoalbuminemia (22 g/l), a urine specific gravity of 1.023 with 3+ protein and a benign sediment, and a UPCR of 5.1.

1 What is your interpretation of the radiographs?
2 What is your assessment of the laboratory findings?

CASE 34 Case 34 is the same dog as in cases 32 and 33. Echocardiography (**34a**, **34b**) was performed and showed a dilated right ventricle, tricuspid regurgitation with a velocity of 4.2 m/s (70 mmHg pressure gradient), and dilated pulmonary arteries. Pulsed wave Doppler flow in the pulmonary artery below the pulmonic valve was 1.8 m/s.

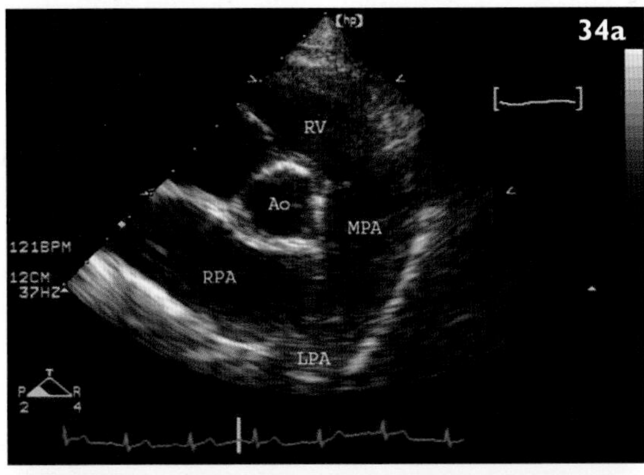

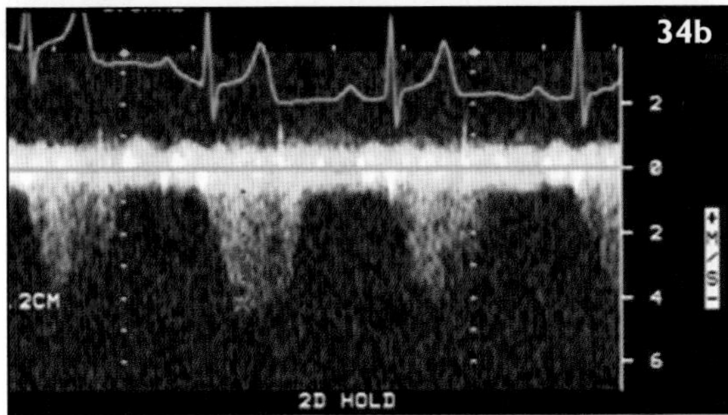

1 What is your interpretation of the echocardiographic examination?
2 What further tests would you recommend?
3 What is the likely underlying pathophysiology for proteinuria in this dog?
4 What is your treatment plan?

CASE 35 A 7-month-old intact male Bernese Mountain Dog was evaluated for a 1-week history of progressive small bowel diarrhea. The diarrhea was described as malodorous and progressing from pudding-like to watery consistency. The dog was fed a commercial diet. He had received a full basic vaccination series and was dewormed 4 months ago. He lived in Munich, Germany, with one other dog in the household and had never been out of the country.

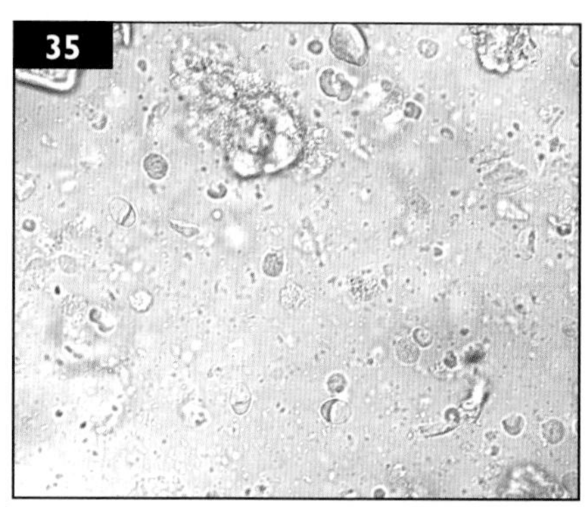

On physical examination, the dog was lethargic. Dehydration was estimated at 6%. Vital signs were within normal limits. Abdominal palpation revealed fluid-filled bowel loops but was otherwise unremarkable. The BCS was 5/9. A fecal flotation was performed (**35**). The owners were concerned about possible detection of fecal parasites, because their two young children and an older mixed-breed dog lived in the same household.

1 What is the diagnosis?
2 If you are not sure about the microscopic interpretation, what additional test(s) could you perform to confirm the diagnosis?
3 Do you think there is a zoonotic risk for the owners and their children?

CASE 36 Case 36 is the same dog as case 35. A fecal SNAP *Giardia* antigen test (IDEXX Laboratories) confirmed the presence of *Giardia* antigen (**36**).

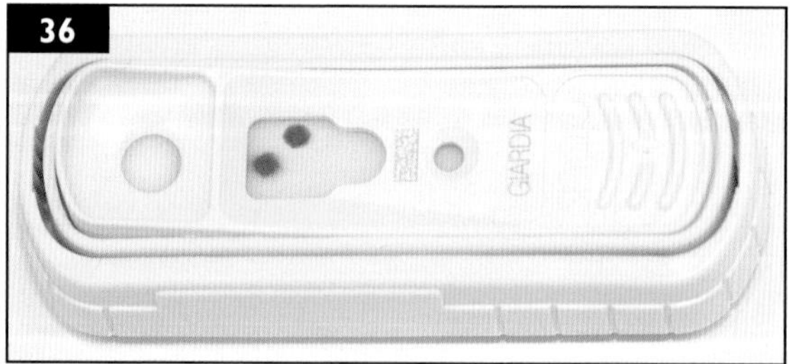

1 What treatment is recommended?
2 Is environmental management indicated, and what recommendations should be made to the owner?

CASE 37 A 4-year-old intact female Labrador Retriever was referred together with two of her 1-week-old puppies (one female and one male) to the emergency service. The bitch had given birth to nine puppies. The owner reported that the birth had been uncomplicated. During the first 4 days of life, the puppies behaved normally. On day 5, the first puppy showed signs of respiratory distress (e.g. tachypnea, gasping for air, and hypersalivation). Other puppies developed the same clinical signs the following day. Affected puppies died 12–24 hours after the onset of clinical signs. Prior to presentation, seven of the puppies had already died. The owner lived in Atlanta, Georgia, USA, and the bitch had never been outside of the area, had received routine vaccinations, and had been treated for endo- and ectoparasites regularly.

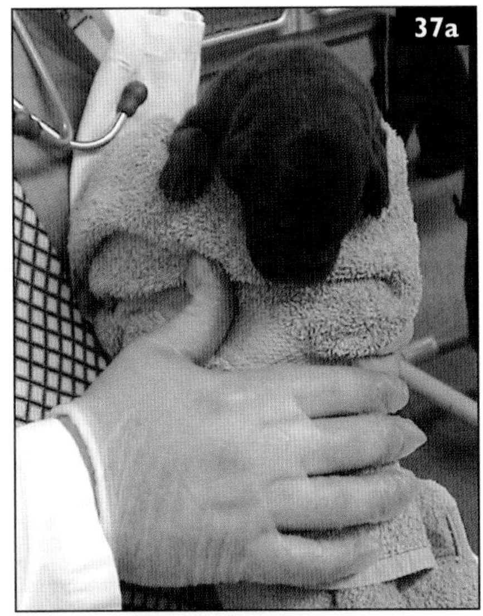

37a

Physical examination of the bitch revealed no significant abnormalities. The genital tract was as expected for the post-whelping period. Both puppies were lethargic with the male being more severely affected (**37a**). They were tachypneic, with vocalization, dyspnea, and hypersalivation. Auscultation of the lungs revealed diffusely increased breath sounds.

Both puppies were euthanized. Necropsy was performed, and findings were similar in both puppies, but more severe in the male pup. On histopathology, multifocal hemorrhage, edema, and increased septal width were found throughout the lungs. Hemorrhage, edema, and necrosis were also found in the liver, kidneys (**37b**), and spleen. Fresh tissue specimens stained positive for canine herpesvirus by IFA.

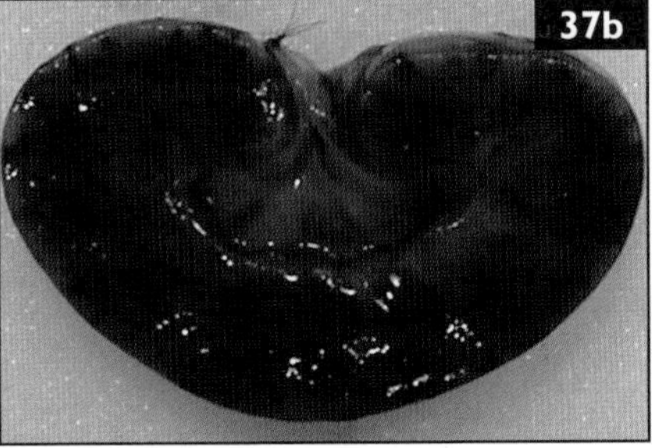

37b

1 How common is canine herpesvirus infection, and how is it transmitted?
2 What clinical signs occur after infection?

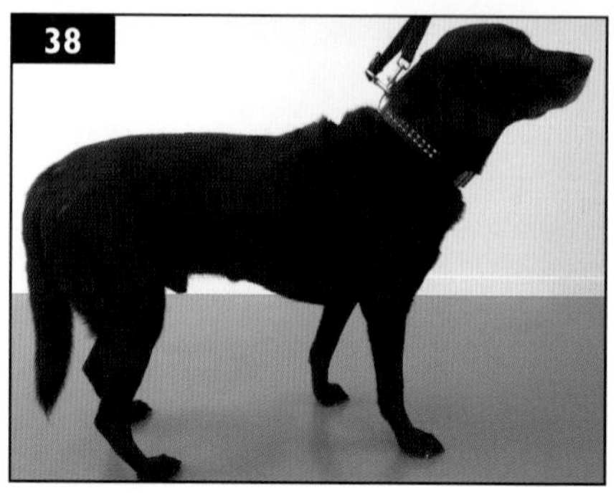

38

CASE 38 An 11-year-old neutered male mixed-breed dog (38) living in Lausanne, Switzerland, was referred for evaluation of possible chronic kidney disease based on the detection of azotemia on bloodwork. The owner reported that the dog had been polyuric and polydipsic for several weeks but was otherwise healthy. The dog had been vaccinated with routine vaccines (distemper virus, adenovirus, parvovirus, *Leptospira* spp., and rabies virus) and was receiving parasiticides on a regular basis. On physical examination, the only abnormalities detected were several subcutaneous masses on the dog's trunk. The results of a CBC, biochemistry panel, and urinalysis with culture (by cystocentesis) are shown below:

Complete blood count	Results	Reference interval
Hematocrit	0.41 l/l	0.42–0.55

Biochemistry panel	Results	Reference interval
Total protein	60 g/l	56–71
Albumin	39 g/l	29–37
Creatinine	122 μmol/l	50–119
Urea nitrogen	6.8 mmol/l	3.8–9.4

Urinalysis	Results	Reference interval
Collection method	Cystocentesis	–
Color, appearance	Yellow, slightly turbid	–
Specific gravity	1.018	1.015–1.045
pH	7.5	5.5–7
Protein	Negative	–
Glucose	Negative	–
Ketone	Negative	–
Bilirubin	+	–
Blood	+	–
Red blood cells	4–8 cells/hpf	0–5
White blood cells	12–20 cells/hpf	0–3
Bacteria	Numerous	0
Urine culture	>10^5 CFU/ml *E. coli* susceptible to amoxicillin	

An abdominal ultrasound revealed no abnormalities.

1 What are your primary differential diagnoses for PU/PD in this dog?
2 How would you interpret the laboratory results?
3 How common are bacterial urinary tract infections in dogs?
4 What are the most common bacterial species causing urinary tract disease in dogs?
5 How would you treat this dog?

CASE 39 A 4-year-old neutered male Cockapoo was evaluated for a 3-week history of anorexia. He had recently developed a non-productive hacking cough. The dog lived in Davis, California, USA, and was employed as a service animal for his disabled owner and traveled on a monthly basis to Hawaii, west Texas, and Arizona. He was regularly vaccinated and on monthly heartworm prophylaxis.

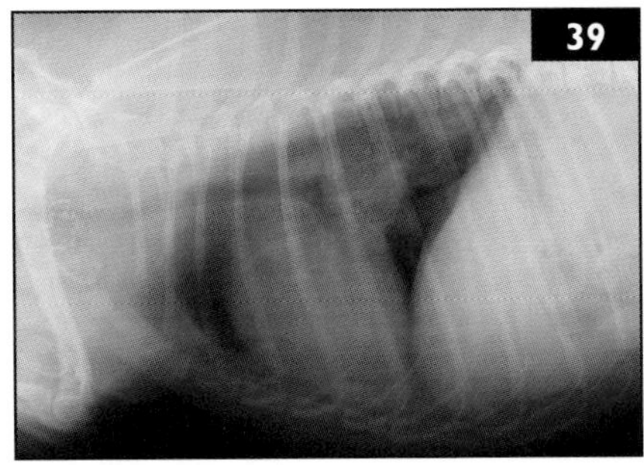

On physical examination, his rectal temperature was 40.1°C (104.2°F), pulse rate was 100 bpm, and respiratory rate was 120 breaths/min. Harsh lung sounds were auscultated bilaterally and a honking cough was elicited on tracheal palpation. Cardiac auscultation was unremarkable. The remainder of the physical examination was normal. A right lateral radiograph had been taken by the veterinarian (**39**).

A CBC was performed:

Complete blood count	Results	Reference interval
Hematocrit	0.388 l/l	0.35–0.58
MCV	66.1 fl	58–72
Platelets	505 × 10^9/l	150–500
White blood cells	24.120 × 10^9/l	5–16
Neutrophils	18.090 × 10^9/l	3–9
Eosinophils	0.555 × 10^9/l	0–1.0
Basophils	0.048 × 10^9/l	0–0.04
Lymphocytes	3.594 × 10^9/l	1–3.6
Monocytes	1.833 × 10^9/l	0.04–0.5

1 How would you interpret the CBC?
2 What imaging abnormalities are present in the radiograph?
3 What differential diagnoses should be considered?
4 What other diagnostic tests should be performed?

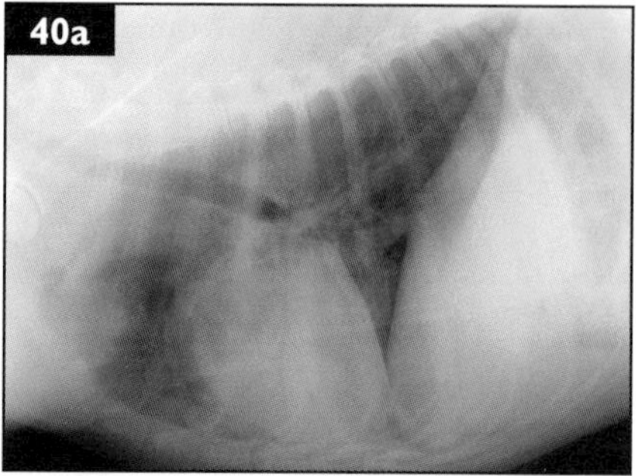

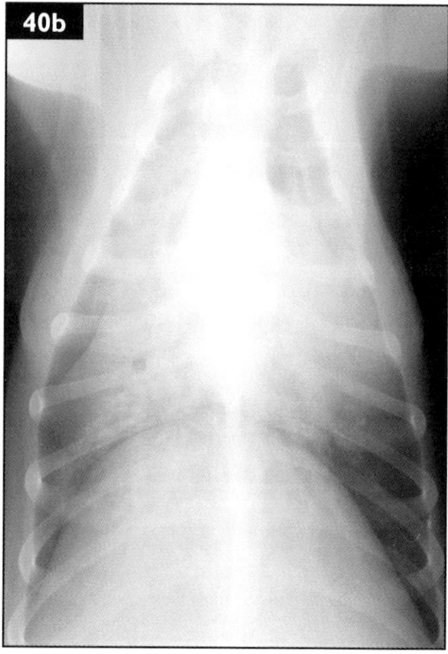

CASE 40 A 5-year-old intact male Weimaraner was evaluated for a 10-day history of cough. Two weeks prior to evaluation, vomiting and diarrhea had been noted but had resolved in 2 days. The owner of the dog lived in Davis, California, USA, and was part of a rescue foundation and frequently admitted new dogs to the household. She was currently caring for six Weimaraners and all had become sick following the last admission. The other dogs had recovered after treatment with amoxicillin and a cough suppressant; however, this dog continued to cough and experienced a 5 kg weight loss. All dogs were vaccinated every 3 years with products purchased from the local supply store. They were also treated with endo- and ectoparasiticides but not on a regular basis.

On physical examination, the temperature was 39.6°C (103.3°F), pulse 108 bpm, and respiratory rate 30 breaths/min with mild expiratory effort. The dog repeatedly exhibited a soft moist cough. Harsh expiratory breath sounds were auscultated dorsally. A CBC and thoracic radiographs (**40a, 40b**) were obtained.

Complete blood count	Results	Reference interval
Hematocrit	0.43 l/l	0.35–0.58
Platelets	365 × 10^9/l	150–500
White blood cells	23.690 × 10^9/l	5–16
Mature neutrophils	19.663 × 10^9/l	3–9
Band neutrophils	0.237 × 10^9/l	0–0.5
Eosinophils	0.474 × 10^9/l	0–1.0
Lymphocytes	0.711 × 10^9/l	1–3.6
Monocytes	2.606 × 10^9/l	0.04–0.5

1 How would you interpret the CBC results and radiographs?
2 Which differential diagnoses are highest on your list?

CASE 41 Case 41 is the same dog as 40. A bronchoscopy was performed (**41a**), and bronchoalveolar lavage fluid was obtained (**41b**).

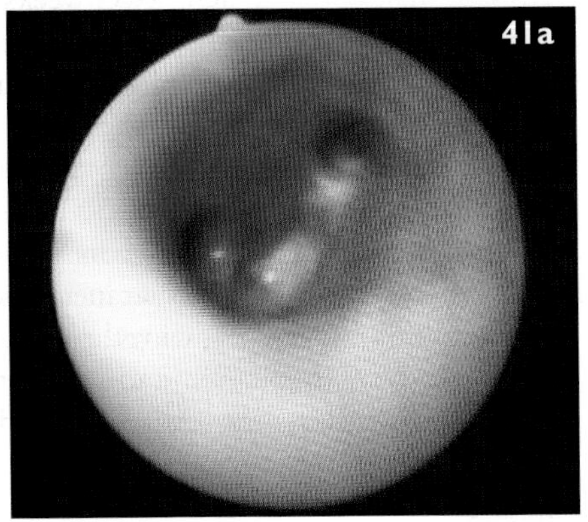
41a

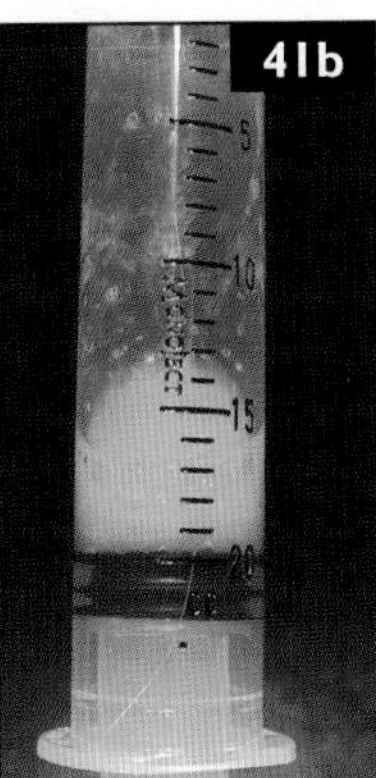
41b

1 What tests would you recommend on this fluid?
2 What underlying diseases should be considered?

CASE 42 A 6-year-old neutered female German Shepherd Dog was admitted to the emergency service of the University Veterinary Teaching Hospital in Munich, Germany, because of lethargy and fever of 2 days' duration. The dog had been bright and alert in the days leading up to this episode, but had been bitten in the cervical area by another German Shepherd Dog 2 weeks previously. The dog had been seen by a veterinarian at that time who had cleaned and closed the wound. The dog was up to date on routine vaccinations and was regularly treated with parasiticides. On physical examination, pulse quality was normal, but an irregular rhythm was noted. No heart murmur was heard on auscultation of the thorax. Temperature was elevated (40.1°C [104.2°F]). The bite wound was identified and appeared to be healing normally. Otherwise the physical examination was unremarkable. An ECG (**42**) was obtained (paper speed 50 mm/s, 1 cm = 1 mV).

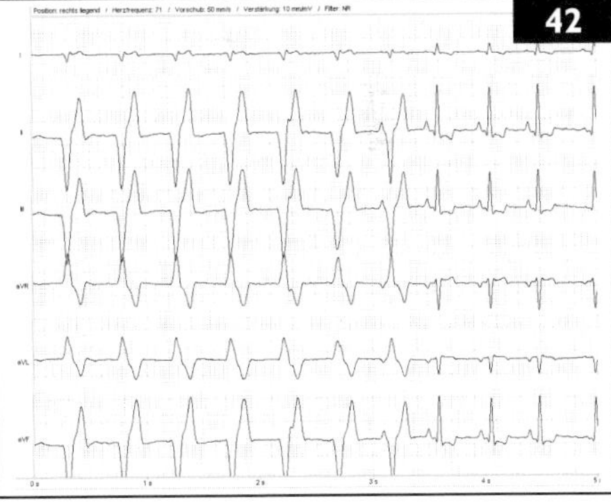
42

1 What is your ECG diagnosis?
2 How would you treat the ECG abnormality?

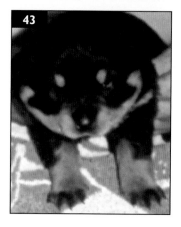

CASE 43 A 3-week-old intact female Rottweiler was evaluated because the owner noted bilateral swelling below the ears (**43**) that appeared over a period of a few hours. No other abnormalities were reported. The puppy otherwise had normal behavior and was suckling. The puppy had not yet been vaccinated or treated for endoparasites. The bitch was 3 years old and was the only adult dog in the household. The owner explained that the pregnancy had been an accident. The owner and his family lived in Warsaw, Poland, and the owner reported that his child had been diagnosed with mumps 6 days previously.

Physical examination revealed a temperature of 38.5°C (101.3°F). Both parotid salivary glands were significantly enlarged, firm, but movable and non-painful on palpation. The skin over the parotid glad was normal. The rest of the physical examination, including an oral cavity examination, was unremarkable.

1 What is the most likely diagnosis?
2 What diagnostic tests could be considered?
3 What is the prognosis?

CASE 44 Case 44 is the same dog as case 43. Mumps is suspected in this puppy. The rest of the litter (nine other puppies) were apparently healthy, and so was the bitch (**44**).

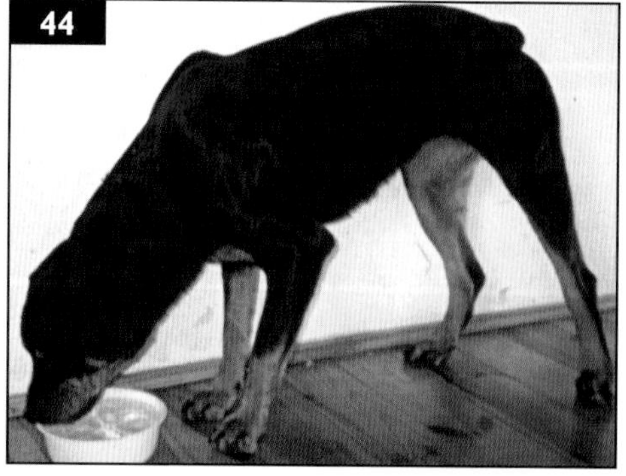

1 What are the possible differential diagnoses?
2 What treatment is needed?
3 What complications can develop in the course of mumps in dogs?
4 Can a dog suffering from mumps transfer this infection to humans or other animals?

CASE 45 A 1-year-old neutered female French Bulldog was evaluated for multiple "wart-like" lesions on the eyelids of its right eye, which had developed within the last 4 weeks. The dog had become increasingly uncomfortable, with a serous ocular discharge from this eye. The owner had also noticed cloudiness at the lateral part of the eye. The dog lived in Atlanta, Georgia, USA, was otherwise healthy, current on all vaccinations, and enrolled in a regular endo- and ectoparasite control program.

Physical examination was unremarkable besides the ophthalmic changes. On ophthalmic examination of the right eye multiple, light-brown pigmented, round, "cauliflower-like" lesions of different sizes were located around the upper and lower eyelids, mainly at the lateral aspect of the eye and the adjacent conjunctiva (45). The conjunctiva was diffusely hyperemic and mildly chemotic. On slit lamp examination, focal corneal edema was found in the lateral quadrant of the cornea, surrounding a deep stromal corneal ulcer. The ulcer stained positive with fluorescein, but a small "clear" area remained in the center of the ulcer. The anterior chamber had very mild flare (positive Tyndall effect). The iris was normal, but the pupil was rather miotic.

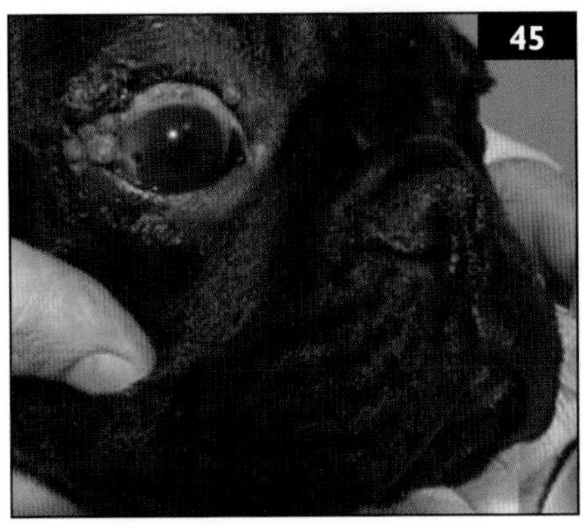
45

Ophthalmic examination	Right eye (OD)	Left eye (OS)
Menace response	Present	Present
Dazzle reflex	Present	Present
Pupillary light reflex	Pupil miotic	Normal
Schirmer tear test	20 mm/min	15 mm/min
Intraocular pressure	10 mmHg	15 mmHg

1 What is your ocular diagnosis?
2 What diagnosis of the eyelid lesions might you suspect based on the clinical presentation?
3 What treatment do you suggest for this dog?

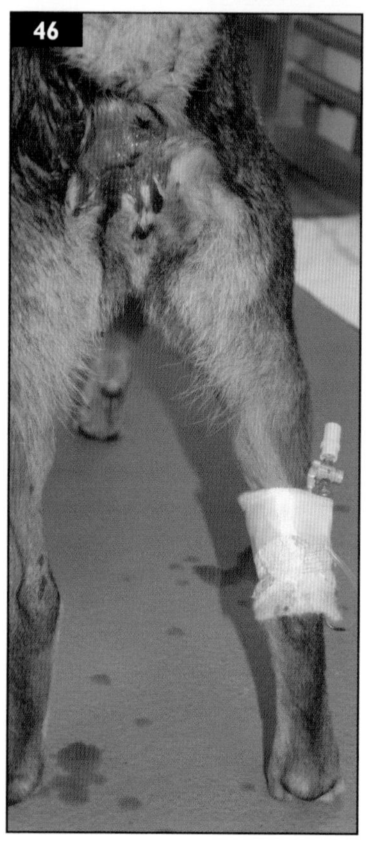

CASE 46 A 5-year-old neutered female mixed-breed dog was evaluated for acute hemorrhagic diarrhea (**46**) of 12 hours' duration. Vomiting had started about 12 hours before the diarrhea was observed. The diarrhea was described as watery with a pale red color, progressing in severity and frequency. Over the last 2 hours, the dog had become lethargic and refused to walk. The dog lived in Munich, Germany, and had never been outside the country. She was regularly vaccinated and dewormed. She also received ectoparasite control on a regular basis. The dog was on a raw meat diet, and this had not been changed for at least 1 year. Intoxication was considered unlikely by the owner.

On physical examination, the dog was lethargic. Heart and respiratory rate were 140 bpm and 54 breaths/min, respectively. The rectal body temperature was 36.7°C (98.1°F). The dog had pale mucous membranes and the capillary refill time was >2 seconds. Dehydration was estimated at 10%. Abdominal palpation revealed a tense but not obviously painful abdomen. The dog had a BCS of 4/9 (30 kg).

1 What are the differential diagnoses for acute hemorrhagic diarrhea, and what diagnostic tests would you perform?
2 What is the definition of hemorrhagic gastroenteritis syndrome?
3 Which dogs are predisposed to hemorrhagic gastroenteritis syndrome?

CASE 47 Case 47 is the same dog as case 46. On evaluation, the dog showed clinical signs that were suggestive of sepsis (e.g. hypothermia, tachycardia, and tachypnea). A blood stream infection with primary enteropathogenic bacteria was considered possible. Therefore, a fecal culture for enteropathogenic bacteria and a blood culture (**47**) were performed.

1 What information from the history is important for interpretation of the fecal culture?
2 What bacterial species are currently considered primary enteropathogenic bacteria?
3 Which bacterial species is believed to play a primary role in dogs with hemorrhagic gastroenteritis syndrome?

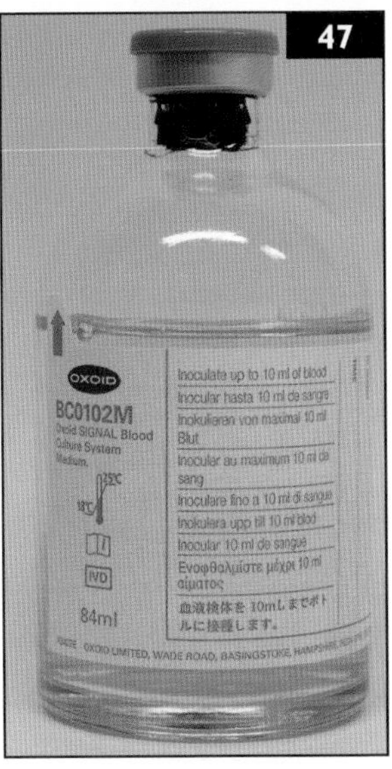

CASE 48 Case 48 is the same dog as cases 47 and 46. During the first 24 hours, a rapid improvement of clinical signs could be observed. Fluid therapy is considered the most important treatment. Different crystalloid and colloid fluids are available (**48**).

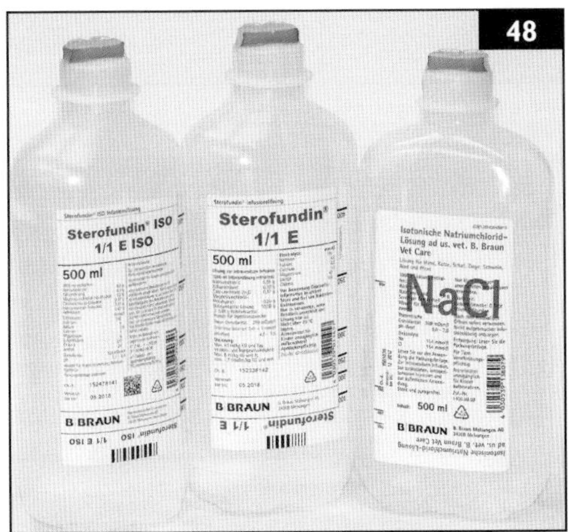

1 Why is fluid therapy considered life saving in this case?
2 How much fluid would you give over the first 24 hours?
3 Would you treat this dog with antibiotics?

CASE 49 A 5-year-old intact male Pointer mix was evaluated for bilateral blindness and bluish-cloudy, red, and painful eyes (**49a, 49b**). Prior to the onset of the ocular symptoms, the dog had been very lethargic with decreased appetite. In addition, intermittent episodes of coughing and lameness were reported. The dog served as an active hunting dog in Helen, Georgia, USA, but the owner often went on hunting trips to the Mississippi and Ohio River valleys. The dog had received regular vaccinations as well as endo- and ectoparasite control.

On physical examination, the mandibular lymph nodes were enlarged and the dog had a rectal body temperature of 39.9°C (103.8°F). The left eye appeared enlarged (**49c**). Otherwise, the physical examination was unremarkable. An ophthalmic examination was performed.

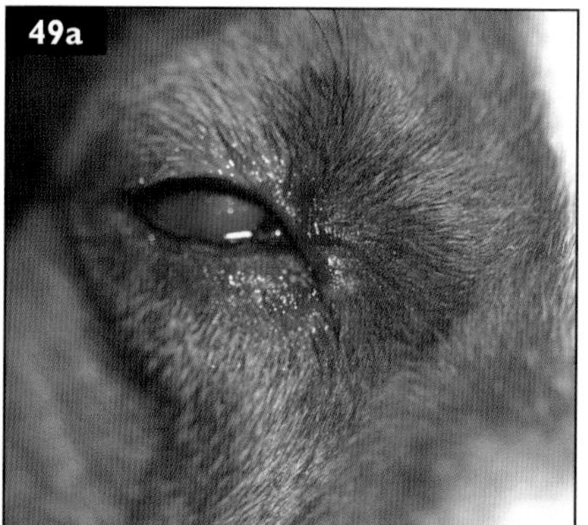
49a

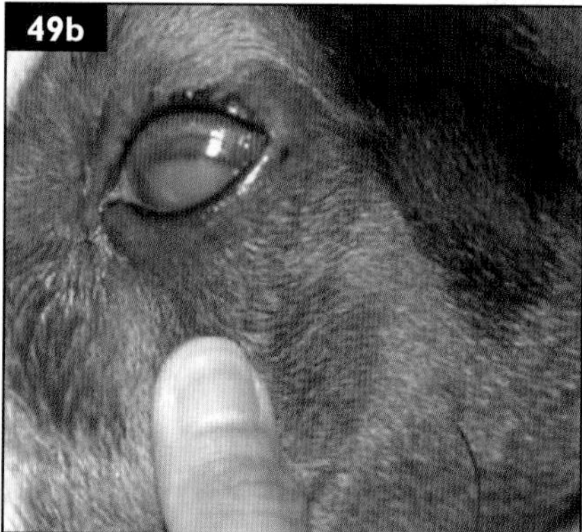
49b

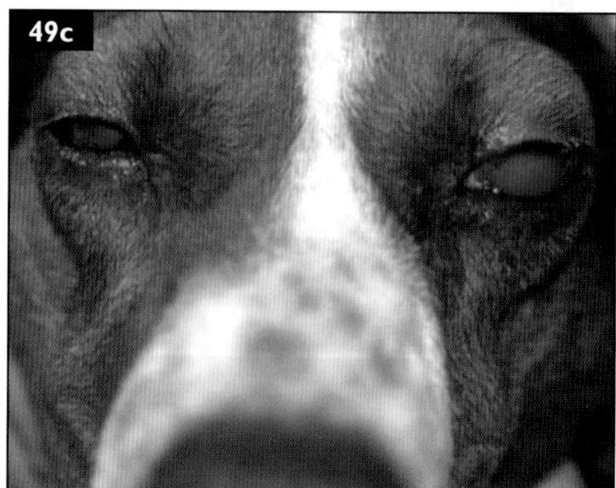
49c

Ophthalmic examination	Right eye (OD)	Left eye (OS)
Menace response	Absent	Absent
Dazzle reflex	Absent	Absent
Pupillary light reflex	Dilated	Cannot assess
Schirmer tear test	15 mm/min	15 mm/min
Intraocular pressure	25 mmHg	58 mmHg

1 What ophthalmic findings are present?
2 What further diagnostic tests would you suggest?

CASE 50 Case 50 is the same dog as case 49. Ocular ultrasound (**50a**) and fine needle aspiration of the right mandibular lymph node with cytologic examination were performed (**50b**).

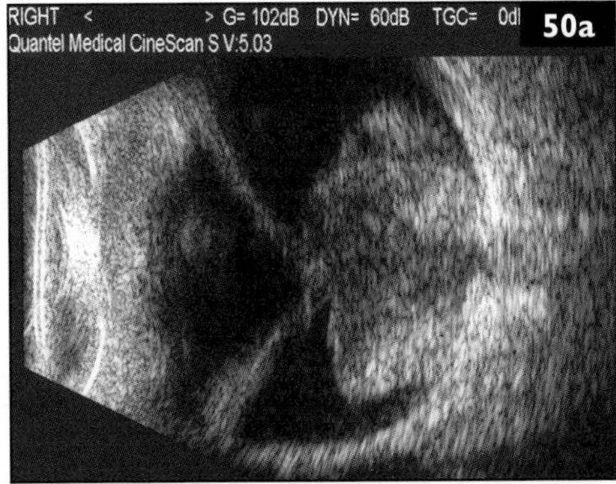

50a

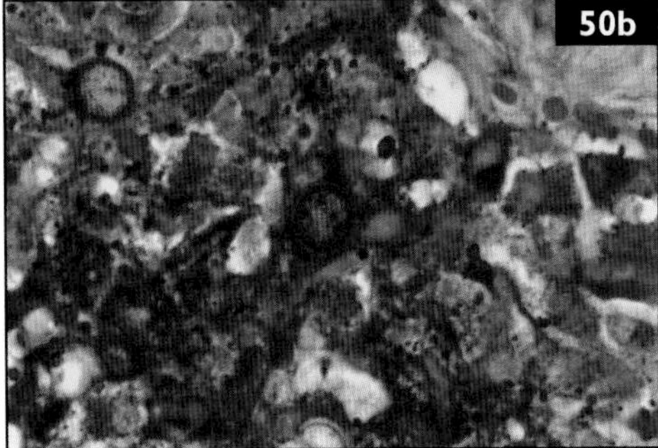
50b

1 What is the diagnosis?
2 What treatment would you suggest?
3 What is the prognosis for vision in this dog?

CASE 51 A 9-year-old neutered female mixed-breed dog living in Augsburg, Germany, was referred for a several-week history of dry cough and lethargy. The owner also noticed exercise intolerance and a decreased activity level. A 10-day course of treatment with enrofloxacin did not improve the clinical signs. The dog had no travel history outside northern Europe. She was up to date on routine vaccinations; preventive treatment for parasites was unknown. On physical examination, the dog was lethargic with normal vital signs. On auscultation of the thorax, slightly harsh lung sounds were noted during inspiration and expiration; the heart sounds were normal. Cutaneous ecchymoses were noted on the ventral and lateral aspects of the abdomen (**51**).

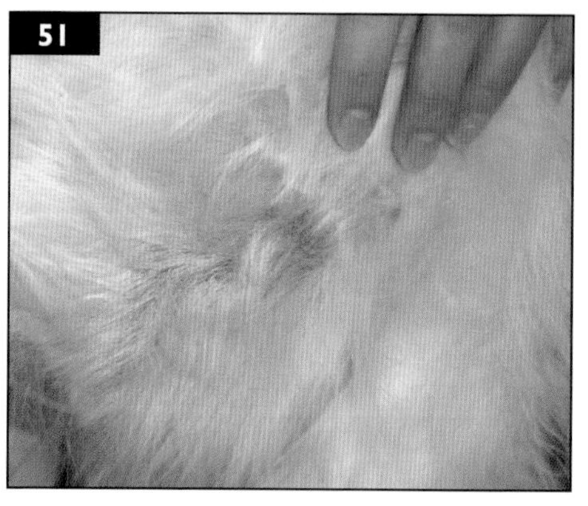
51

1 What are the differential diagnoses for the problems identified?
2 What diagnostic tests would you perform?

CASE 52 Case 52 is the same dog as case 51. Thoracic radiographs (**52a, 52b**), CBC, serum biochemistry analysis, urinalysis, and a coagulation profile were performed. The CBC showed only mild eosinophilia. Serum biochemistry

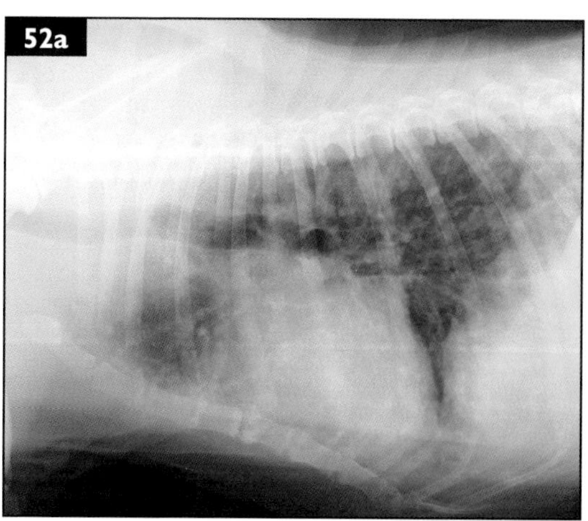
52a

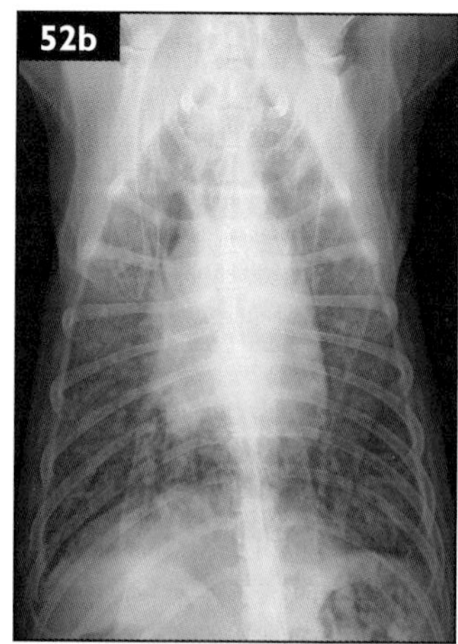
52b

analysis and urinalysis detected no abnormalities. The coagulation profile revealed the following:

Coagulation panel	Results	Reference interval
PT	42 sec	16–27
aPTT	56 sec	10–13
D-dimers	1,000 ng/ml	<250

1 What is your assessment of the diagnostic test results?
2 What additional diagnostic work-up would you suggest?

CASE 53 Case 53 is the same dog as cases 51 and 52. Baermann fecal examination was negative. Cytologic examination of bronchoalveolar lavage fluid revealed larvae of *Angiostrongylus vasorum* (53).

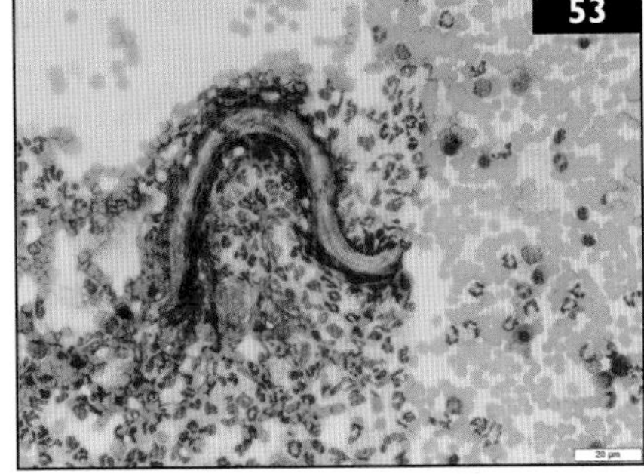
53

1 What treatment would you suggest for this dog?
2 What should you recommend to the owner to prevent reinfection?

CASE 54 A 7-year-old neutered male Golden Retriever was evaluated because of a 2-month history of serous right-sided nasal discharge and sneezing. He walked and ran daily in the fields and woods around the owner's house. The dog lives in Davis, California, USA. The dog was up to date on core vaccinations and was receiving monthly heartworm prophylaxis. The photograph was taken on physical evaluation (54).

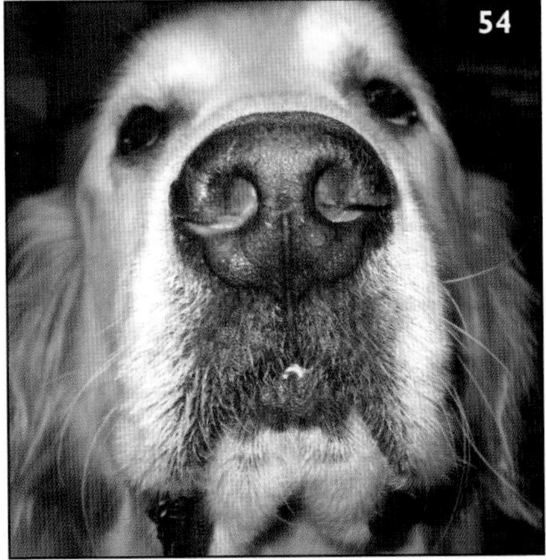
54

1 What is the most likely diagnosis?
2 What physical examination features would be expected in this dog?

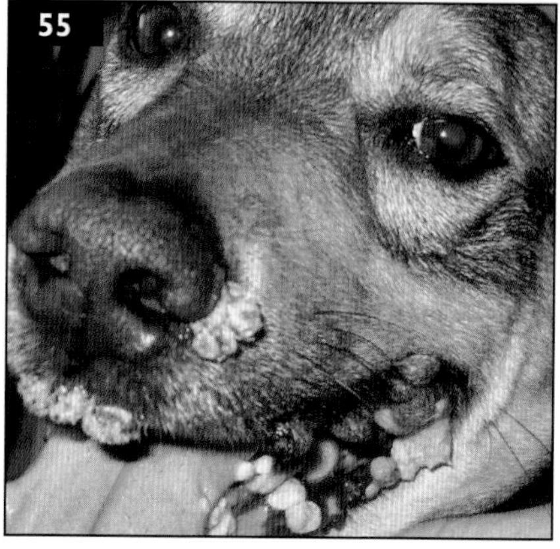

CASE 55 A 1.5-year-old intact male mixed-breed dog was evaluated for wart-like lesions in the mouth, which had been present for at least the last 3 weeks. The dog lived in Katowice, Poland, had never traveled outside the country and had received regular vaccinations (distemper virus, adenovirus, parvovirus, and rabies virus) and prophylactic treatment for ectoparasites and endoparasites.

On physical examination, the dog was bright and alert and in good body condition. The only abnormalities noted were multiple, variably sized, firm, white–gray cauliflower-like lesions on lips, buccal mucosa, palate, tongue, gingiva, and mucocutaneous junctions around the mouth (**55**).

1 What is the most likely diagnosis?
2 Are there other differential diagnoses?
3 How can the diagnosis be confirmed?

CASE 56 Case 56 is the same dog as case 55. Canine oral papillomatosis was diagnosed, based on the appearance of the lesions (**56**).

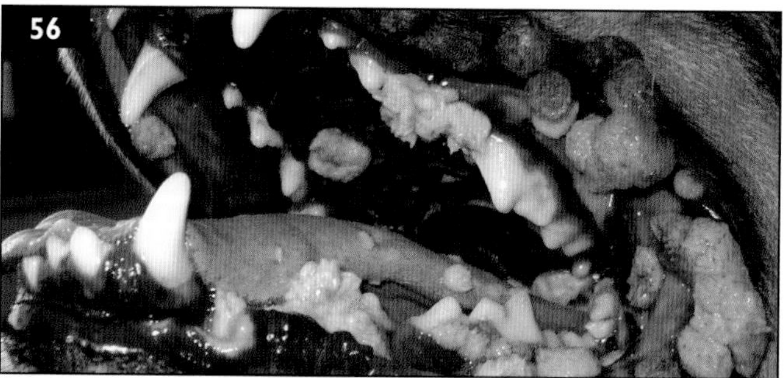

1 What is the prognosis?
2 What treatment is indicated?
3 Can dogs be vaccinated against oral papillomatosis?

CASE 57 Case 57 is the same dog as cases 55 and 56. Laser surgery was performed to remove prominent warts (57).

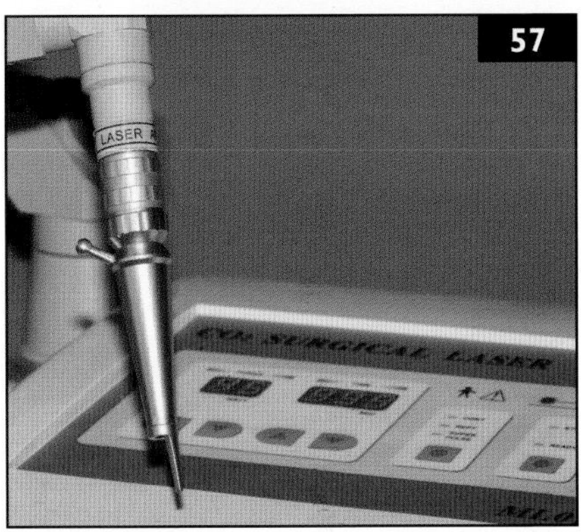

1 Can this dog spread the disease to other dogs?
2 Are other animals and humans at risk of becoming infected?

CASE 58 A 5-year-old intact male Rhodesian Ridgeback was evaluated for non-ambulatory tetraparesis, reduced mentation, and a mild head tilt to the right (58). Further questioning of the owner revealed a 3-month history of chronic progressive ataxia with hypermetria. Sudden worsening of the dog's clinical condition occurred 1 week after treatment with prednisolone (1 mg/kg/day) was initiated.

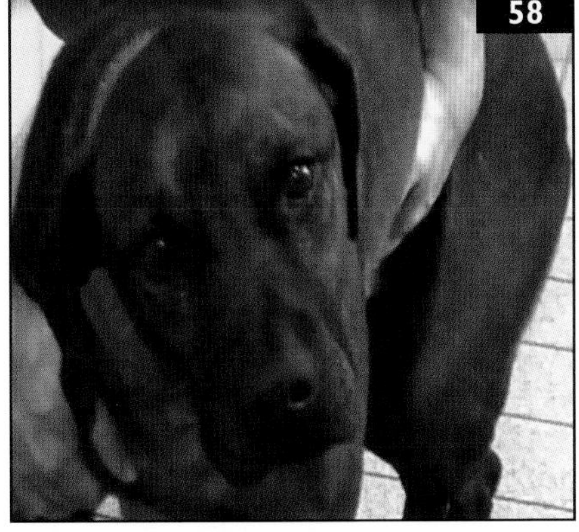

The dog came from Munich, Germany, had never traveled outside the country, and had received regular vaccinations. He had not received any antiparasitic treatment within the last 2 years.

On neurologic examination, masticatory muscle atrophy and mild cervical pain were noted as additional findings. Besides the neurologic changes, the physical examination was unremarkable.

Further work-up with MRI and cerebrospinal fluid examination showed cerebellar atrophy and a lymphohistiocytic CSF pleocytosis.

1 What further diagnostic tests should be performed?
2 What treatment should be started while results of diagnostic tests are pending?
3 Why might glucocorticoids be contraindicated for treatment of this disease?

CASE 59 A 6-year-old neutered male Pug was evaluated for labored breathing, cough, lethargy, anorexia, and pale mucous membranes. These signs had progressed over the previous 2 weeks (**59**). No ocular or nasal discharge, cough, sneezing, polyuria, or polydipsia was present. Urination was normal. The dog had no significant past medical history. The dog lived indoors only and currently lived in Montreal, Canada, but traveled with his owners every summer to the Gulf coast of the United States. The dog was up to date on vaccinations. The clients did not use any preventive treatments for parasites because the dog did not have outdoor access.

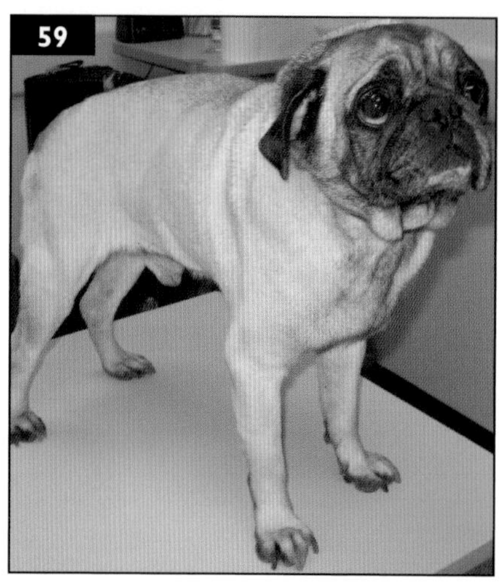

Physical examination revealed a temperature of 38.3°C (100.9°F), increased bronchovesicular lung sounds in the caudodorsal region of the thorax, tachypnea with a deep labored breathing pattern, pale mucous membranes, a grade III/VI right apical systolic murmur, and an irregular cardiac rhythm with pulse deficits.

1 How would you initially manage this case?
2 The client is concerned about costs; therefore, what diagnostic tests would you perform?
3 What are the primary differential diagnoses for the problems?

CASE 60 Case 60 is the same dog as case 59. Lateral and ventrodorsal thoracic radiographs were obtained (**60a, 60b**).

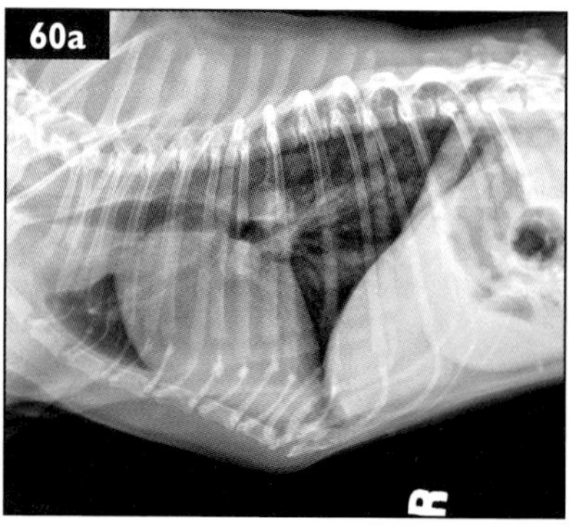

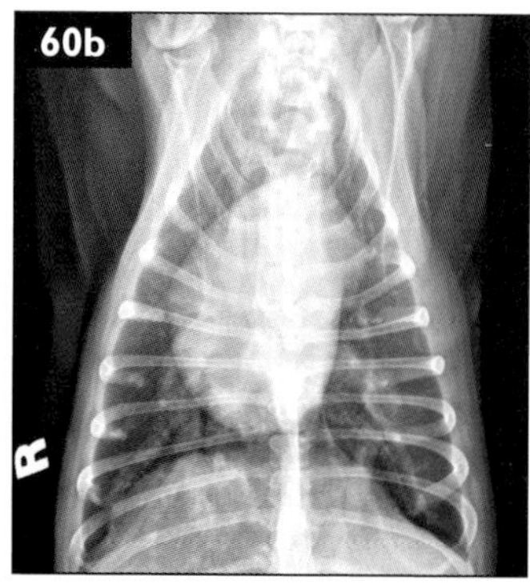

1 Describe the thoracic radiographic findings.
2 How do these findings affect the differential diagnoses list in this case?
3 What is your diagnostic plan?

CASE 61 Case 61 is the same dog as cases 59 and 60. The ECG indicated a sinus tachycardia (156 bpm) with atrial premature complexes and right-shift deviation of the mean electrical axis, suggestive of right ventricular hypertrophy and atrial disease. An echocardiogram showed severe thickening of the right ventricle, with concentric hypertrophy and mild dilation. Pulmonic and tricuspid valvular regurgitation was identified. The right ventricular systolic pressure was estimated via Doppler interrogation of the pulmonic regurgitation gradient as approximately 90 mmHg, consistent with severe pulmonary arterial hypertension. Multiple heartworms were present, which moved from the right ventricle to the right atrium during diastole (**61a**, white arrow). An in-clinic ELISA test was positive for *Dirofilaria immitis* antigen. Microfilariae were detected in blood smears (**61b**). Diagnosis of heartworm disease was confirmed.

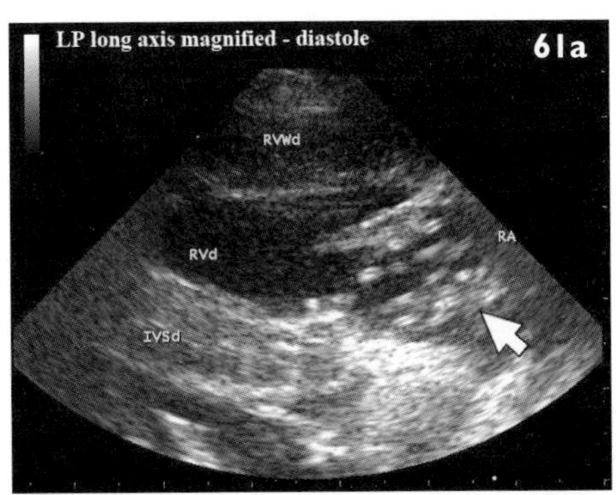

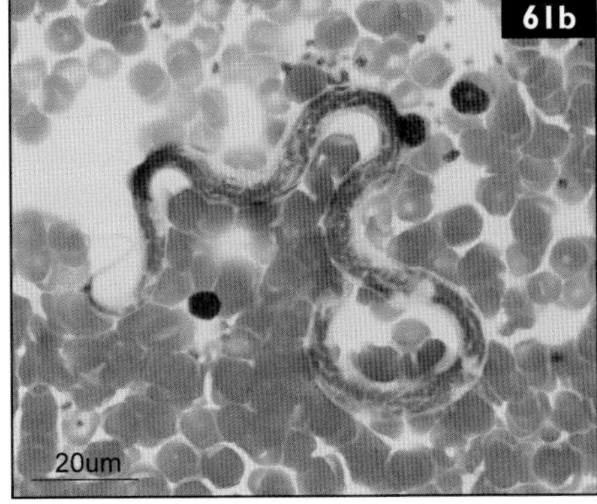

1 What are other important consequences of infection with this parasite?
2 How would you classify the stage of heartworm disease in this case?
3 How would you treat this dog?
4 What is the prognosis?

CASE 62 A 9-year-old neutered female mixed-breed dog from Zurich, Switzerland, was evaluated for a second opinion regarding recurrent cystolithiasis. Over the last 2 years, stones had been surgically removed three times. On abdominal radiography before the first surgery, bladder stones were visible (**62**). Aerobic bacterial urine culture prior to the first surgery was negative. No further urine cultures were performed. Although the dog is currently clinically normal, the owner wanted to make sure that the stones did not recur. Physical examination was unremarkable.

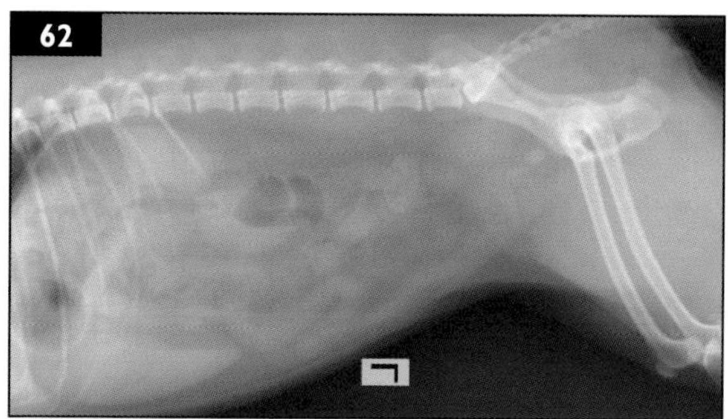

1 What is the most common composition of uroliths in dogs?
2 What further tests would you recommend in this dog?

CASE 63 Case 63 is the same dog as case 62 (**63**). For further diagnostic work-up, cystocentesis was performed for urinalysis including urine culture:

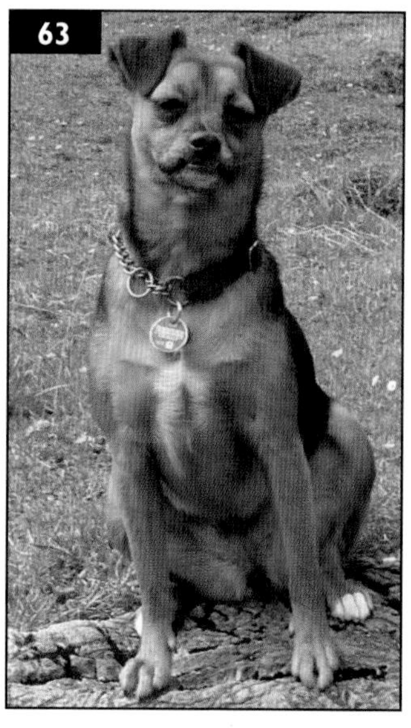

Urinalysis	Results
Color, appearance	Light yellow, medium
Specific gravity	1.026
pH	6.0
Protein	+
Glucose	Negative
Ketone	Negative
Bilirubin	+
Blood	++
Protein to creatinine ratio	0.19
Red blood cells	8–12 cells/hpf
White blood cells	Too numerous to count
Bacteria	Many cocci
Urine culture	Large numbers of coagulase-negative *Staphylococcus* spp.

Abdominal radiographs and ultrasound showed no evidence of cystoliths.

1 Considering the results of the urinalysis, how would you treat this dog?
2 What methods of stone removal other than surgical cystotomy after laparotomy would be possible in this dog?
3 The dog was stone free but bacteriuria was present. What is the difference between bacteriuria and urinary tract infection? List possible reasons for recurrent urinary tract infections in dogs.

CASE 64 A 2-year-old intact male German Shepherd Dog was evaluated for a 2-day history of inappetence and stiff gait, followed by rapidly progressive muscular rigidity and several generalized seizures. A week before the onset of these signs, the owner had taken the dog to another veterinary clinic for a 3-day history of mild lameness. The owner had also noticed a small amount of blood on the left front footpad just before the onset of lameness. Rest was recommended, and the lameness disappeared. The dog lived in a rural area outside Warsaw, Poland, with two other adult dogs and a litter of puppies. The dog had never been vaccinated or treated for parasites. On admission, lateral recumbency and extensor rigidity were present (**64**). The dog was hypersensitive to external stimuli, which resulted in tonic convulsions with opisthotonus, trismus, contraction of the facial musculature (risus sardonicus), enophthalmos with prolapse of the third eyelid, and erect ears. Severe respiratory dysfunction (periods of apnea followed by gasping) and hyperthermia were present. Generalized tetanus was diagnosed, based on the history and clinical signs.

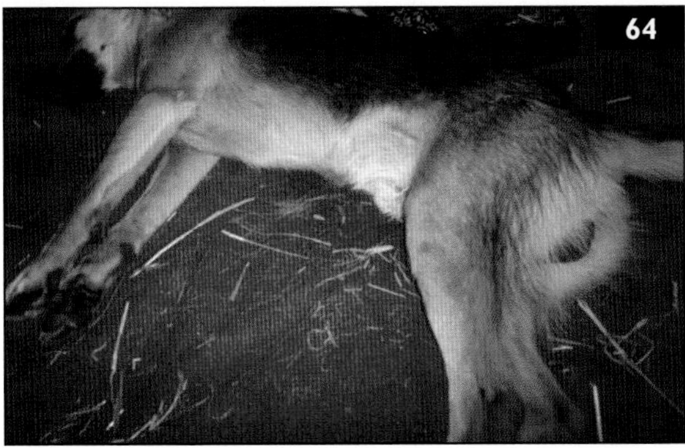
64

1 What is the risk of infection to other animals and humans?
2 Should dogs be vaccinated to prevent tetanus?
3 How can tetanus be prevented in dogs?

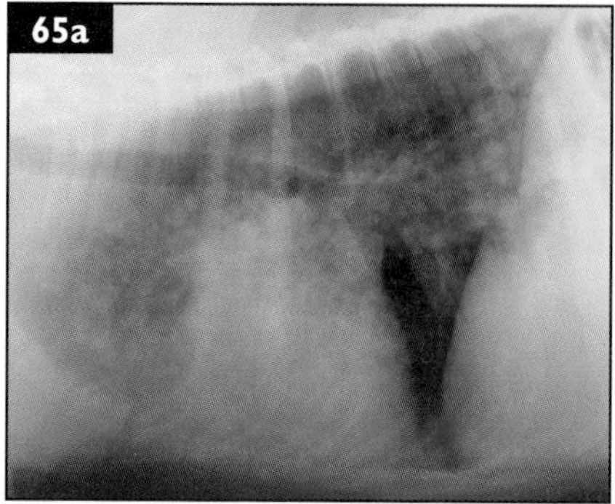

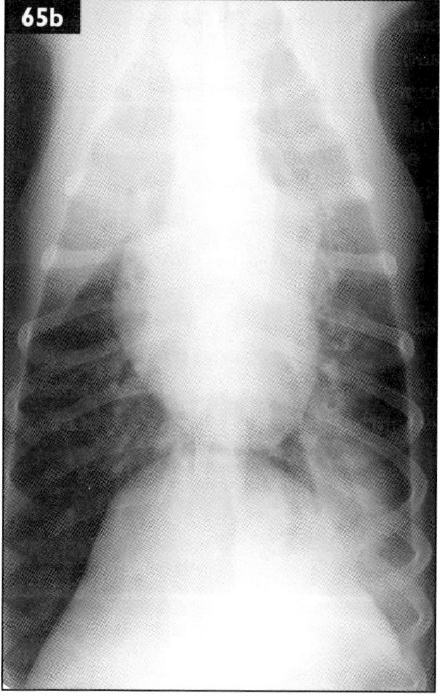

CASE 65 A 2-year-old neutered male Golden Retriever was evaluated because of lethargy and anorexia of 1 week's duration. He lived in the Sierra Nevada Mountains of northern California, USA, and had recently traveled to Ontario in Canada, Vermont in the northeastern USA, and Carmel on the coast of northern California. The dog was up to date on vaccinations and was on heartworm prophylaxis.

On physical examination, the temperature was 39.1°C (102.4°F), pulse 120–160 bpm, and the dog panted continually. The dog demonstrated marked flaring of the nostrils during respiration, and open-mouth breathing. Harsh breath sounds heard bilaterally over the thorax obscured the heart sounds, but no pulse deficits were detected. A dry cough was elicited on tracheal palpation. With minor exertion, marked respiratory difficulty with cyanosis was noted. The remainder of the physical examination was unremarkable. Thoracic radiographs were obtained (**65a, 65b**).

1 What is your interpretation of the thoracic radiographs?
2 What differential diagnoses should be considered?
3 What diagnostic tests should be performed?

CASE 66 Case 66 is the same dog as case 65. Tracheal wash fluid cytology showed a marked pyogranulomatous inflammation and yeast structures that were 15–30 μm in diameter, consistent with infection by the dimorphic fungus *Blastomyces* spp. (**66**).

1 Given the tissue tropism of this organism, what other examinations might be indicated?
2 What treatment options should be considered?

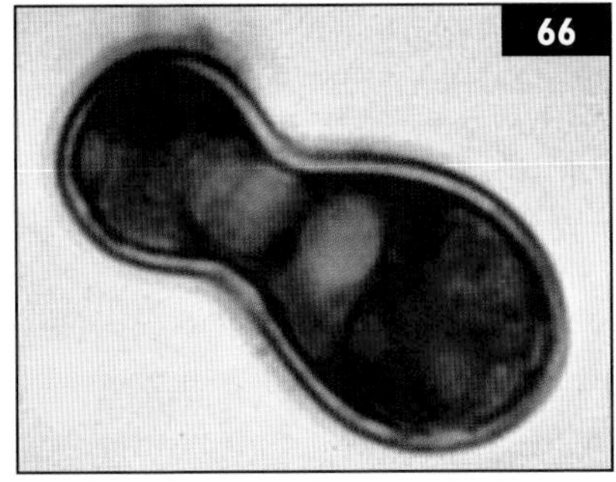
66

CASE 67 A 2-year-old neutered female Pug was evaluated for skin lesions in the region of the right carpus. Erythema, scaling, alopecia, and crusting were present (67). The dog was bright and alert and not very pruritic. It was regularly vaccinated and treated for endoparasites. The dog lived in Ausgburg, Germany, and had never been outside the country.

Physical examination revealed no abnormalities besides the skin lesions described. Skin scrapings were negative. An impression smear was made, stained with a modified Wright's stain, and revealed numerous macrophages and some neutrophils with only a few extracellular bacteria.

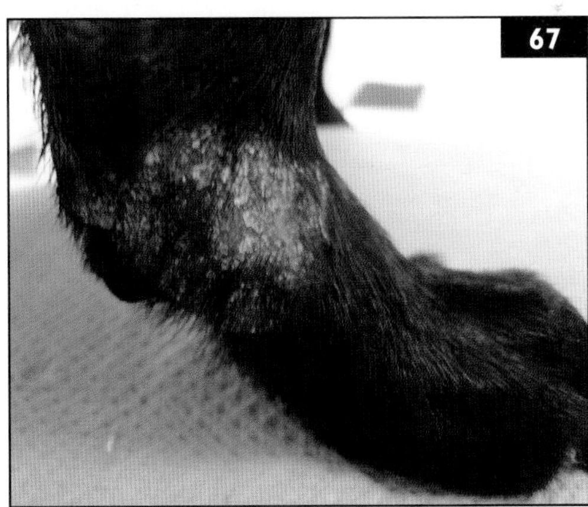
67

1 What is your most likely diagnosis?
2 What further tests are indicated in this dog?
3 How would you treat this dog based on your most likely diagnosis?

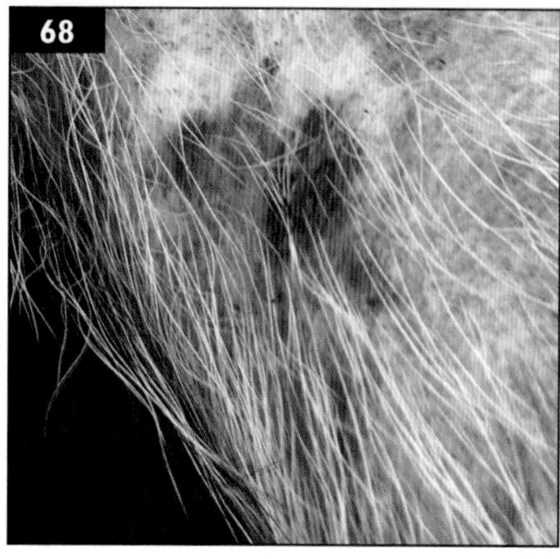

CASE 68 A 6-month-old intact male mixed-breed stray puppy was presented to the University Veterinary Teaching Hospital in Messina, Italy, with severe acute diarrhea and vomiting a few days after he was rescued by an animal shelter. No previous history was available.

On physical examination, abnormal findings included pale mucous membranes, prolonged capillary refill time (3 sec), 7–8% dehydration, pain on abdominal palpation, and increased temperature (40.1°C [104.2°F]). A fecal parvovirus in-house antigen test was positive and CBC revealed a lymphopenia. The dog was kept in isolation and received intensive care, including intravenous fluids, antiemetics, and a parenteral third-generation cephalosporin. Subsequently, there was a progressive improvement of the dog's clinical condition. However, on day 6 the dog again became very lethargic and vomited. In addition, pyrexia and ecchymotic hemorrhages on the skin and mucosal surfaces were observed (**68**).

1 What are your primary differential diagnoses for the new clinical presentation?
2 What diagnostic tests should be done first?

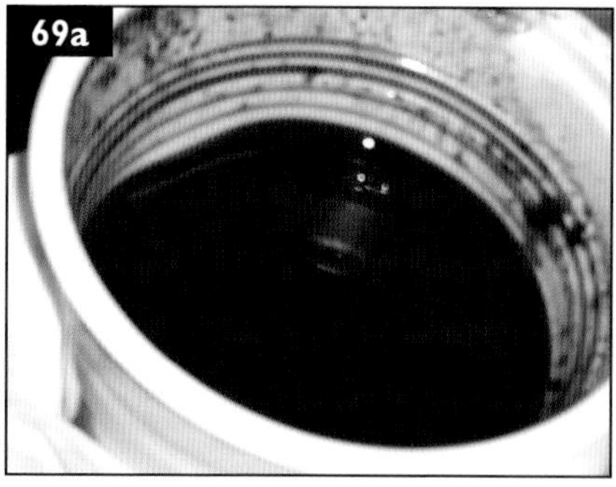

CASE 69 Case 69 is the same dog as case 68. Leukopenia with lymphopenia and neutropenia, a low platelet count, very high ALT activity (7,423 U/l), as well as high aPTT and D-dimers were found on CBC, biochemistry panel, and coagulation profile. One day later, the dog developed hematemesis, melena, and dark orange urine (**69a**). Abdominal and thoracic radiographs were unremarkable.

1 What is the most likely diagnosis in this puppy?
2 What tests could be performed to confirm the diagnosis?
3 Why are confirmatory tests necessary?
4 What is the prognosis for this dog?

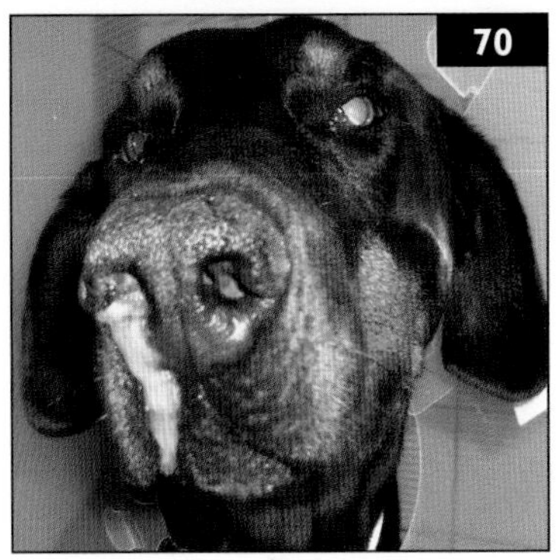

CASE 70 A 3-year-old intact male Doberman Pinscher from Munich, Germany, was evaluated for a 6-month history of mucopurulent nasal discharge (**70**), mainly on the right side. The dog was regularly vaccinated and treated with intestinal parasite preventives. Except for the nasal discharge, the owner did not report any other problems; the dog was bright, alert, and eating well. The dog had received several courses of antimicrobials (including first amoxicillin, later enrofloxacin). During antimicrobial treatment, the nasal discharge improved only slightly. A sample of the nasal discharge had been submitted for bacterial culture and susceptibility testing and yielded *Pasteurella multocida*. The isolate was susceptible to all tested antibiotics. Physical examination revealed purulent right-sided nasal discharge and a slightly enlarged right mandibular lymph node. Otherwise the physical examination was unremarkable.

1 What differential diagnoses should be considered for nasal discharge in this patient?
2 Why did the patient not respond to antimicrobial treatment?
3 How would you proceed to work-up the case?

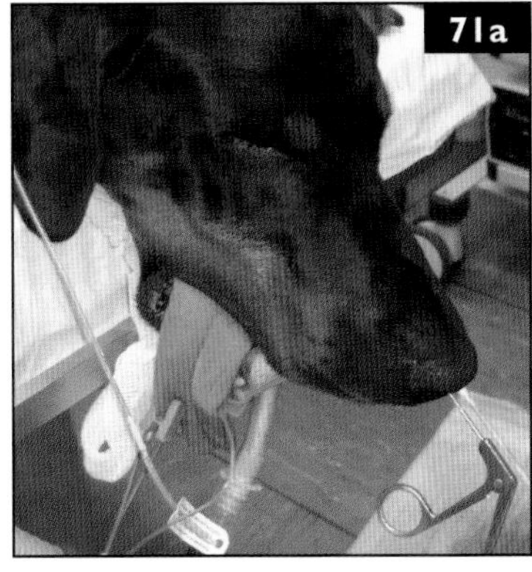

CASE 71 Case 71 is the same dog as case 70. A diagnostic work-up was performed as described. A CBC and serum biochemistry were unremarkable, and coagulation times were normal. CT revealed severe destruction of the turbinates in the right nasal cavity, moderate destruction on the left side, and thickening of the frontal and maxillary bones. The frontal sinuses were filled with abnormal soft tissue on both sides. The cribriform plate was intact. On rhinoscopy with a rigid endoscope (**71a**), white fungal plaques could be visualized on the mucosal surfaces, and there was destruction of the turbinates bilaterally. The right frontal sinus could be accessed with a flexible endoscope and fungal plaques could be visualized in this area as well. Several biopsies were taken of the plaques and submitted for histopathology and fungal culture.

1 What is your diagnosis?
2 What do you recommend for treatment in this case?

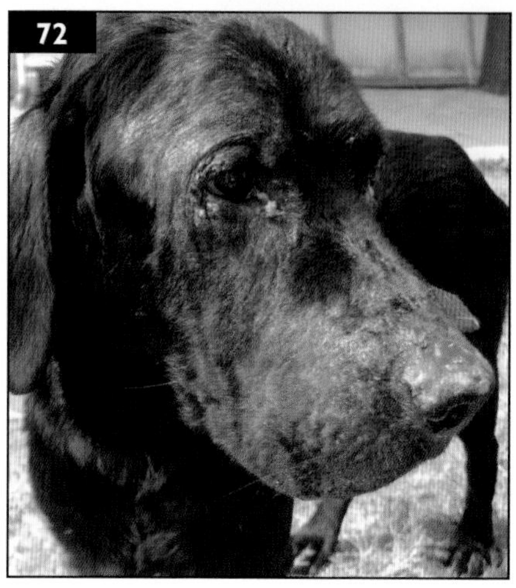

CASE 72 A 6-year-old male Labrador Retriever from Bristol, UK, that had lived in Spain in recent years before returning to the UK 6 months ago was evaluated for a skin problem that included alopecia, crusts, scaling, and hyperpigmentation around the face, ears, limbs, and dorsum (72). Over the last 2 months, the dog had developed progressive inappetence, lethargy, polydipsia, and weight loss. The dog had regularly received core vaccines (distemper virus, adenovirus, parvovirus, rabies virus, and *Leptospira* spp.) and was treated regularly for intestinal parasites.

Physical examination revealed a thin body condition (BCS 2–3/9), mucoid ocular discharge, generalized peripheral lymphadenomegaly, splenomegaly, mild pyrexia, and pale mucous membranes. A CBC, biochemistry panel, and urinalysis were performed.

Complete blood count	Results	Reference interval
Hematocrit	0.26 l/l	0.35–0.58
Reticulocytes	0×10^9/l	0–60
Platelets	50×10^9/l	150–500

Biochemistry panel	Results	Reference interval
Total protein	95 g/l	55.5–77.6
Albumin	21 g/l	31.3–43
Globulin	74 g/l	24.2–34.6
Creatinine	175 μmol/l	44–125
Urea nitrogen	64.2 mmol/l	3.52–10.78
Calcium	2.55 mmol/l	2.2–2.8

Urinalysis revealed a specific gravity of 1.015, with 3+ protein and a benign sediment. The UPCR was 1.5 (RI <1.5).

1 What are the most likely differential diagnoses in this dog?
2 What diagnostic tests should be done next?

CASE 73 Case 73 is the same as case 72. Serum was submitted for *Leishmania* spp. antibody detection. Cytologic examination of a fine needle aspirate of the right popliteal lymph node (73) was performed.

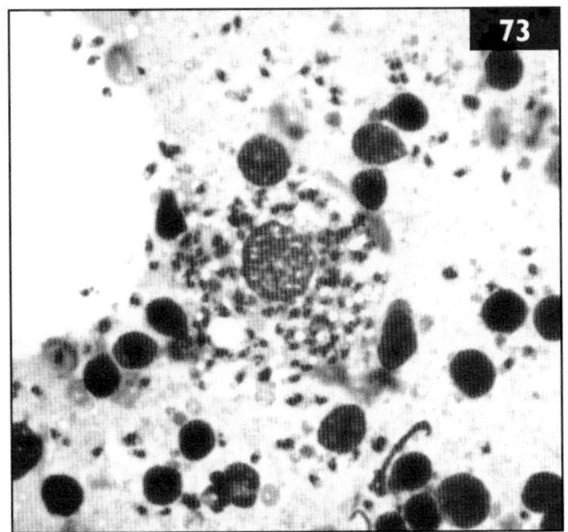

1 Describe the cytologic findings in the lymph node aspirate.
2 What factors can influence the results of *Leishmania* spp. antibody tests?

CASE 74 Case 74 is the same as cases 72 and 73. An indirect fluorescent antibody test revealed a high antibody titer to *Leishmania* spp. (74). The clinical stage of the patient was classified as grade III (severe disease).

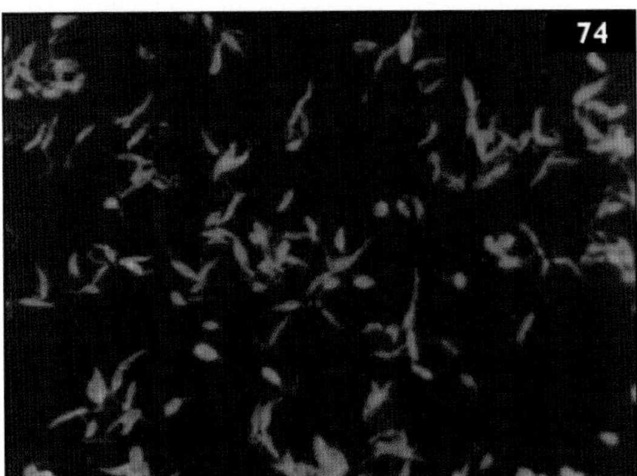

1 What are the treatment options, and what is the prognosis for this dog?
2 The owner has two other dogs and three young children. What actions are indicated to prevent human infection in this situation?

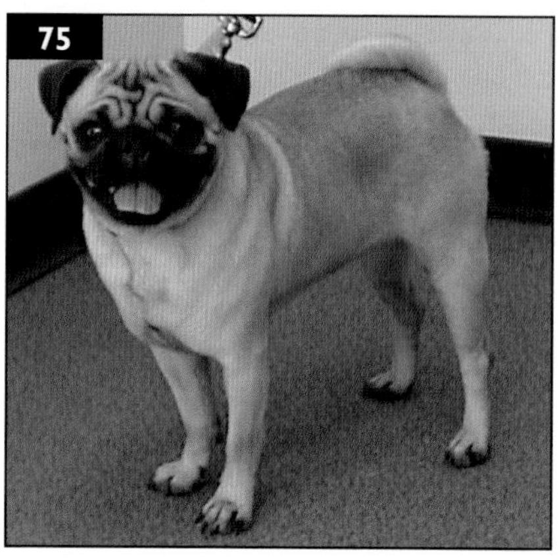

CASE 75 A 4-year-old intact female Pug (75) was referred for evaluation of a 6-week history of cough, respiratory difficulty, and exercise intolerance. The referring veterinarian had previously performed echocardiography and had suspected right ventricular hypertrophy. The dog was up to date on vaccinations (distemper virus, adenovirus, parvovirus, rabies virus, and *Leptospira* spp.), but had not been treated with parasiticides within the last 2 years. The dog lived in Munich, Germany, and had never left the country. On physical examination, the dog was in respiratory distress, lung sounds were harsh on thoracic auscultation, especially during expiration, and the respiratory rate was 80 breaths/min. No cardiac murmur was heard. The heart rate was 160 bpm, but pulses were strong and synchronous. The mucous membranes were pink with a normal capillary refill time. Physical examination otherwise was unremarkable.

1 What is your first assessment of this dog's problems?
2 What diagnostic steps should you perform next?

CASE 76 Case 76 is the same dog as case 75. Thoracic radiographs were performed (**76a**, **76b**) and echocardiography was repeated. Color-flow Doppler showed no evidence of aortic, tricuspid, pulmonic, or mitral valve insufficiency. Figure **76c**

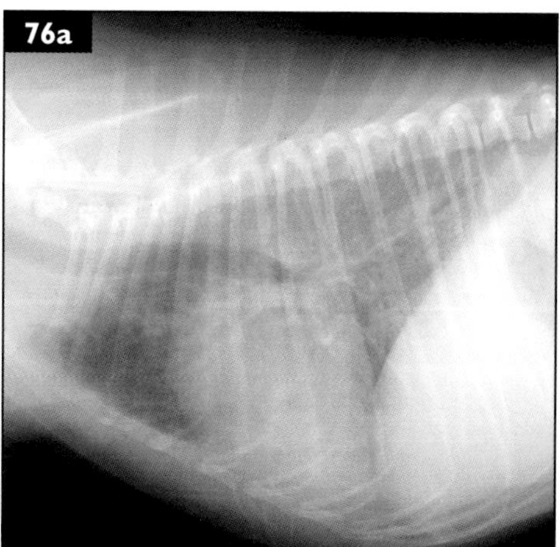

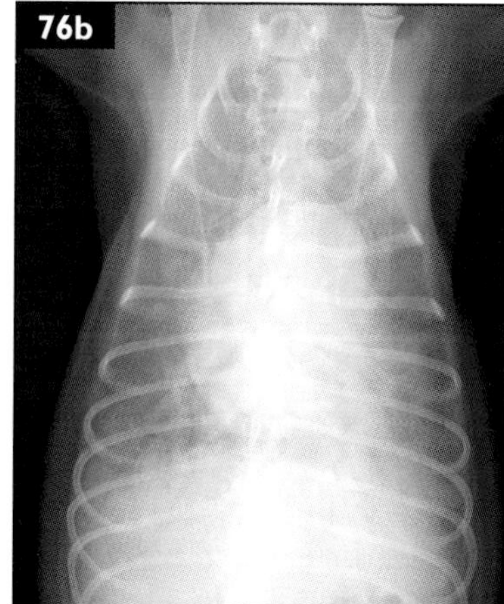

shows a right parasternal long axis view; figure **76d** shows a short axis view with left atrium, aorta, and pulmonary artery.

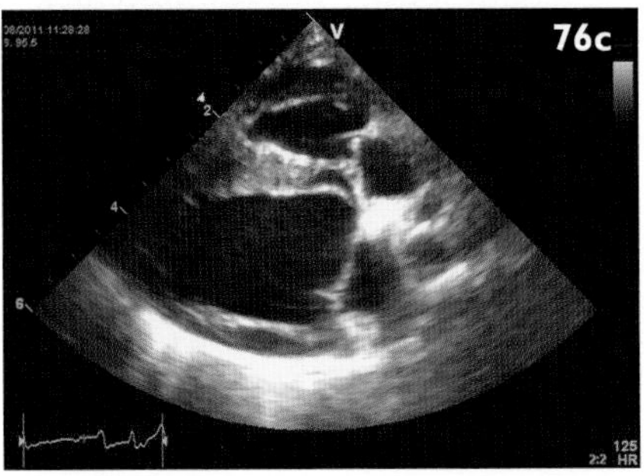

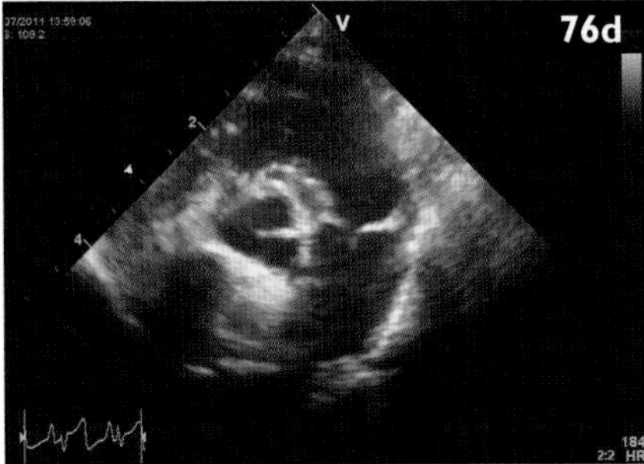

1 What is your assessment of the radiographic findings, and what is the differential diagnosis?
2 What is your assessment of the echocardiographic study?

CASE 77 Case 77 is the same dog as cases 75 and 76 (77). The owners agreed to a further work-up. The echocardiographic study raised suspicion for pulmonary hypertension.

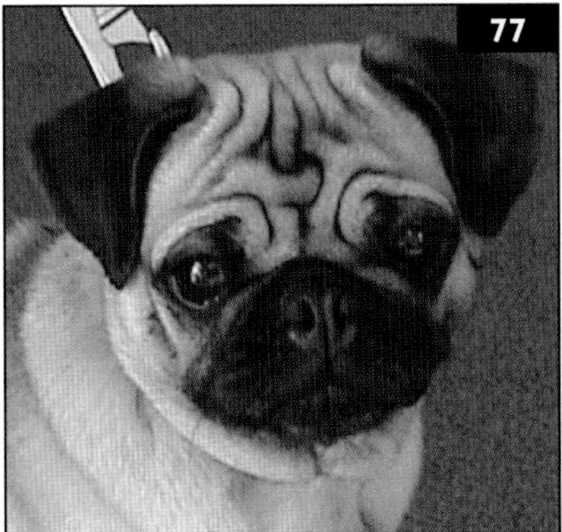

1 How can pulmonary hypertension be confirmed by echocardiography?
2 What other tests are available to identify pulmonary hypertension?
3 What are the main differential diagnoses for pulmonary hypertension?
4 What further tests do you recommend?

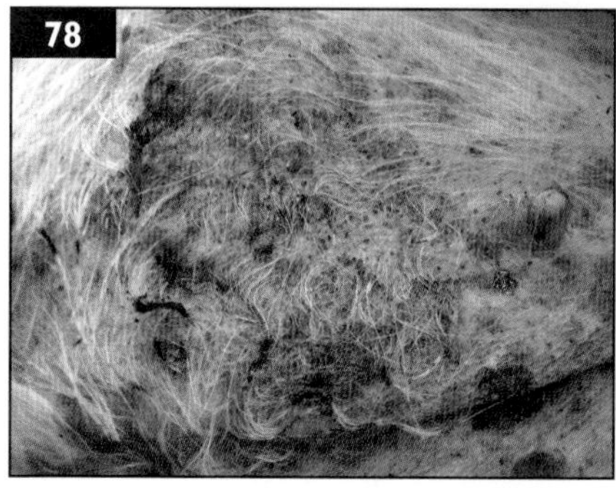

CASE 78 A 10-year-old intact female Old English Sheepdog was evaluated for a 6-month history of skin disease that initially started with hypotrichosis and then gradually deteriorated. The dog had generalized skin lesions (papules, pustules, crusts, and alopecia) that were most pronounced on the abdomen (78) and limbs. An injection with glucocorticoids did not seem to alleviate the clinical signs. A 2-week course of cephalexin at 25 mg/kg PO q12h improved the clinical signs, but did not lead to remission. In the last month, pruritus had become a more prominent feature, and over the last 2 weeks the dog had become lethargic and showed a reduced appetite. The dog came from Munich, Germany, had never traveled outside the country, and had received regular vaccinations. It had not received any antiparasitic treatment within the last 2 years.

Besides the skin changes, the physical examination was unremarkable.

1 What are the three most likely differential diagnoses for this dog, based on your review of the image provided?
2 What diagnostic tests should be done immediately?

CASE 79 Case 79 is the same dog as case 78. Cytology (**79a**) and deep skin scrapings (**79b**) were performed.

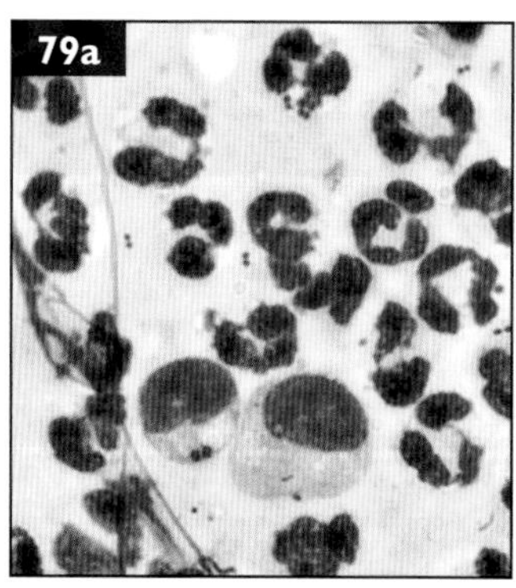

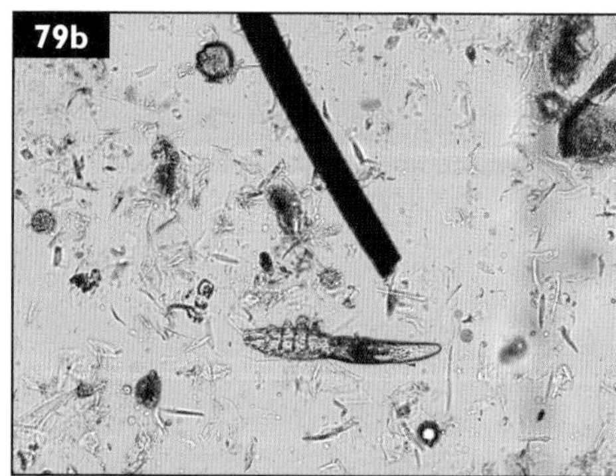

1 What questions need to be asked to guide your further diagnostic testing?
2 If there are no additional clues in the history, what other diagnostic tests should be considered for this patient?

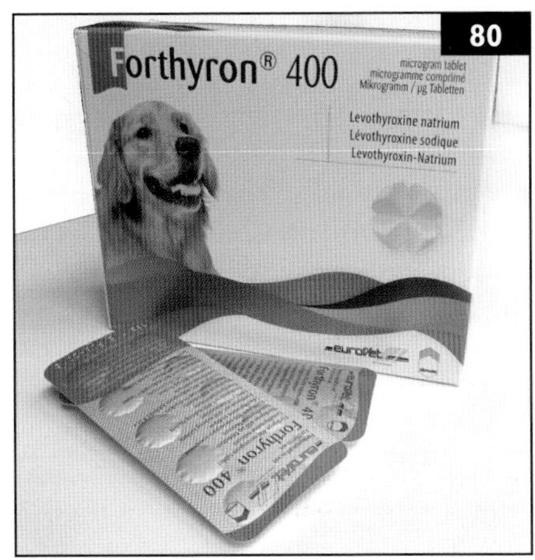

CASE 80 Case 80 is the same dog as cases 78 and 79. The dog had low thyroxine concentrations (3 nmol/l, RI 11–60 nmol/l) and high TSH concentrations (8.2 pg/ml, RI <5 pg/ml), supporting a diagnosis of underlying hypothyroidism. Levothyroxine (20 µg/kg PO q12h) was prescribed (**80**).

1 How would you treat the dog's demodicosis?
2 How would you monitor and adjust the thyroid hormone supplementation?

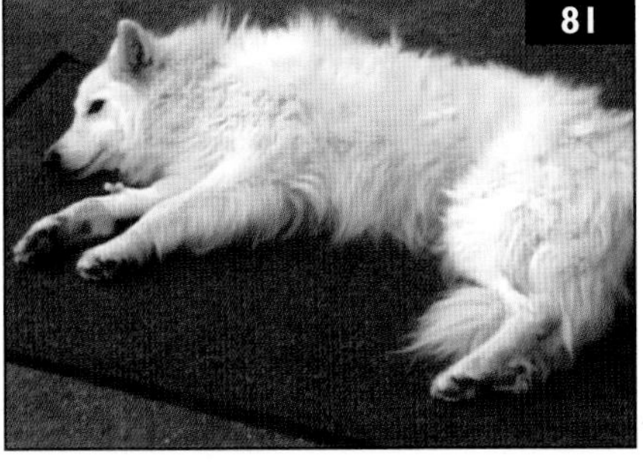

CASE 81 A 2-year-old neutered male Kuvasz was evaluated for acute onset of lateral recumbency. The day before evaluation, the dog had been lethargic but otherwise normal. The dog belonged to a group of three dogs that had consumed a dead animal carcass 3 days ago. The other two dogs also showed signs of paresis, although less severe. There was no trauma or relevant previous illness in any of the dogs. All the dogs were up to date on vaccinations, and tick and flea preventives were used regularly. The three dogs came from Ingolstadt, Germany, and none of them had traveled outside of the country.

General physical examination was unremarkable apart from lateral recumbency. Neurologic examination revealed inability to lift the head or move the limbs. Spinal reflexes (patellar reflexes, flexor withdrawal reflexes) were absent in all limbs (**81**). The dog was responsive to pain stimuli as assessed by eye movements and his ability to wag the tail. Cranial nerve examination showed slightly mydriatic pupils with a decreased pupillary light reflex, but was otherwise unremarkable. Fundic examination was unremarkable. Neuroanatomic localization in this dog was a generalized lower motor neuron disorder.

1 What are your differential diagnoses in this dog?
2 What are the next diagnostic steps?
3 What treatment is indicated?

CASE 82 A 2-year-old neutered female mixed-breed dog was evaluated for lethargy and difficulty in walking. The dog had trouble rising from recumbency over the last 2 months. Occasionally, she scuffed the left pelvic limb while walking. Over the last 5 days, she had become paraplegic. The dog was still eating and drinking normally. The dog was picked up as a stray and admitted to a shelter about 1.5 years previously. She was neutered during her residency at that shelter. The dog had been obtained from the shelter by the owners about 1 year previously. The dog now lived in Atlanta, Georgia, USA, and had no travel history within the last year. The dog was currently vaccinated and received parasiticides on a regular basis.

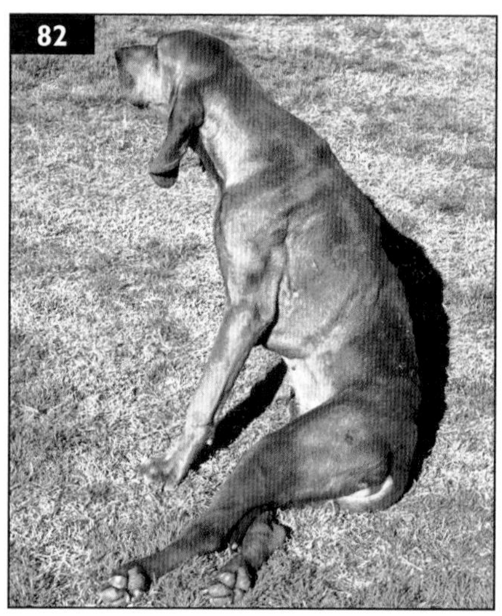

On physical examination, mild lymphadenomegaly was evident in the palpable superficial lymph nodes. The dog was dragging her pelvic limbs (82). She had an arched back, and paraspinal hyperesthesia was evident during muscle palpation of the dorsal mid-lumbar region. When her weight was supported, proprioceptive deficits were evident bilaterally and were most severe in the left pelvic limb. Myotatic reflexes were normal to increased in both limbs. Miosis was present in the right eye and aqueous flare was seen in the anterior chamber.

1 What would be the next diagnostic steps to further work-up the dog's major problems?
2 What are the differential diagnoses for generalized lymphadenomegaly, and what is the first step in a diagnostic work-up?
3 What disease processes can be associated with miosis and aqueous flare?

CASE 83 Case 83 is the same dog as case 82. A complete neurologic examination confirmed postural reaction deficits (hopping, conscious proprioception, extensor postural thrust) in the pelvic limbs, which were worse on the left side. Flexor and myotatic reflexes were present in both pelvic limbs, with slightly increased reflex responses noted in the left limb. Ophthalmic examination showed fundic abnormalities including aqueous flare and hyphema in the right eye. Retinal lesions were found in the ocular fundus of this eye indicative of chorioretinitis.

The CBC was unremarkable. In the biochemistry profile, hyperproteinemia with hyperglobulinemia was present (total protein 88.6 g/l, albumin 36.3 g/l, globulin 52.3 g/l). A serum protein electrophoresis was performed (**83**).

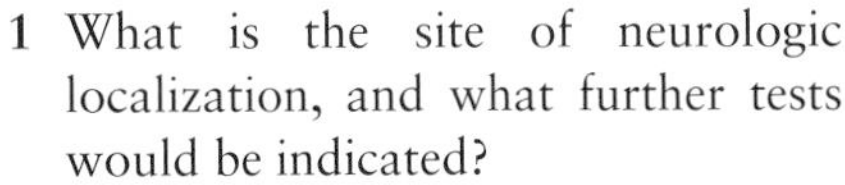

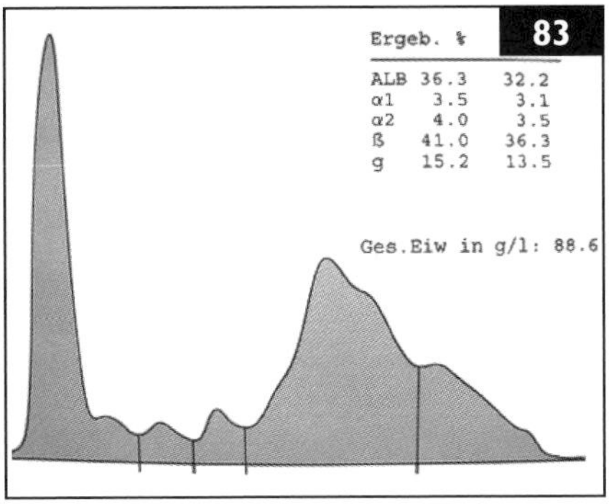

1 What is the site of neurologic localization, and what further tests would be indicated?

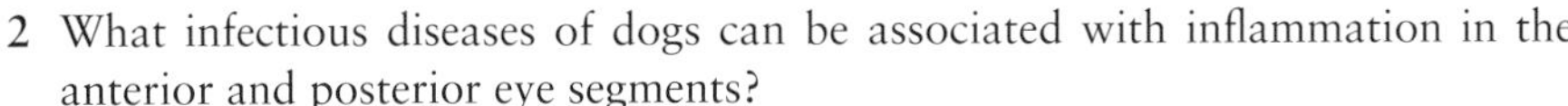

2 What infectious diseases of dogs can be associated with inflammation in the anterior and posterior eye segments?
3 What further diagnostic tests would you suggest to confirm one of these infections?
4 What does electrophoresis suggest about the cause of the globulin increase?

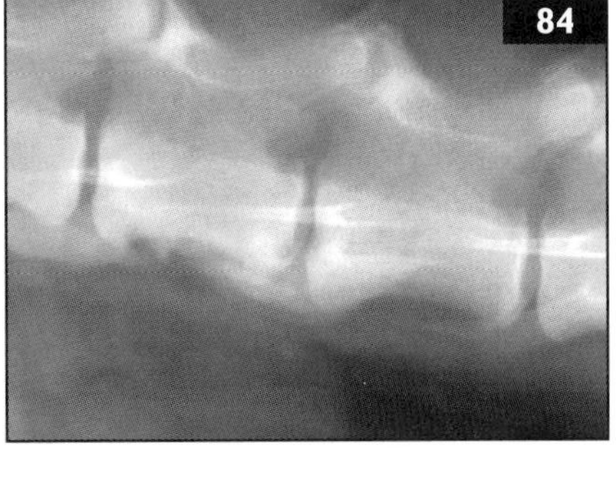

CASE 84 Case 84 is the same dog as cases 82 and 83. Radiography of the lumbar spine revealed an osteoproliferative and osteolytic lesion at the L3–L4 disc space (**84**). The osteoproliferative and lytic lesion at the disc space was interpreted as discospondylitis. A myelogram was performed and the spinal cord was compressed at this point, more severely on the left side. CSF was collected and analyzed for protein and cell count and type at the time of the myelogram, and no abnormalities were detected.

Results of a *Brucella canis* screening test (slide agglutination) were positive in this dog, and a tube agglutination titer was 200.

1 What are the most common etiologic agents that cause discospondylitis in dogs?
2 How would you interpret the *Brucella canis* test results?
3 What other signs would be expected in a neutered or intact dog with brucellosis?

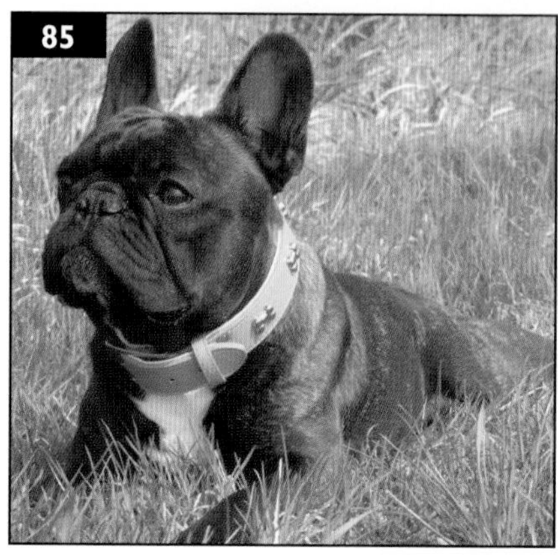

CASE 85 An 8-month-old intact male French Bulldog (85) was referred because of a 12-week history of chronic diarrhea. The dog had tenesmus, and the owner frequently observed mucus and sometimes fresh blood on the feces. The dog had been treated by a veterinarian over the last 10 weeks for this problem. The veterinarian had detected coccidian oocysts (*Isospora* spp.) on fecal flotation and had treated the dog for coccidiosis three times without clinical improvement. There was partial improvement in the gastrointestinal signs when the dog was fed a hypoallergenic diet in combination with oral amoxicillin for 7 days. After cessation of the antibiotics, the clinical signs had worsened and the dog began to defecate in the house. The owners commenced a new elimination diet (duck and potato based), which was fed for 2 weeks without any other foods. There was no improvement in clinical signs with this treatment. The dog lived in Nurnberg, Germany, and had never been outside the country. He had received a full basic vaccination series and had been treated with fenbendazole several times. He had never received medications to prevent ectoparasites.

On physical examination, the dog was bright, alert, and responsive. He was in a good body condition. Rectal body temperature was 38.4°C (101.1°F), pulse was 104 bpm, and respiratory rate was 32 breaths/min. Mucous membranes were pink. On palpation, the abdomen was tense, but not painful.

1 What are the typical clinical signs of large and small intestinal diarrhea, and how would you categorize the diarrhea in this dog?
2 Do you think coccidiosis is a likely explanation for the chronic diarrhea in this dog?
3 What part of the physical examination is missing, but absolutely indicated in this case?

CASE 86 Case 86 is the same dog as case 85. On rectal examination, an irregular and rough mucosa could be palpated, and mucoid feces could be seen on the glove.

A CBC, biochemistry panel, urinalysis, and fecal flotation were performed. No abnormal laboratory findings were present, and no parasites could be detected in the feces. Abdominal radiographs were unremarkable. On abdominal ultrasound, a thickened colonic wall (3 mm) was detected (86).

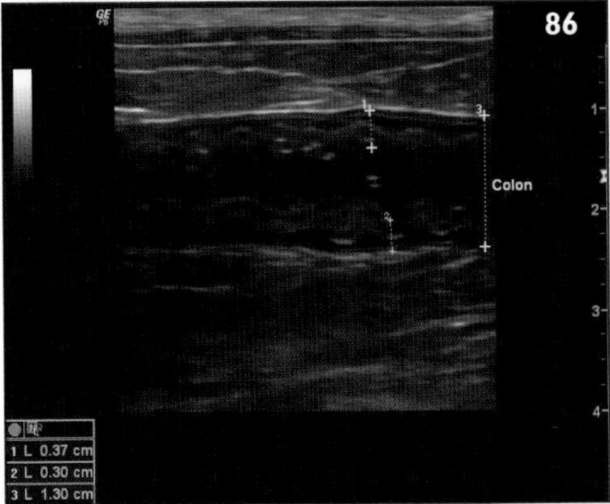

1 What causes of large bowel diarrhea are still on your differential diagnosis list?
2 How would you manage an idiopathic inflammatory bowel disease involving the large intestine?
3 Why might colonic biopsies be indicated before starting immunosuppressive therapy, especially in this case?

CASE 87 Case 87 is the same dog as cases 85 and 86. A colonic biopsy was performed endoscopically. Histologic changes showed a moderate to severe colitis with a predominance of neutrophils (87). In addition, erosions and crypt hyperplasia could be detected.

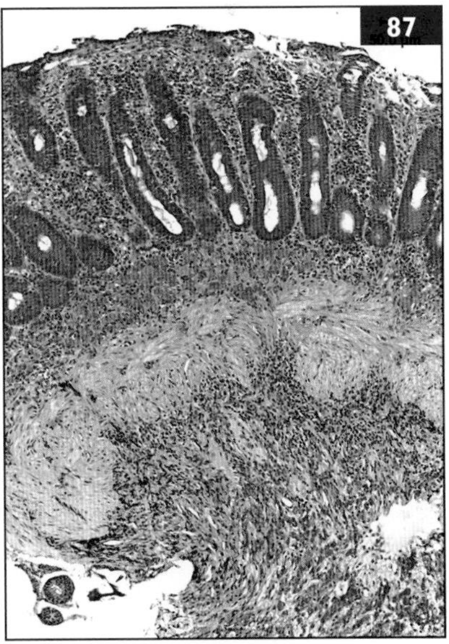

1 What test would you perform to differentiate idiopathic neutrophilic inflammatory bowel disease from histiocytic colitis?
2 What is the cause of histiocytic ulcerative colitis?
3 How would you treat a dog with histiocytic ulcerative colitis, in contrast to idiopathic inflammatory bowel disease?

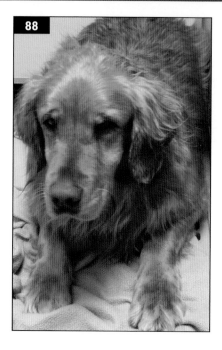

CASE 88 A 6-year-old neutered male Golden Retriever was evaluated for a history of weight loss and progressive inappetence for 1 month (**88**). The owner reported weakness, anorexia, and moderately labored breathing over the last 2 days. No vomiting, diarrhea, cough, polyuria, or polydipsia was reported. The dog was from San Diego, California, USA, had supervised outdoor access, and was up to date on vaccines. The last healthcare visit had been 4 months ago, and the dog had been clinically normal. The owners used flea and tick preventives only during spring and summer.

Physical examination revealed lethargy, pyrexia (38.7°C [100.0°F]), a grade III/VI diastolic decrescendo murmur at the left heart base, and bounding pulses. Otherwise, the physical examination was unremarkable. Bloodwork revealed leukocytosis, thrombocytopenia, elevated liver enzymes, and hypoalbuminemia with hyperglobulinemia.

1 What is the most likely cause of the cardiac murmur?
2 Are the other abnormalities in this case associated with the cardiac disease?
3 What are the next diagnostic steps?

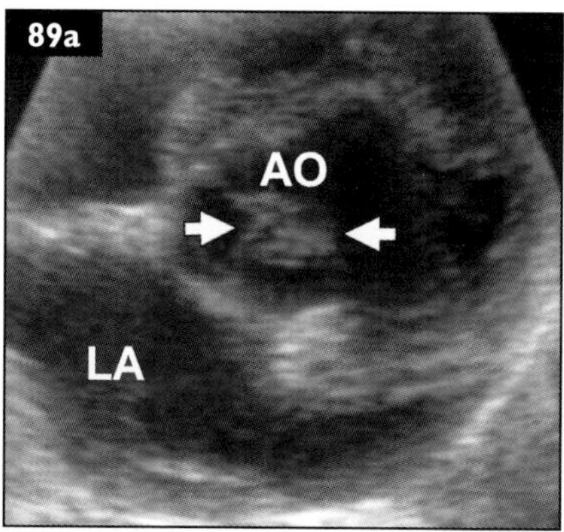

CASE 89 Case 89 is the same dog as case 88. Thoracic radiographs did not reveal any parenchymal or vascular abnormality in the lungs. The systolic blood pressure was increased, but the diastolic pressure was decreased, which explained the bounding pulses. An echocardiogram documented a large vegetative lesion on the aortic valve (**89a, 89b**), causing moderate obstruction and significant regurgitation.

1 How are the valvular vegetations formed, and how do they cause cardiac murmurs?
2 What factors predispose to endocarditis?
3 What are other systemic signs of endocarditis?
4 Should any therapy be considered pending microbiologic tests?

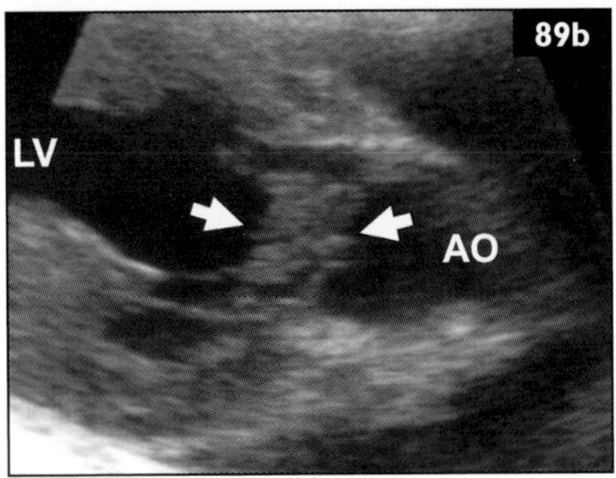

CASE 90 Case 90 is the same dog as cases 88 and 89. Pre-enrichment blood culture in BAPGM (*Bartonella* alpha-proteobacteria growth medium) for 2 weeks followed by culture in blood agar for another 2 weeks (**90**) yielded growth of a gram-negative coccobacillus suggestive of *Bartonella* spp. Specific PCR assay amplified *Bartonella* spp. DNA from the plate isolates, and DNA sequencing confirmed infection with *Bartonella vinsonii* subspecies *berkhoffii*.

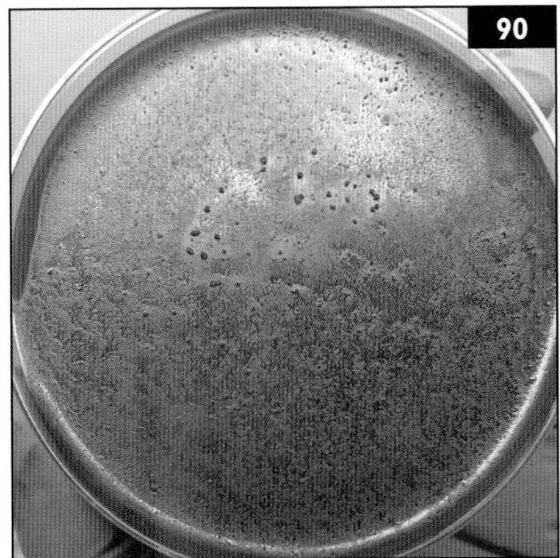

1 How did this dog become infected with *B. vinsonii* subspecies *berkhoffii*?
2 What are the most common *Bartonella* species that infect dogs, and what are their reservoir hosts?
3 What are other signs of *Bartonella* spp. infection in dogs?
4 What is the recommended therapy for endocarditis caused by *Bartonella* spp.?
5 What are the public health implications of this diagnosis?

CASE 91 A 10-month-old intact male German Shepherd Dog from Bari, Italy, was brought to a veterinarian for a routine wellness examination and vaccination. On physical examination, a solitary depigmented papule with scaling margins was identified adjacent to the left nostril (**91**). The owner had noticed the lesion about 2 months previously.

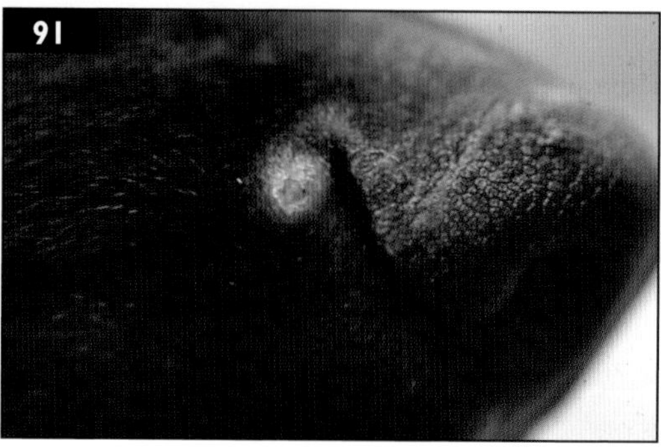

1 What is your assessment of the dermal lesion?
2 What further diagnostic tests are indicated?

CASE 92 Case 92 is the same dog as case 91. A few *Leishmania* amastigotes were detected in fine needle aspiration smears (**92**, arrows), and a *Leishmania infantum* PCR was positive. Therefore, a diagnosis of papular dermatitis associated with *L. infantum* infection was made.

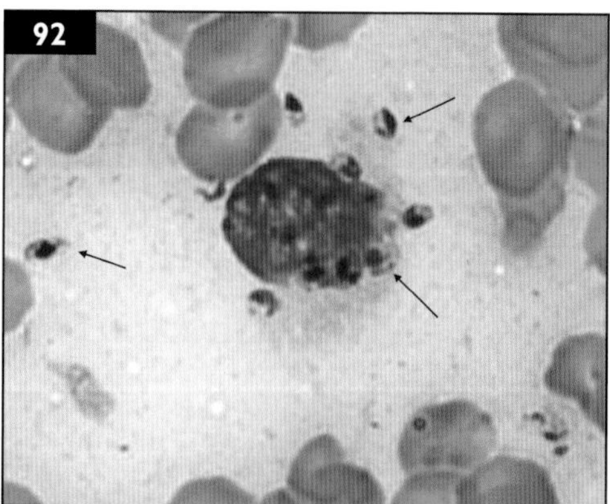

1 What treatment do you recommend for this dog?
2 How should the dog be monitored in the future?

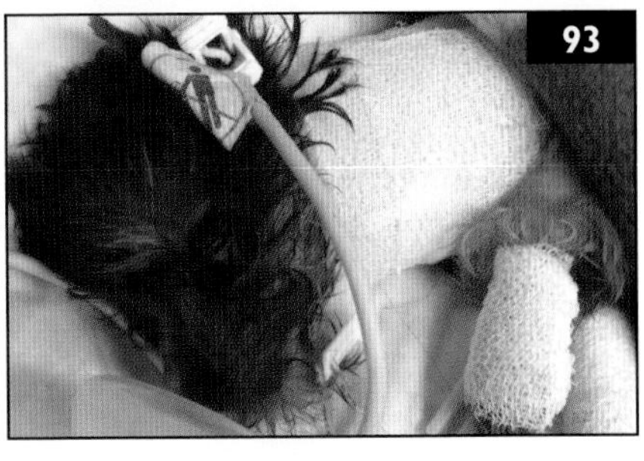

CASE 93 A 12-week-old intact male Yorkshire Terrier (**93**) was evaluated for a 1-day history of vomiting, diarrhea, and anorexia. The owners lived in Munich, Germany, and had purchased the dog over the internet 3 days previously. Therefore, the dog's origin was obscure and whether he had received vaccinations and antiparasitic treatment was unknown. On physical examination, the dog was recumbent and dull but reacted to acoustic stimuli. The heart rate was 220 bpm, pulse was weak, capillary refill time was 5 seconds, mucous membranes were pale, peripheral limbs were cold, and respiratory rate was 32 breaths/min. The dog weighed 0.5 kg. A fecal parvovirus antigen test was performed and was positive.

1 What is the dog's most life-threatening problem?
2 What initial treatment would you perform to address this problem?
3 What laboratory parameters should be assessed in order to optimize treatment?

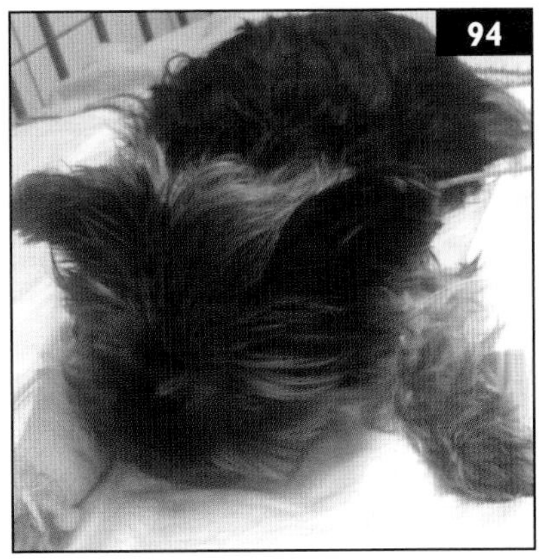

CASE 94 Case 94 is the same dog as case 93. After initial shock fluid therapy, heart rate was 140 bpm, mucous membranes were pink, capillary refill time was 2 seconds, pulse was regular, but the dog was still obtunded (**94**). Mucous membranes were tacky, and skin turgor was reduced. The dog was vomiting about once an hour and had severe diarrhea about four times per hour.

Initial laboratory work-up revealed a hematocrit of 0.45 l/l (RI 0.35–0.58 l/l), a total white blood cell count of 1.4 × 10^9/l (RI 5–16 × 10^9/l), a neutrophil count of 0.2 × 10^9/l (RI 3–9 × 10^9/l), glucose of 1.2 mmol/l (RI 3.8–6.6 mmol/l), potassium of 2.8 mmol/l (RI 3.8–5.5 mmol/l), creatinine of 54 µmol/l (RI 45–125 µmol/l), total protein of 65 g/l (RI 56–78 g/l), and albumin of 32 g/l (RI 31–43 g/l).

1 What should be the fluid therapy plan for the next 10 hours?
2 What should be the nutritional plan when the vomiting is under control?

CASE 95 A 3-year-old neutered male German Shepherd Dog was evaluated for a cloudy and painful right eye (**95**) with increased redness and ocular discharge. The dog had appeared a little more lethargic over the last week. The owners lived in two places, and traveled regularly between Munich, Germany, and Ravenna, Italy. In Italy, the house was located near a wooded area close to dense shrubs, and the owners took their dog for frequent walks. The dog had been properly vaccinated and never had any previous health issues. He had received his last treatment for endoparasites and flea preventive about 6 months ago.

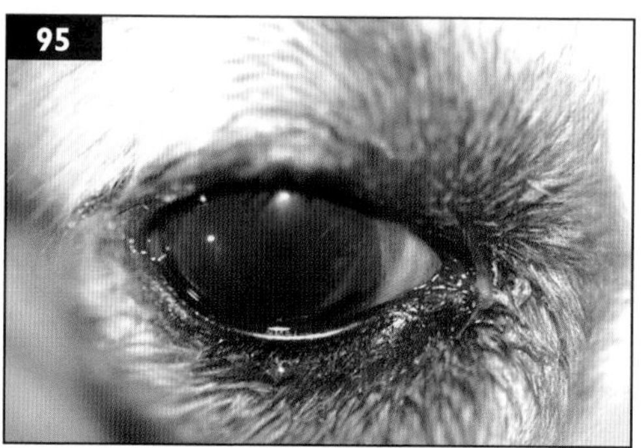

Physical examination was unremarkable besides the ocular changes. An ophthalmic examination was performed. In the right eye, blepharospasm, photophobia, and ocular discharge were observed. The cornea did not stain with fluorescein. Slit lamp examination of the anterior chamber revealed a moderate amount of aqueous flare (positive Tyndall effect). The surface of the iris was hyperemic and mildly swollen (rubeosis iridis), and the pupil was miotic.

Ophthalmic examination	Right eye (OD)	Left eye (OS)
Menace response	Positive	Positive
Dazzle reflex	Positive	Positive
Pupillary light reflex	Complete	Complete
Schirmer tear test	15 mm/min	15 mm/min
Intraocular pressure	6 mmHg	15 mmHg

1 What is the ocular diagnosis based on the clinical findings?
2 What further tests would you recommend?

CASE 96 Case 96 is the same dog as case 95. For fundic examination, the pupils of both eyes were dilated with 1% tropicamide. The examination of the right fundus was difficult owing to the flare in the anterior chamber, but in the left eye the retina was visible (**96**). A CBC and a biochemistry panel were performed.

Complete blood count	Results	Reference interval
Red blood cells	7.3×10^{12}/l	5.5–9.3
Hematocrit	0.45 l/l	0.35–0.58
Platelets	23×10^{9}/l	150–500
White blood cells	7.30×10^{9}/l	5–16
Neutrophils	5.18×10^{9}/l	3–9
Eosinophils	0.22×10^{9}/l	0–1.0
Basophils	0×10^{9}/l	0–0.04
Lymphocytes	1.46×10^{9}/l	1.0–3.6
Monocytes	0.44×10^{9}/l	0.04–0.50

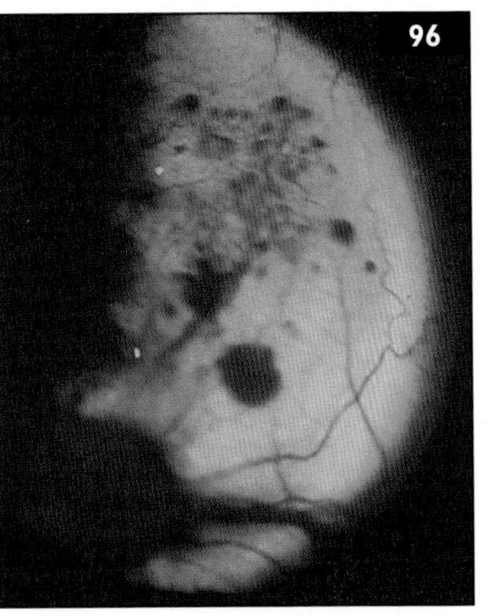

Biochemistry panel	Results	Reference interval
ALT	21 U/l	0–110
ALP	21 U/l	0–152
Total protein	80 g/l	55–77
Albumin	26 g/l	31–43
Bilirubin	0.1 µmol/l	0–5.3
Creatinine	79.6 µmol/l	35.4–159.1
BUN	6.6 mmol/l	2.6–9.9
Glucose	5.2 mmol/l	3.8–6.6
Sodium	144 mmol/l	139–163
Potassium	4.1 mmol/l	3.8–5.5
Chloride	112 mmol/l	105–118
Calcium	2.5 mmol/l	2.0–3.1
Phosphorus	1.4 mmol/l	0.7–2.0

1 What is your interpretation of the findings in the left retina?
2 What is your interpretation of the laboratory findings?
3 What underlying disease would you suspect, based on the physical examination, the ophthalmic findings, and the laboratory results? What additional diagnostic tests would you recommend?

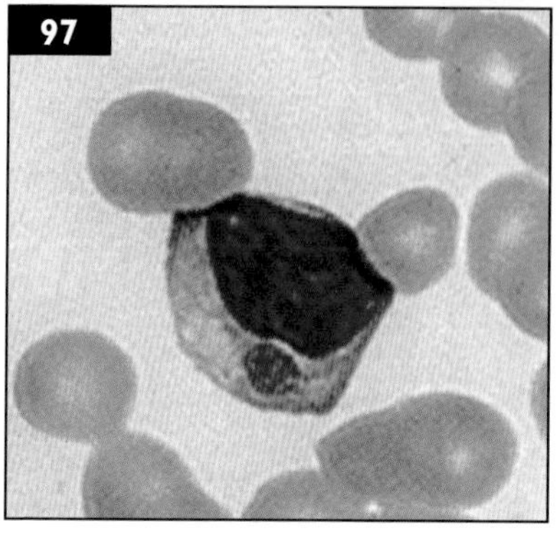

CASE 97 Case 97 is the same dog as cases 95 and 96. Rickettsial morulae were detected on the blood smear (**97**), and the dog was positive for *Ehrlichia canis* by PCR.

1 What *Ehrlichia* species infect dogs, and how are they transmitted?
2 Describe the different phases of canine monocytic ehrlichiosis, including the typical clinical signs.
3 What is the most common ocular finding in dogs with canine monocytic ehrlichiosis, and what is the pathogenesis?
4 What systemic and ophthalmic treatment would you recommend?

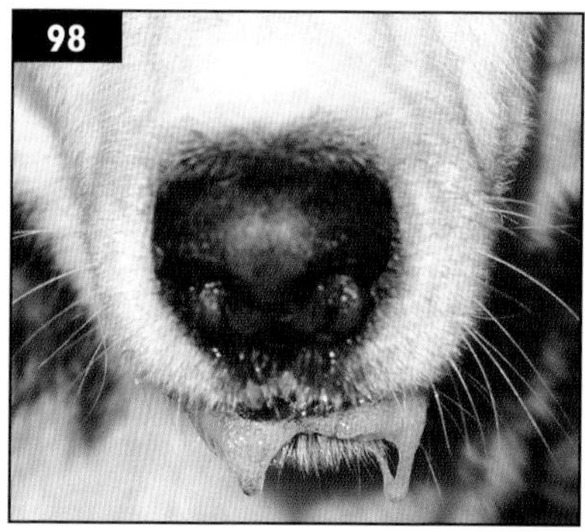

CASE 98 A 5-year-old intact female Siberian Husky was evaluated for a 4-day history of progressive anorexia, restlessness, irritability, and vocalization. On the day of evaluation, the dog had become aggressive toward the household members and developed hypersalivation (**98**). The dog lived in Budapest, Hungary, in an apartment and was walked regularly next to the house only. One month previously, the owner had returned from vacation in the countryside in the area of Debrecen, Hungary, near the Romanian border, where the dog had escaped several times and roamed in the forest area. The owner was not aware of any exposure to toxins or trauma. The dog had been vaccinated against distemper, parvovirus infection, and canine infectious hepatitis twice as a puppy; the last dose was at 13 weeks of age. There was no other history of illness or medications.

On physical examination, pyrexia (40.5°C [104.9°F]), hypersalivation, and mydriasis were seen in addition to the neurologic signs described above.

1 How likely is rabies in this dog, considering that a bite wound was not seen?
2 How can a diagnosis of rabies be made?
3 How would you treat a dog suspected to have rabies?

CASE 99 A 3-year-old neutered female Jack Russell Terrier was evaluated for multifocal areas of erythema, scaling, and mild crusting on the distal front limbs (**99**). The disease had begun 2 weeks previously with mild hair loss. The affected areas gradually increased and lesions became more prominent, but pruritus was marginal. The dog otherwise was bright and alert and showed no other clinical signs. The dog lived in Ingolstadt, Germany, was used for hunting, had never been outside the country, and was regularly vaccinated and treated with antiparasitic drugs. Physical examination showed no abnormalities besides the skin lesions.

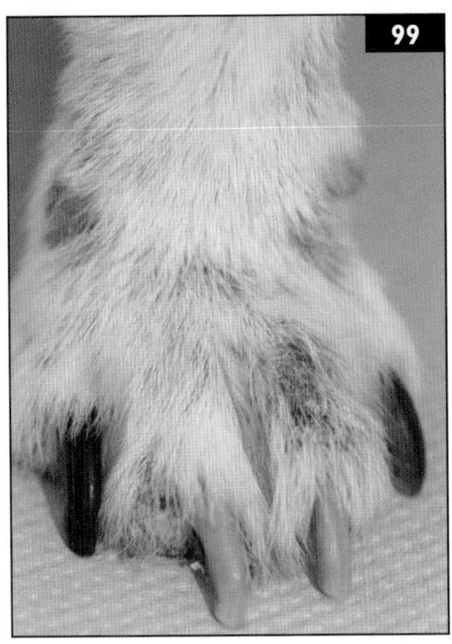

1 What is the most likely diagnosis?
2 Name three other differential diagnoses.
3 What diagnostic tests are indicated in this dog?

CASE 100 Case 100 is the same dog as case 99. A fungal culture was positive for *Microsporum gypseum* (**100**).

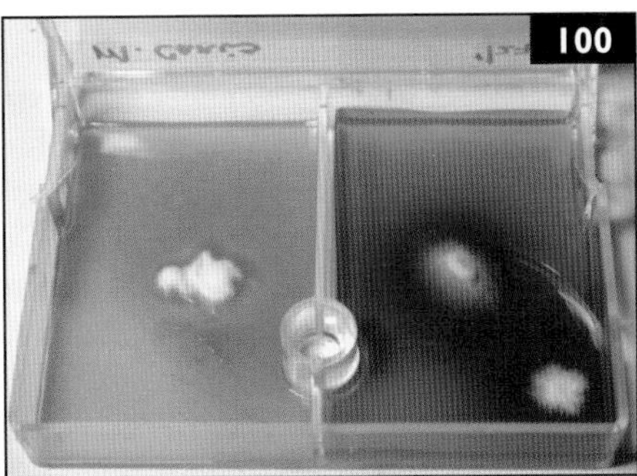

1 How should this dog be treated?
2 How would you treat the environment around this dog?
3 What recommendations should be provided to the owner to minimize the chance of zoonotic transmission?

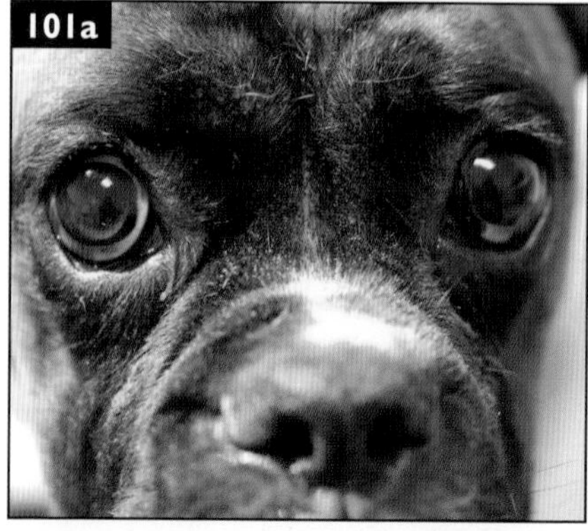

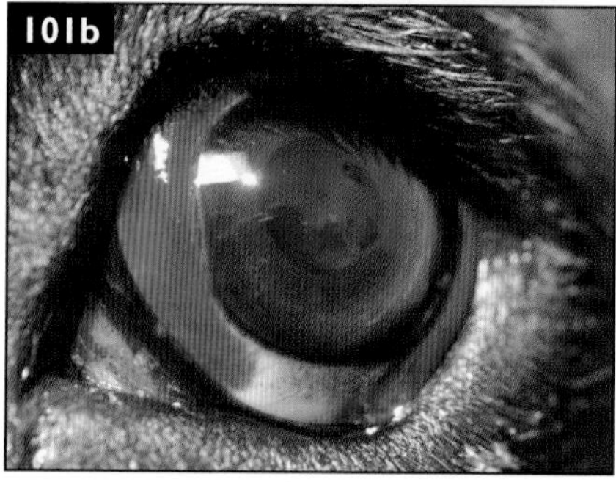

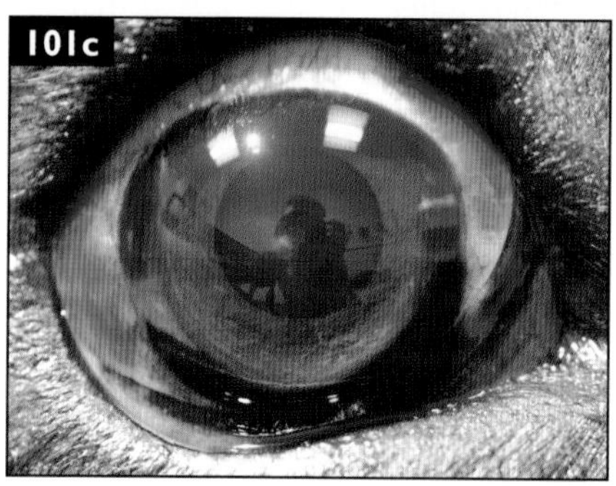

CASE 101 A 1-year-old neutered female Boxer dog was evaluated for ocular changes, lethargy, and pain in the back, neck, and head. The dog had a slightly hunched posture and kept the head lowered during walking. The owner had observed color changes in both eyes (**101a**). The dog lived in Brighton, UK, and had never traveled outside the country. The dog was fully vaccinated, but deworming had not been performed since puppy age and she was not on any ectoparasite control program.

Physical examination was normal besides the neurologic and ophthalmic changes. The neurologic examination showed reduced postural reactions in the pelvic limbs, weakness in the right thoracic and pelvic limbs, positional nystagmus, severe neck pain, kyphosis, low head carriage, and lethargy. The ophthalmic examination showed scleral hemorrhage bilaterally (**101b, 101c**). Retropulsion of the right eye was painful for the dog. Further diagnostic work-up included a CBC, a biochemistry panel, urinalysis, and a coagulation profile. In the CBC, a mild thrombocytopenia was noted. The coagulation profile showed prolonged prothrombin and activated partial thromboplastin clotting times.

Ophthalmic examination	Right eye (OD)	Left eye (OS)
Menace response	Absent	Present
Dazzle reflex	Present	Present
Pupillary light reflex	Normal (direct and indirect)	Normal (direct and indirect)
Schirmer tear test	15 mm/min	15 mm/min
Intraocular pressure	15 mmHg	17 mmHg

An MRI (**101d, 101e**) was performed and revealed a lesion with irregular margins within the left occipital lobe, which measured 2.2 cm in length, 2.6 cm in height, and 7 mm in width. The lesion was markedly hyperintense on T2-weighted images with a hypointense rim; on T1-weighted images it was hypointense. On T2 it showed a heterogeneous signal void. It had a mass effect, causing a mild right midline shift. There was white matter hyperintensity surrounding the lesion. There was a linear signal void within the third and the central aspect of the left lateral ventricle. A pinpoint T2 signal void was visible within the rostral aspect of the left occipital lobe, the central aspect of the left occipital lobe, and left lateral to the caudal aspect of the vermis.

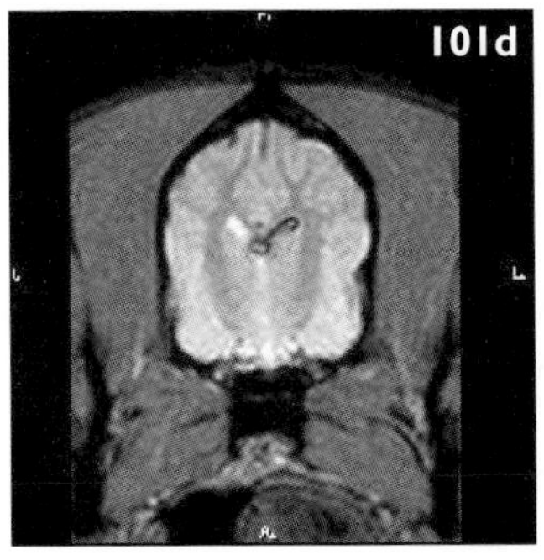
101d

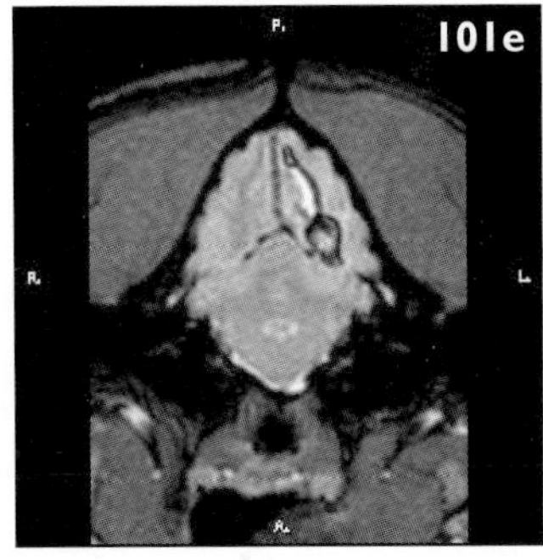
101e

1 What is your assessment of the ocular lesions?
2 What is the MRI diagnosis?
3 What would be the primary infectious agent to test for, and what is the test of choice?

CASE 102 Case 102 is the same dog as case 101. Baermann faecal flotation (**102**) showed *Angiostrongylus vasorum* larvae.

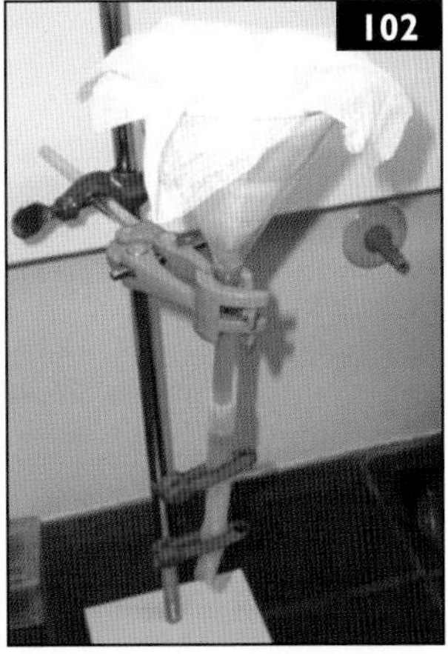
102

1 What is the epidemiology and pathophysiology of angiostrongylosis?
2 What treatment would you suggest?

CASE 103 An 8-year-old neutered male mixed-breed dog was evaluated for a long-term history of chronic recurrent cough. The dog had been seen repeatedly by several different veterinarians and managed using various courses of different antimicrobial drugs. Over the past 2 months, the cough had become progressively more frequent despite treatment with antibiotics and cough suppressants. The dog lived in Sacramento, California, USA, and had no travel history outside California. He had received core vaccinations every 3 years for the last 6 years, but had never been administered prophylaxis for parasitic infections.

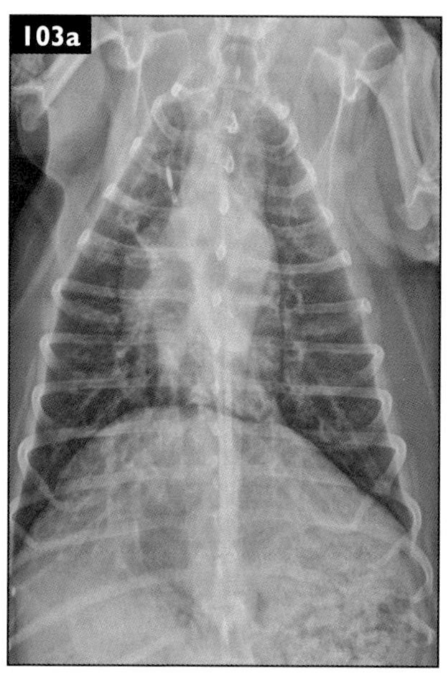

103a

On physical examination, the dog had a temperature of 38.9°C (102.0°F), pulse of 136 bpm, and respiratory rate of 28 breaths/min. Harsh crackles (expiratory louder than inspiratory) were auscultated in all lung fields. Increased airway sounds were apparent on tracheal auscultation and a harsh cough was easily elicited on tracheal palpation. Thoracic radiographs were obtained (**103a, 103b**).

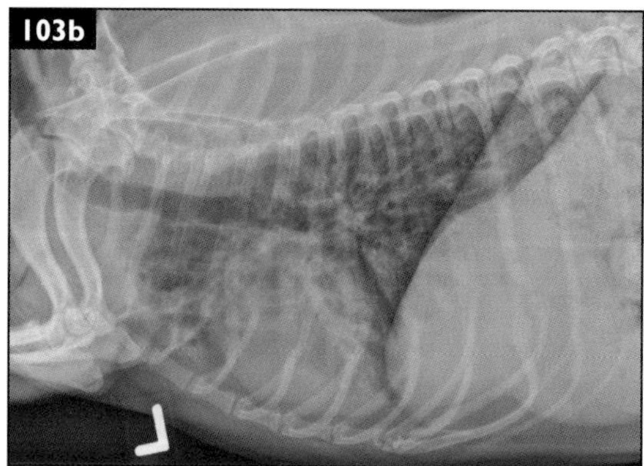

103b

1 How would you interpret the radiographic findings?
2 What underlying disease process could be present?
3 What complications are possible?

CASE 104 Case 104 is the same dog as case 103 (**104**). Pulse oximetry revealed an oxygen saturation of 87%. A CBC was obtained:

Complete blood count	Results	Reference interval
Hematocrit	0.528 l/l	0.35–0.58
MCV	70.2 fl	58–72
Platelets	414 × 10^9/l	150–500
White blood cells	12.450 × 10^9/l	5–16
Neutrophils	8.217 × 10^9/l	3–9
Eosinophils	1.494 × 10^9/l	0–1.0
Basophils	1.494 × 10^9/l	0–0.04
Lymphocytes	0.747 × 10^9/l	1–3.6
Monocytes	0.498 × 10^9/l	0.04–0.5

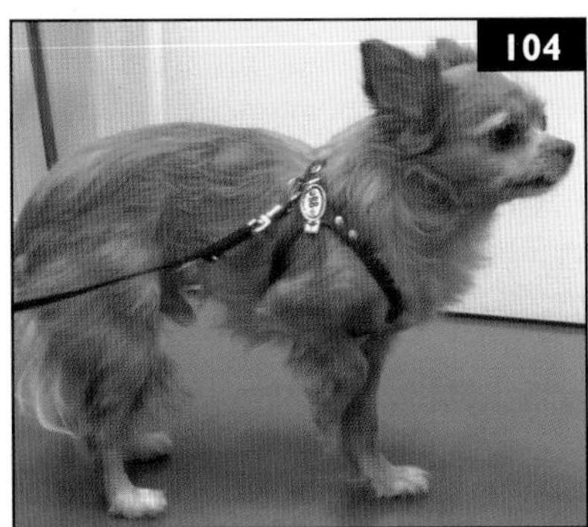
104

1 How would you interpret the pulse oximetry reading?
2 How would you interpret the CBC?

CASE 105 A 6-year-old neutered male Rottweiler living in Davis, California, USA, was evaluated for a bilateral nasal discharge. The dog was otherwise healthy, had been vaccinated regularly, and was on heartworm prophylaxis.

Physical examination revealed no abnormalities besides bilateral mucoid nasal discharge. Rhinoscopy and a brush cytology were performed (**105a, 105b**).

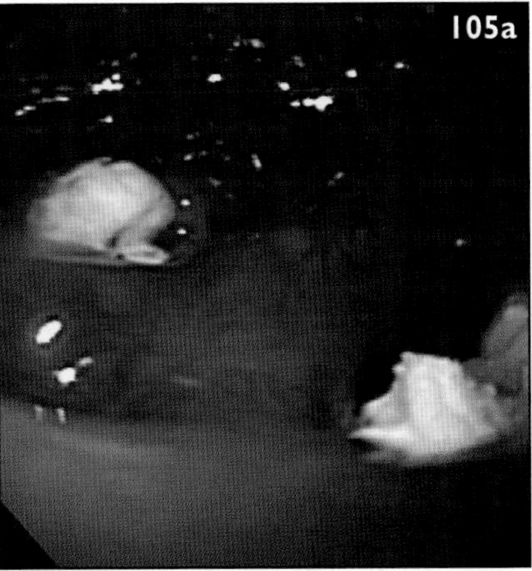
105a

1 How would you interpret the rhinoscopy findings?
2 How would you interpret the cytologic findings in this dog?
3 What treatment should be considered?

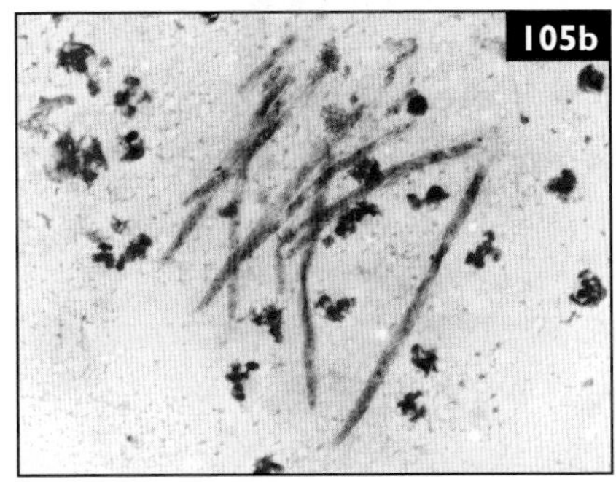
105b

CASE 106 An 8-year-old neutered female Dachshund mix (**106a**) was referred for evaluation of a non-healing bite wound. Seven months previously, the owner had witnessed a dog fight between this dog and one of his other five dogs. Multiple deep puncture wounds were noted immediately afterwards on the Dachshund mix's caudal dorsum. A veterinarian anesthetized the dog, the wounds were cleaned and debrided, and two Penrose drains were placed. The dog was then treated with cephalexin (30 mg/kg PO q12h). Although an Elizabethan collar was placed on the dog, the owner removed it 2 days later and the dog started to lick the wounds. The owner (who was a nurse) removed the drains 3 weeks later, but the wounds continued to drain and a new wound appeared in the left axilla. Two months later, the veterinarian performed exploratory surgery of the region. All necrotic tissue was excised, and the dog was treated with clindamycin (20 mg/kg PO q12h). Although there appeared to be initial improvement, draining lesions then recurred and intermittent pyrexia was noted (39.4–40.1°C [102.9–104.2°F]) over the next 4 months. Shortly after, a new draining tract appeared on the left thorax. Throughout the entire 7-month period, the dog otherwise was bright, alert, and eating normally. There was no other significant medical history. The dog lived in Fresno, central California, USA, and had not traveled to other places. The dog was regularly vaccinated and on endo- and ectoparasite control.

On physical examination, the dog was bright and alert. The temperature was 39.6°C (103.3°F), while other vital signs were normal. The BCS was 7/9. The caudal aspect of the dog's dorsum was concave in appearance on the left side and had multifocal to coalescing linear ulcerated lesions that were draining purulent material (**106b**). Soft tissue in the left inguinal region was firm and painful. A draining tract was also noted on the right side of the dorsal abdomen, and surrounding soft tissue was enlarged and firm. The soft tissue in the left axilla

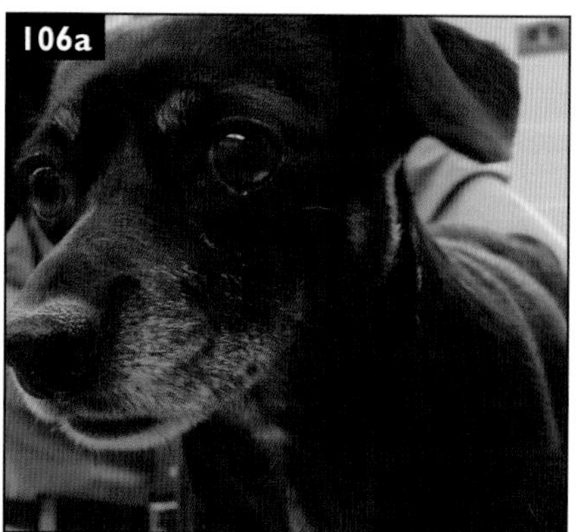
106a

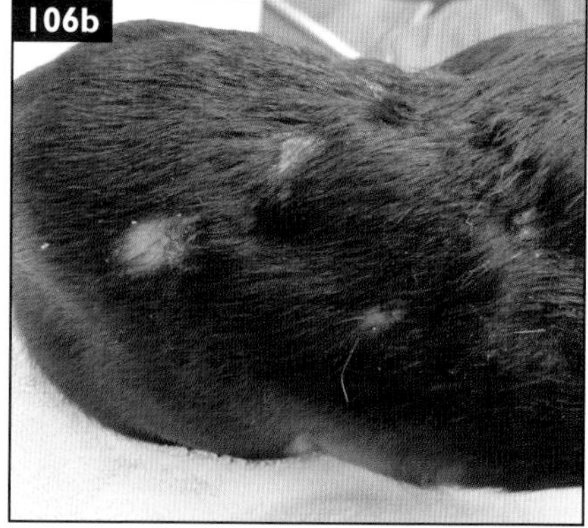
106b

was firm with two healing draining tracts. There was no evidence of peripheral lymphadenopathy.

1 What is your differential diagnosis for the non-healing wounds?
2 What diagnostic tests would you recommend for this dog?

CASE 107 Case 107 is the same dog as case 106. The CBC showed a moderate mature neutrophilia (31.85 × 10^9 cells/l) with a mild left shift (2.54 × 10^9 band neutrophils/l, RI 0–0.3 × 10^9/l). A biochemistry panel showed mild hypoalbuminemia (30 g/l, RI 34–43 g/l) and hypoglobulinemia (32 g/l, RI 17–31 g/l). Ultrasound of the region showed no large fluid pockets or foreign material, only heterogeneous, hyperechoic, and disorganized tissue. Histopathology of a biopsy revealed marked multifocal chronic pyogranulomatous cellulitis (**107**). All special stains were negative for organisms. Culture revealed small numbers of *Enterococcus faecalis* from enrichment broth (likely a contaminant) and very small numbers of a rapidly growing mycobacterial species. The mycobacterial culture was sent to a specialized laboratory for further identification of the species, which was found to be *Mycobacterium abscessus* (by *rpoB* gene sequencing).

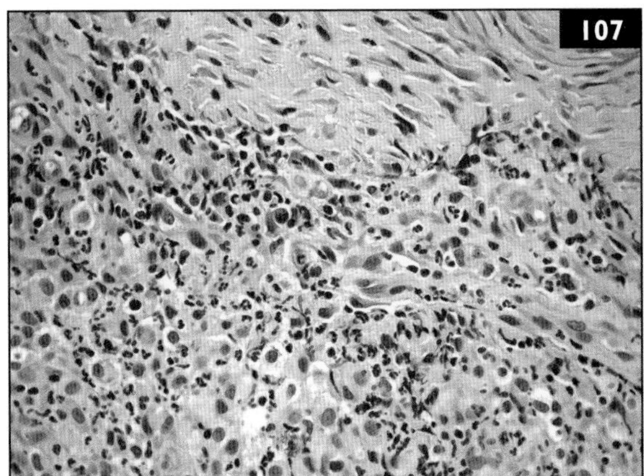

1 Which other rapidly growing mycobacterial species can infect dogs and cats?
2 How does the clinical presentation of disease caused by rapidly growing mycobacteria differ from that caused by *Mycobacterium avium*?
3 What is the zoonotic potential of this organism?
4 How should this infection be treated?

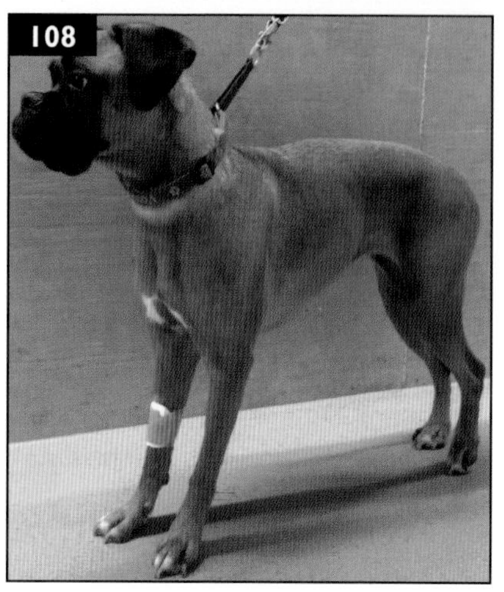

CASE 108 A 6-year-old neutered female Boxer mix from Bern, Switzerland, was evaluated for PU/PD, reduced appetite, and weight loss of several months' duration. Previously, increased serum urea nitrogen concentration was detected on bloodwork and, thereafter, the dog had been fed a prescription renal diet. The dog had received regular vaccinations (distemper, hepatitis, parvovirus) and regular treatment for internal parasites. On physical examination, the dog appeared lethargic and had a body condition score 3/9 (**108**). Otherwise, the physical examination was unremarkable. A CBC, biochemistry panel, and urinalysis were performed:

Complete blood count	Results	Reference interval
Hematocrit	0.37 l/l	0.42–0.55
MCV	71 fl	64–73
MCH	23 pg	23–26
MCHC	34 g/dl	34–36

Biochemistry panel	Results	Reference interval
Total protein	50 g/l	56–71
Albumin	21 g/l	29–37
Creatinine	247 μmol/l	50–119
Urea nitrogen	19.4 mmol/l	3.8–9.4
Cholesterol	6 mmol/l	3.5–8.6

Urinalysis	Results	Reference interval
Collection method	Cystocentesis	–
Color, appearance	Light yellow, slightly turbid	–
Specific gravity	1.021	–
pH	5	5.5–7
Protein	++++	–
Glucose	Negative	–

Continued

Urinalysis	Results	Reference interval
Ketone	Negative	–
Bilirubin	+	–
Blood	+	–
Protein to creatinine ratio	9.67	0–0.5
Red blood cells	12–20 cells/hpf	0–5
White blood cells	12–20 cells/hpf	0–3
Casts	Several/hpf	0
Bacteria	Large quantities/hpf	0

1 How would you interpret the laboratory results?
2 What further work-up would you suggest?

CASE 109 Case 109 is the same dog as case 108. Further work-up revealed the presence of *Leishmania* spp. antibodies by ELISA (**109**). An immunofluorescent antibody test was also performed and a high titer was obtained considered consistent with infection.

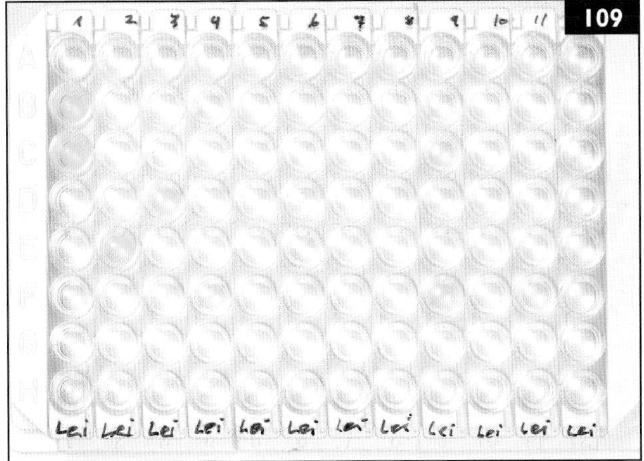

1 Does leishmaniosis explain the clinical abnormalities in this dog?
2 How would you treat this dog?
3 What is the prognosis?

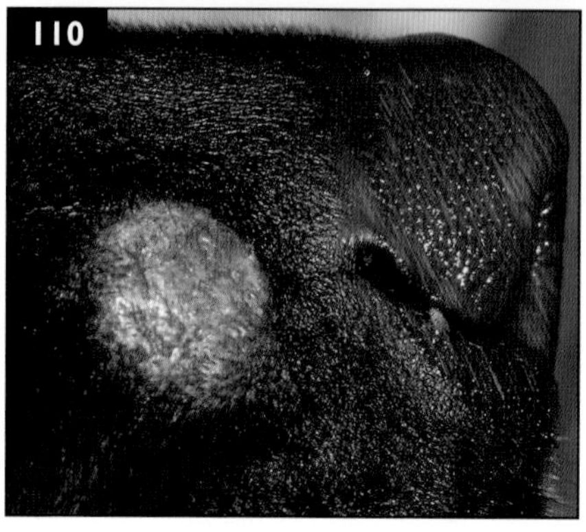

CASE 110 A 1-year-old intact male Labrador Retriever was evaluated for an alopecic annular lesion on the nose of about 1 cm in diameter (**110**). The owner had noticed this lesion about a week previously and it seemed not to have increased in size. There had been no signs of pruritus. The owner was concerned about ringworm. The dog lived in Warsaw, Poland, had received a complete basic vaccination series, and had been treated for endoparasites and ectoparasites every 3 months. The owner reported that, about 4 weeks before the appearance of the lesion, a healthy stray kitten had been adopted from a shelter. The kitten and the dog had been playing together. On physical examination, slight erythema and scaling were noted in association with the lesion. No other lesions were detected. The dog appeared otherwise healthy.

1 Is this lesion consistent with dermatophytosis?
2 What is a "dermatophyte"?
3 What tests should be done if dermatophytosis is suspected?

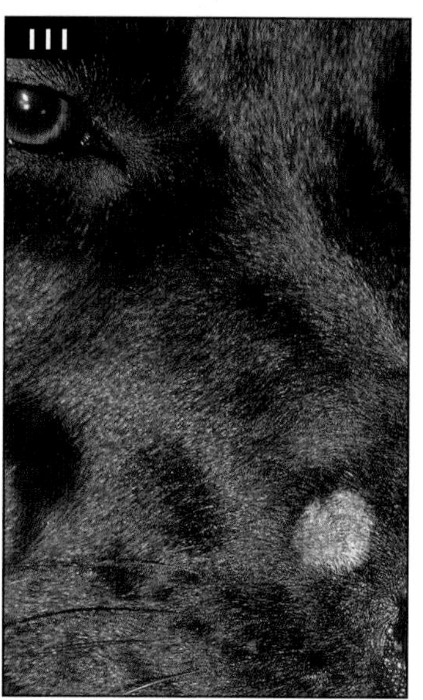

CASE 111 Case 111 is the same dog as case 110. *Microsporum canis* was cultured from the hairs and skin scrapings of this lesion (**111**).

1 What was the likely source of *Microsporum canis* infection in this dog?
2 What is the prognosis?
3 Can the dog transmit this disease to other animals or humans?

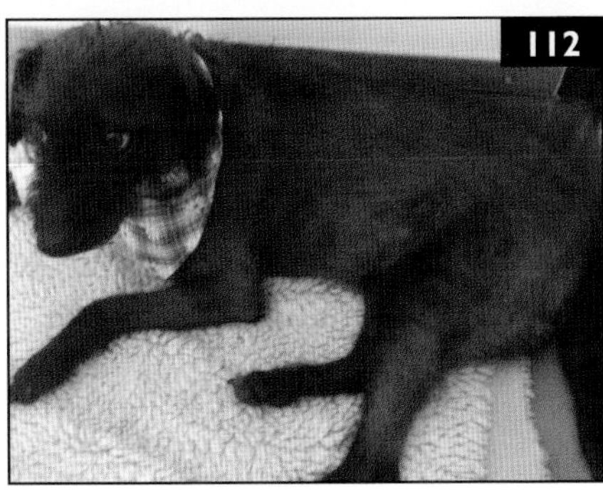

CASE 112 A 12-year-old neutered female 10 kg mixed-breed dog (**112**) was evaluated for weakness and pale mucous membranes. The dog lived in Munich, Germany, and had returned 2 days previously from a vacation in Salerno, Italy. The dog had only been vaccinated as a puppy and had not received any antiparasitic treatment or preventives within at least the last 5 years.

On evaluation, the dog was lethargic, had very pale mucous membranes, a capillary refill time of 2 seconds, a heart rate of 186 bpm, bounding pulses, and a rectal body temperature of 39.6°C (103.3°F). No other abnormalities were noted.

1 What differential diagnoses should be considered for mucosal pallor, and what is your assessment for this dog?
2 What are the next diagnostic steps?

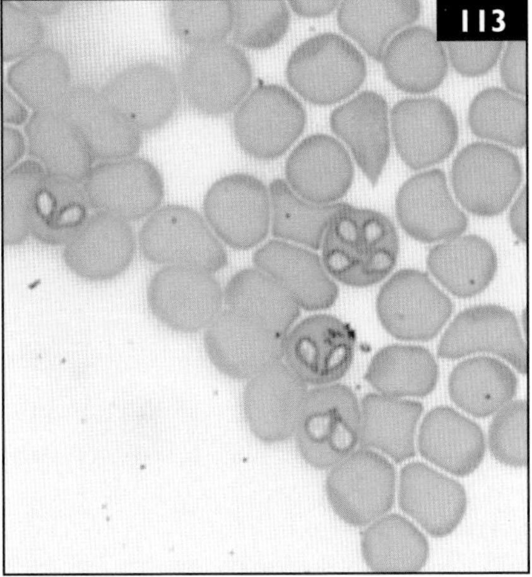

CASE 113 Case 113 is the same dog as case 112. The dog had a hematocrit of 0.15 l/l. A blood smear was obtained (**113**). The dog (10 kg) needed a blood transfusion, but no stored blood was available. However, the owner offered to bring in a 5-year-old Rottweiler (50 kg), which belonged to the son of the owner, as a blood donor. This dog was healthy, completely vaccinated, and received preventive treatment for parasites regularly.

1 What is your diagnosis?
2 What factors have to be addressed and kept in mind before and during a blood transfusion?

CASE 114 A 10-year-old neutered female Miniature Poodle was referred for signs of increasing pain and discomfort that had become progressively worse in the last 2 months. She had become reluctant to jump up on furniture, as previously accustomed to doing. The dog was evaluated by a veterinarian, and generalized lymphadenomegaly and elevated rectal temperatures that ranged from 38.5 to 41.0°C (101.3 to 105.8°F) were noted. The dog lived in Savannah, Georgia, USA, had never traveled. She had an irregular vaccination history. Parasiticides had not been applied for at least the last 2 years.

On presentation, the dog appeared stiff with a dorsally arched spine (**114**). The dog was mentally alert. Postural reactions were assessed, and the limbs had normal initiation on hopping reaction with delayed or stiff follow through. There were no deficits in any of the limbs with respect to conscious proprioceptive testing. Myotatic and flexor reflexes were present but weak motor movements were noted. The dog was painful on palpation of muscles in the extremities and paraspinal regions and on flexion and extension of the limbs. The remainder of the physical examination was unremarkable.

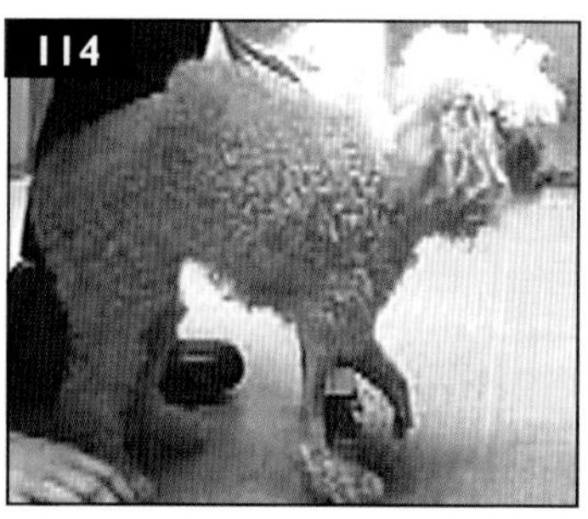
114

1 What are the two underlying pathophysiologic processes associated with hyperesthesia?
2 Are the four anatomic structures associated with diffuse hyperesthesia?
3 What are two underlying pathophysiologic processes associated with elevated rectal temperature?

CASE 115 Case 115 is the same dog as case 114. Ophthalmologic examination, including fundic examination, was performed and showed no lesions.

A CBC, biochemistry profile, and urinalysis were done, and revealed a marked leukocytosis (50.5×10^9/l) with neutrophilia (42.3×10^9/l), a left shift (5.3×10^9/l), and a mild increase in creatine kinase activity (2,547 U/l). Radiographs of the axial and appendicular skeleton revealed periosteal proliferation of the pelvis and proximal aspects of the pelvic limbs (**115a**). The results of CSF analysis were normal. Muscle biopsy findings showed a purulent and eosinophilic myositis. In some areas of the musculature, cysts with an “onion skin”-type appearance were found (**115b**).

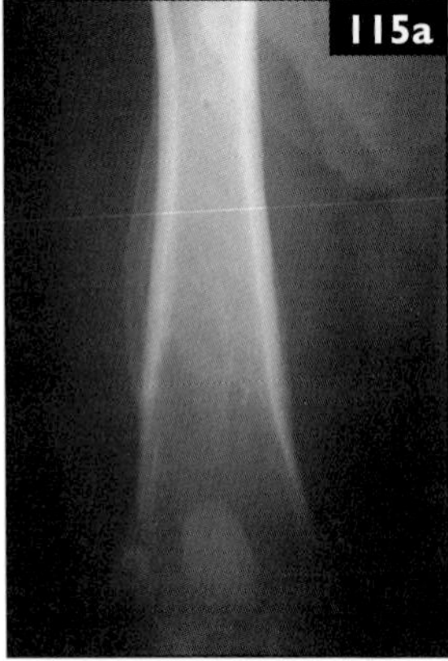

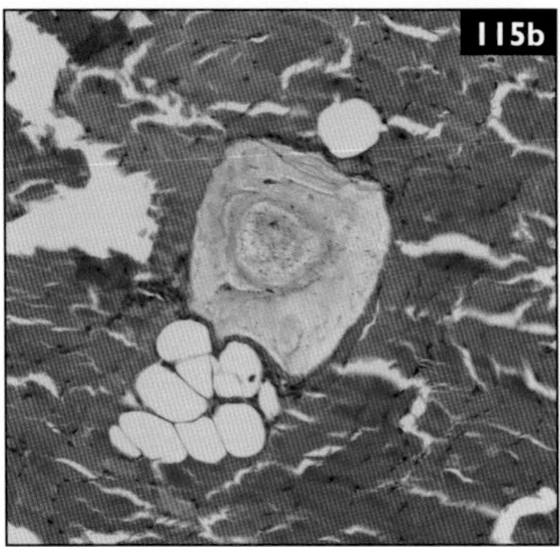

1 Which organ systems are likely to be responsible for the hyperesthesia in this dog, and how can this be associated with fever?
2 Which type of organism is seen in the muscle biopsy (e.g. virus, bacterium)?
3 What infectious diseases caused by these types of organisms are associated with polymyositis?
4 Which of these organisms can additionally cause polyperiostitis?

CASE 116 Case 116 is the same dog as cases 115 and 114. The dog was treated for hepatozoonosis and her gait improved during the course of 6 months of continuous therapy (**116**).

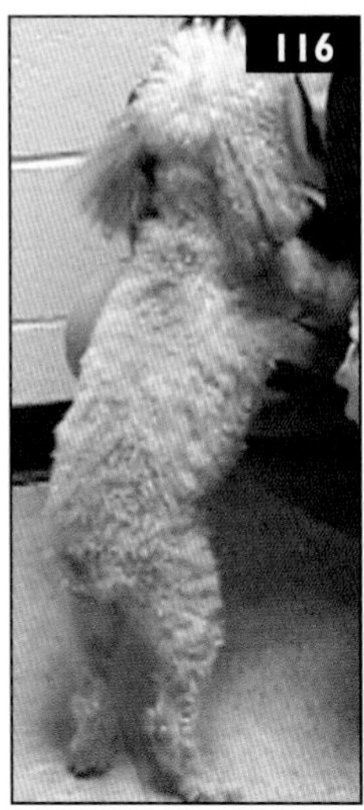

1 What drugs are used in the treatment of hepatozoonosis, and how long must treatment be continued?
2 How do the clinical manifestations and diagnostic findings differ between *Hepatozoon canis* and *Hepatozoon americanum* infection?

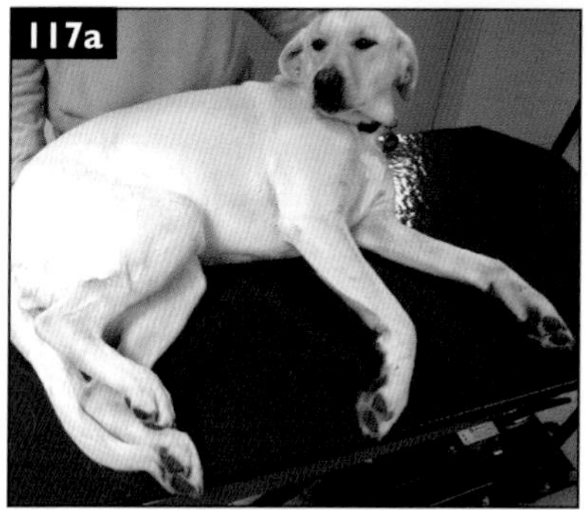

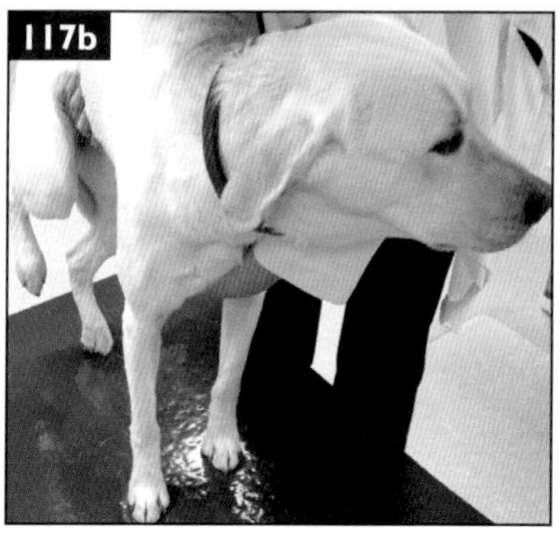

CASE 117 A 3-year-old neutered male Labrador Retriever from Minneapolis, Minnesota, USA, was evaluated for a 3-day history of inappetence, lethargy, shifting-leg lameness, and reluctance to walk. There was no history of trauma or recent travel. The dog frequently hiked with the owner. The dog was regularly vaccinated with core vaccines, but had not been treated for endoparasites in the last year. According to the owner, ectoparasite preventives were only used during the "tick season". No other medications had been administered to the dog.

On arrival at the veterinary clinic, the dog refused to walk and had to be transported on a gurney (**117a**). On physical examination, the body temperature was 40°C [104°F], and the popliteal lymph nodes were slightly enlarged and firm on palpation. Joints were painful when manipulated, especially the pelvic limb joints, but joint effusion was not detectable. Neurologic examination was within normal limits, but the dog was reluctant to bear weight with his pelvic limbs (**117b**). No other abnormalities were detected during physical examination, and no ectoparasites were noted.

1 What are the most likely differential diagnoses for this case?
2 What diagnostic testing should initially be performed?

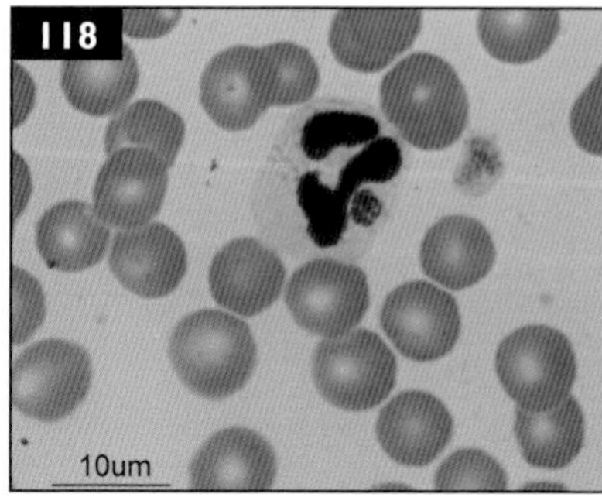

CASE 118 Case 118 is the same dog as case 117. A CBC showed a mild non-regenerative anemia, lymphopenia (0.5×10^9 lymphocytes/l, RI $1–5 \times 10^9$/l), and thrombocytopenia (85×10^9 platelets/l, RI $150–400 \times 10^9$/l). A blood smear was obtained (**118**). A serum biochemistry profile and urinalysis were within normal limits. Radiographs of affected limbs did not show evidence of erosive disease in

any joint. Arthrocentesis of both stifle and tarsal joints was performed bilaterally. Cytologic examination of synovial fluid revealed decreased viscosity, 6,500 nucleated cells/µl (RI <3,000 cells/µl) with 75% non-degenerate neutrophils (RI <5%), 37 g/l protein (RI <25 g/l), and absence of bacteria.

1 What is the structure seen in the neutrophil?
2 What conclusions can be made from the results of the synovial fluid analysis?

CASE 119 Case 119 is the same dog as cases 117 and 118. An in-clinic ELISA assay (SNAP 4Dx Plus, IDEXX Laboratories) was negative for antibodies to *Borrelia burgdorferi* and *Ehrlichia canis*, (and *Ehrlichia ewingii*), and for antigens of *Dirofilaria immitis*, but it was positive for *Anaplasma* spp. antibodies (**119**).

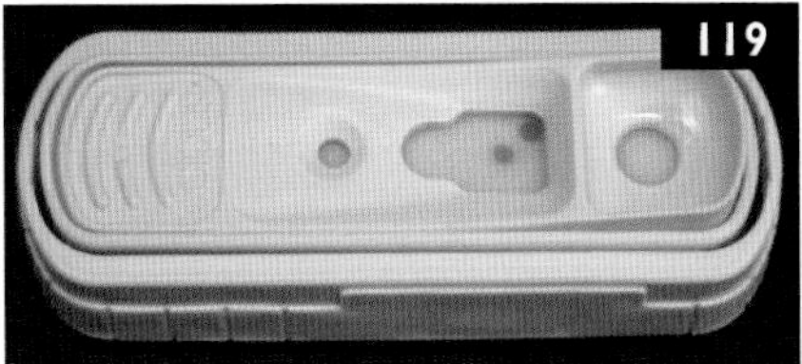
119

1 Does this result alone confirm a diagnosis of granulocytic anaplasmosis?
2 What other tests could be performed?
3 What is the treatment for this disease in dogs?
4 What is the prognosis in this case?

CASE 120 A 10-year-old neutered male Retriever mix (**120**) was presented to a veterinary clinic for a consultation. The owner of the dog had died from tuberculosis 1 week previously. Throughout the last 3 months, the dog had stayed almost constantly in the bedroom in close contact with the owner, who did not leave his bed. The son's family now needed to decide whether they would keep the dog, and wanted to know whether the dog could have contracted infection with *Mycobacterium tuberculosis*. The family had a 2-month-old baby. The dog had lived in Regensburg, Germany, and now had moved to Munich, Germany. Previous travel history as well as vaccination and parasite control status of the dog were unknown.

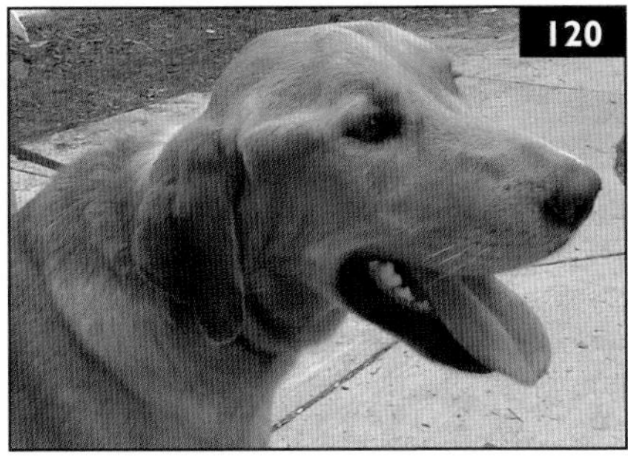
120

On physical examination, the dog was unremarkable apart from some dental tartar and a slightly thin body condition (3.5/9).

1 What is the likelihood that the dog was infected with *Mycobacterium tuberculosis*?
2 Are there diagnostic tests that can rule out the possibility of infection in this dog?

CASE 121 A 12-week-old intact male English Bulldog was evaluated for acute onset of respiratory difficulty followed by vomiting yellow to clear fluid. The dog lived in San Francisco, California, USA, had been acquired from a breeder 4 weeks previously, and had visited his local veterinarian 1 week previously for examination and vaccinations. He was being regularly treated for internal parasites and the second vaccination in the series was scheduled in 4 weeks. On physical examination, he had a temperature of 38.7°C (101.7°F), pulse of 160 bpm, and respiratory rate of 80 breaths/min with marked abdominal effort. Mild mucoid nasal and ocular discharges were present and inspiratory and expiratory stertor was audible without a stethoscope. Crackles were auscultated diffusely across all lung fields. The remainder of the physical examination was unremarkable. Thoracic radiographs were obtained (**121a, 121b**).

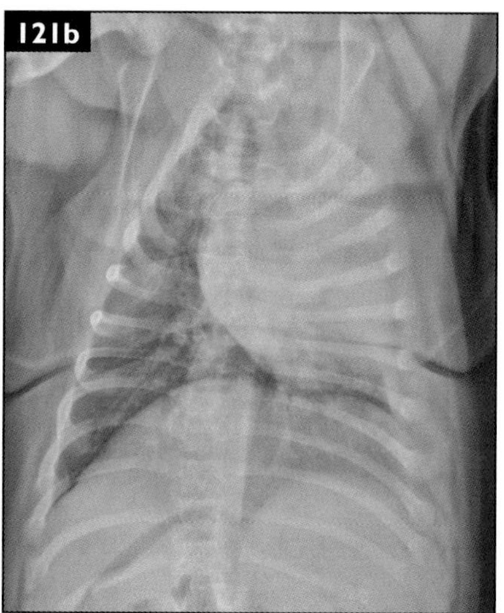
121b

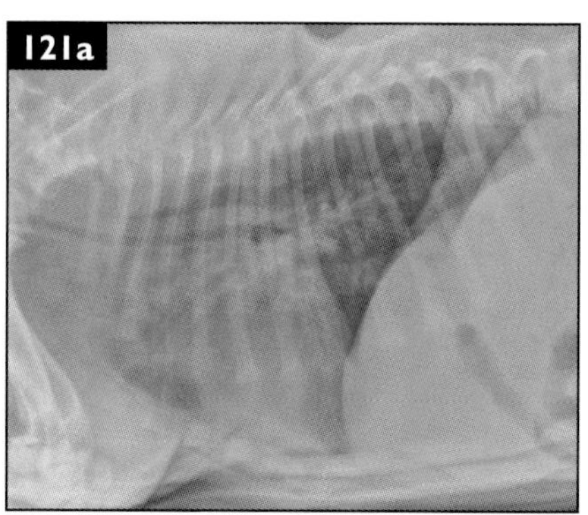
121a

1 What is your interpretation of the thoracic radiographs?
2 What differential diagnoses should be considered?
3 What diagnostic tests should be performed?

CASE 122 Case 122 is the same dog as case 121. A CBC was performed. A biochemistry panel showed hyperphosphatemia of 2.9 mmol/l (RI 1–1.6 mmol/l) and a slightly elevated ALP of 190 U/l (RI 0–152 U/l) (consistent with a growing puppy). The dog was closely monitored (**122**). Pulse oximetry results varied from 93 to 94%. PCR of blood, urine, and conjunctival scrapings for canine distemper virus was negative.

Complete blood count	Results	Reference interval
Hematocrit	0.328 l/l	0.35–0.58
MCV	69.3 fl	58–72
Reticulocytes	66.0×10^9/l	–
Platelets	800×10^9/l	150–500
White blood cells	33.780×10^9/l	5–16
Mature neutrophils	24.322×10^9/l	3–9
Band neutrophils	5.0×10^9/l	0–0.5
Eosinophils	0.0×10^9/l	0–1.0
Basophils	0.0×10^9/l	0–0.04
Lymphocytes	1.013×10^9/l	1–3.6
Monocytes	2.702×10^9/l	0.04–0.5

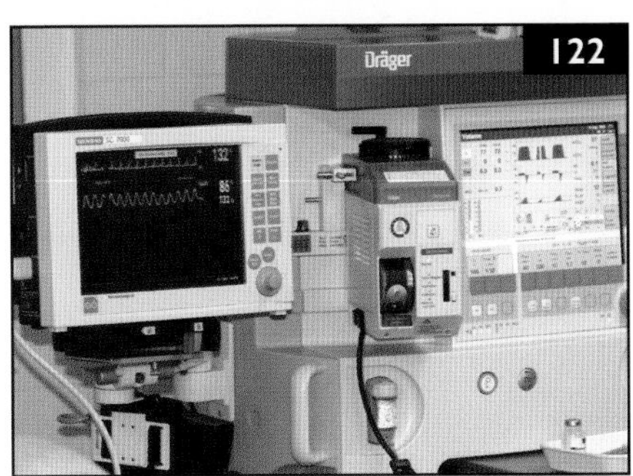

122

1 How would you interpret the CBC?
2 What stabilizing treatment should be provided?
3 What follow-up tests should be considered?

CASE 123 A 10-year-old neutered male mixed-breed dog (**123**) was referred for evaluation of progressive limb edema. The dog had been diagnosed with leishmaniosis 5 years ago and was on allopurinol treatment. He had not been vaccinated within the last 5 years, but received parasite prevention on a regular basis. The dog originally came from Rome, Italy, but for the last 6 years had lived in Munich, Germany, without any additional travel history. Physical examination revealed edema that involved all four limbs. No other abnormalities were noted.

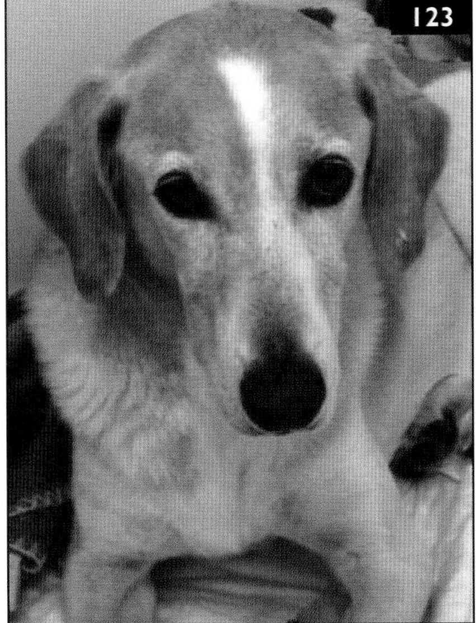
123

1 What is a likely explanation for the edema, based on the history?
2 How could the problem and its clinical consequences be addressed?

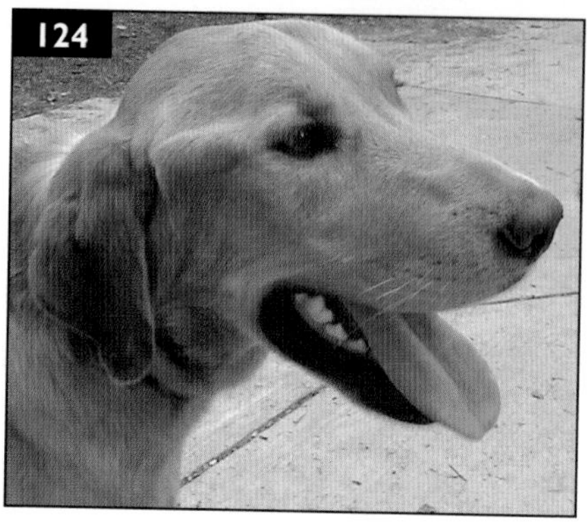

CASE 124 A 6-year-old neutered male, 20.6 kg mixed breed dog (**124**) was referred for a cardiac work-up, because the referring veterinarian had heard a new continuous heart murmur. The dog was known to have had a systolic murmur for several years. Along with dental prophylaxis, a grade I mast cell tumor had been surgically removed from the right thoracic limb 1 year previously. There was no history of exercise intolerance or other clinical signs. The dog lived in Ingolstadt, Germany, and was current on vaccinations and treated regularly with parasiticides. He had never traveled outside Germany.

Physical examination revealed that the dog was active, alert, and responsive. The rectal temperature was 38.9°C (102.0°F), mucosal membranes were moist and pink, capillary refill time was <2 seconds, all lymph nodes were of normal size, and abdominal palpation was unremarkable. Lung sounds were physiologic, and the respiratory rate was 36 breaths/min. A left basal continuous heart murmur with an intensity of V/VI was audible. The regular heart rate was 128 bpm. Pulse quality was normal, without pulse deficit or evidence of jugular vein distension/pulsation. The remainder of the physical examination was unremarkable.

1 What is your interpretation of the physical examination, and what are the differential diagnoses for the described heart murmurs?
2 What further diagnostic procedure should be recommended?

CASE 125 Case 125 is the same dog as case 124. Echocardiography was performed. A left apical five-chamber view (**125a**), a colour Doppler image (**125b**), and a CW Doppler image (**125c**) are shown.

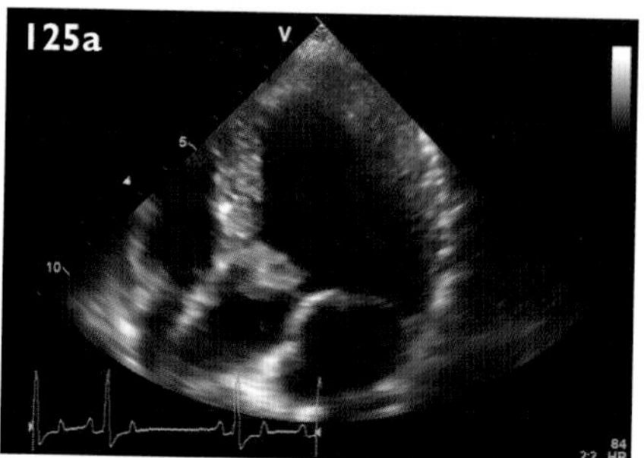

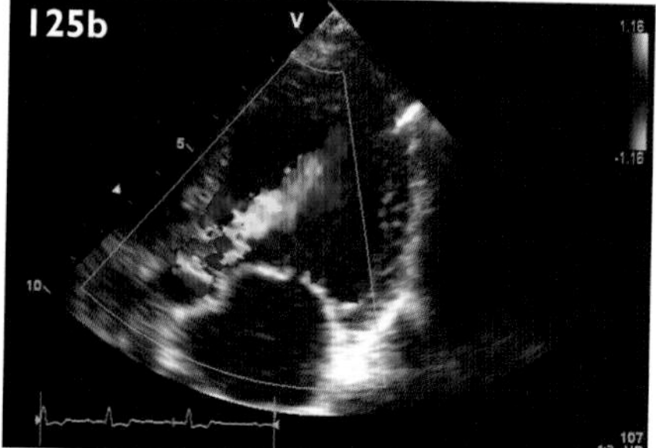

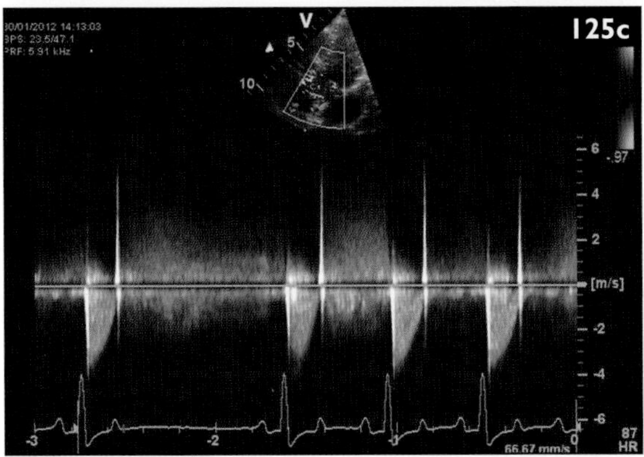

1 What is your interpretation of the echocardiographic images?
2 What is your main differential diagnosis?
3 What further tests would you recommend?

CASE 126 Case 126 is the same dog as cases 124 and 125. *Erysipelothrix rhusiopathiae* was grown from all three blood cultures taken from the jugular and peripheral veins. While culture was pending, antimicrobial drug treatment was commenced with a combination of amoxicillin–clavulanic acid and enrofloxacin. The *E. rhusiopathiae* isolate was susceptible to amoxicillin–clavulanic acid but resistant to enrofloxacin, so enrofloxacin treatment was discontinued. The dog remained alert and responsive during treatment (**126**); however, he died suddenly 2 weeks later, possibly as a result of a thromboembolic event or an arrhythmia.

1 What are the suggested criteria for diagnosis of infective endocarditis?
2 What are known predisposing factors for endocarditis?
3 What is the general prognosis for dogs with endocarditis?

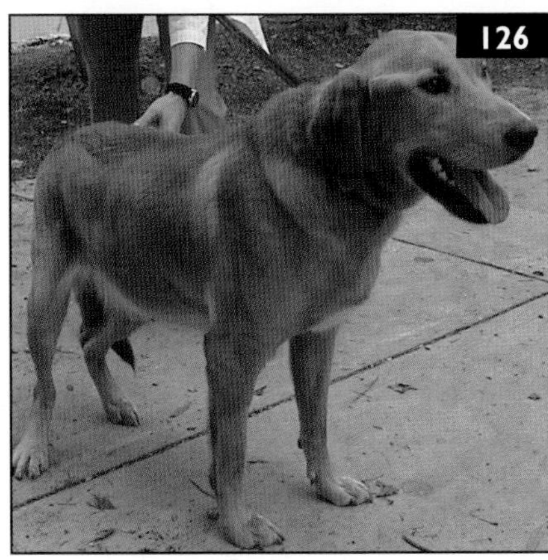

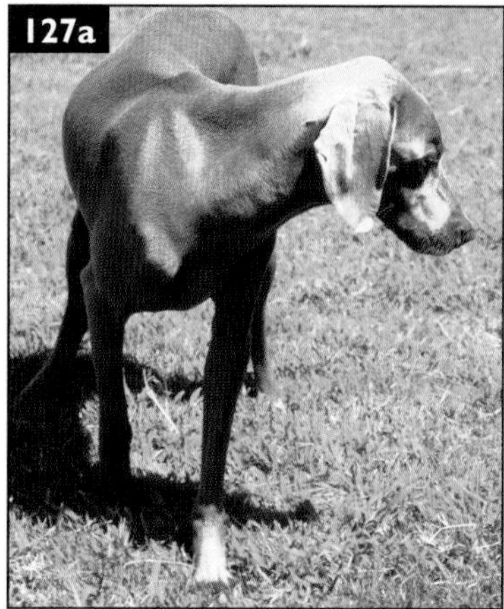

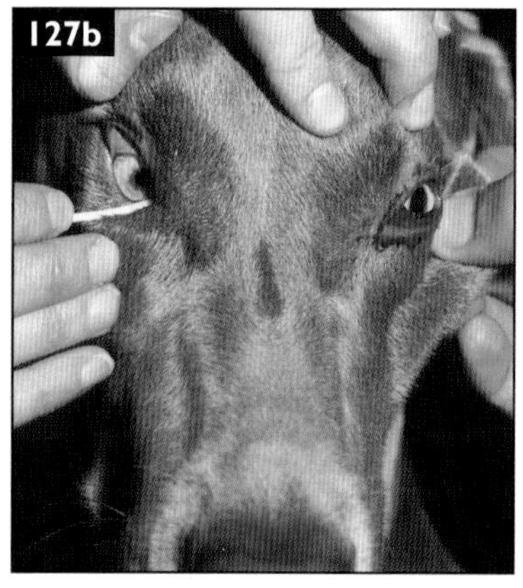

CASE 127 A 2-year-old neutered male Weimaraner was evaluated for a history of intermittent diarrhea that had been occurring over the last 2 months. The diarrhea was characterized by small volumes of feces with tenesmus, and intermittent hematochezia. One week prior to examination, the dog had a grand mal seizure and began to circle to the left side. The owner observed a reduced mental awareness. The dog also appeared to have lost visual acuity as he was observed to bump into objects in his environment and could not visually track silently moving objects. This visual dysfunction was recognized to be separate from and despite the dog's neurologic impairments. The dog lived in Atlanta, Georgia, USA, and had no travel history. He was fully vaccinated and received regular endoparasite and ectoparasite control.

Physical examination was unremarkable besides the neurologic and ophthalmologic abnormalities. The dog had a depressed mental status and would stand with his head and neck flexed to the left (**127a**). He had reduced noxious perception of pain with stimulation of the right nares. The left eye had a mydriatic pupil with cloudiness of the anterior chamber. There was a reduced menace response in both visual fields of the left eye. The right pupil was miotic, the left pupil was mydriatic (**127b**). Pupillary light reflexes were present bilaterally, although pupillary constriction was slow when the light was directed into the left eye.

1 What are the body systems in which problems were identified in this dog?
2 Where would you suspect the neurologic localization?
3 What would be your diagnostic plans for the various problems?

CASE 128 Case 128 is the same dog as case 127. Rectal scraping cytology was performed (**128**; Diff-Quik stain ×1,000). Ophthalmoscopic findings included aqueous flare in the anterior chambers of both eyes. Multifocal granulomatous white to gray lesions were observed on the retinas of both eyes and there was almost complete retinal detachment on the left side.

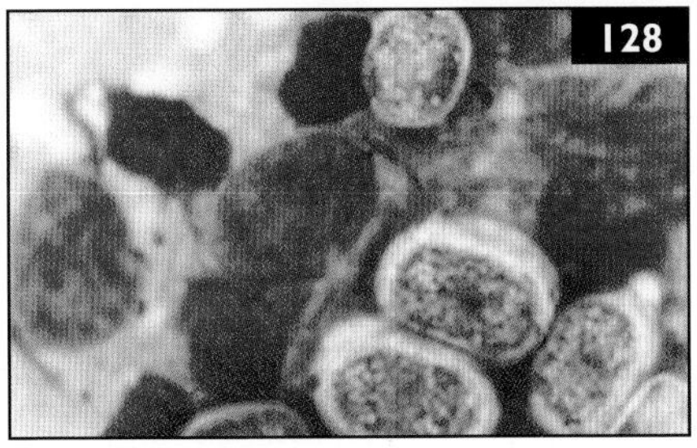

In this dog, abnormal findings on analysis of CSF from the cerebellomedullary cisterna were an increased total nuclear cell count of 1,150/µl (reference value <5/µl) and a total protein concentration of 1,240 mg/dl (reference value <30 mg/dl). The diferential cell count on a cytocentrifuged Wright–Giemsa-stained preparation showed many nucleated cells and few erythrocytes. Nucleated cells consisted of 50% eosinophils 40% non-degenerative neutrophils, 10% small lymphocytes, and occasional macrophages. Some macrophages showed erythrophagocytosis and hemosiderin pigment granules. Rare variably stained 15–20 µm basophilic organisms, with a granular texture and a clear unstained halo, were surrounded by phagocytic cells.

1 What organisms can be seen on the rectal scraping cytology?
2 What diagnostic tests could be performed for definitive diagnosis of this disease?
3 Are there any treatment options for this disease?

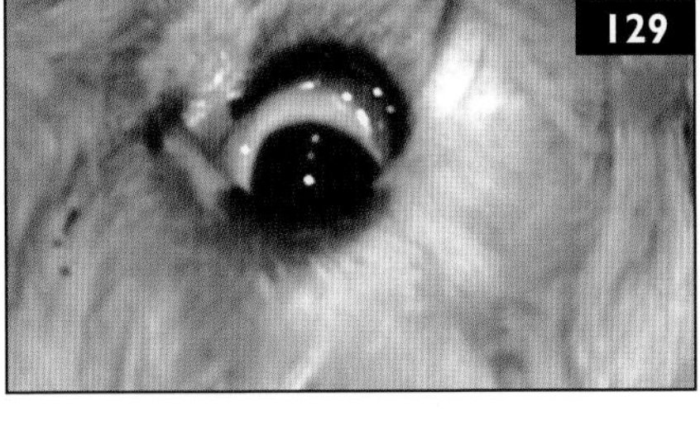

CASE 129 A 2-year-old intact male Old English Sheepdog was evaluated for a 4-day history of lethargy, inappetence, vomiting, and occasional cough. The dog had been adopted as a stray, 3 weeks before the onset of clinical signs, in Poznan, Poland. It had been vaccinated against rabies and treated for endoparasites and ectoparasites at the time of adoption, but no other vaccines had been administered.

On physical examination, the dog was febrile (40.3°C [104.5°F]), lethargic, icteric (**129**), had a stiff gait, abdominal pain, and appeared dehydrated with a capillary refill time of 3 seconds. A CBC revealed neutrophilia with a left shift, thrombocytopenia, high serum urea nitrogen and creatinine concentration, increased liver enzyme activities, and hyperbilirubinemia. Leptospirosis was suspected. Subsequent to hospitalization, a microscopic agglutination test (MAT) to detect antibodies against different *Leptospira* serovars was performed. The resulting titers were as follows: serovar Canicola 1:200, Icterohaemorrhagiae negative, Grippotyphosa 1:800, Australis 1:100.

1 Can such titers result from previous vaccination with *Leptospira* vaccines?
2 What is the diagnostic significance of MAT results in a non-vaccinated dog?
3 What other tests could help to confirm or rule out leptospirosis?

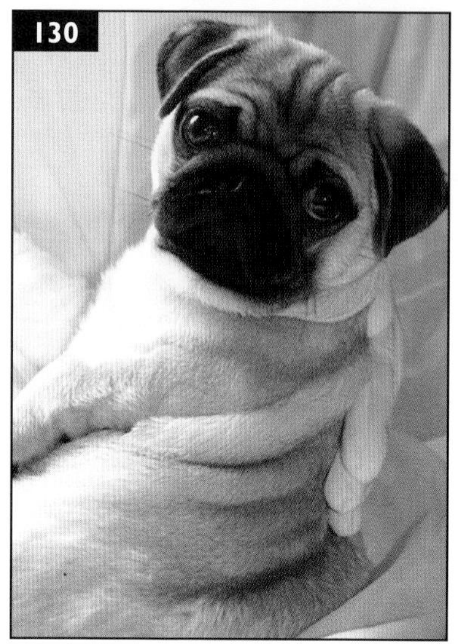

CASE 130 A 6-month-old intact male Pug (**130**) was evaluated for a 3-day history of vomiting, lethargy, and anorexia. The dog had been purchased from a breeder in Nurnberg, Germany, at the age of 10 weeks, and lived now in Munich, Germany. He had never been outside Germany. There were no other dogs in the household, but there were two cats. The dog had been vaccinated against parvovirus and distemper virus twice, at the age of 6 and 10 weeks. The dog had been dewormed at the age of 6 weeks but never since. He had not received any ectoparasite control.

On physical examination, the dog was very lethargic and slightly dehydrated. The abdomen was tense and the bowel loops appeared fluid-filled. A CBC was performed.

Complete blood count	Results	Reference interval
Red blood cells	5.6×10^{12}/l	5.5–9.3
Hemoglobin	7.53 mmol/l	7.45–12.5
Hematocrit	0.36 l/l	0.35–0.58
Platelets	440×10^9/l	150–500
White blood cells	3.53×10^9/l	5–16
Mature neutrophils	1.80×10^9/l	3–9
Band neutrophils	0.35×10^9/l	0–0.5
Eosinophils	0×10^9/l	0–1.0
Basophils	0.04×10^9/l	0–0.04
Lymphocytes	1.03×10^9/l	1–3.6
Monocytes	0.31×10^9/l	0.04–0.5

1 What is your differential diagnosis for the leucopenia?
2 Can a vaccinated dog develop parvovirosis?
3 Could a dog become infected with parvovirus from a cat?

CASE 131 Case 131 is the same dog as case 130. The results of a fecal SNAP parvovirus antigen test (IDEXX Laboratories) supported the diagnosis of parvovirosis (**131**).

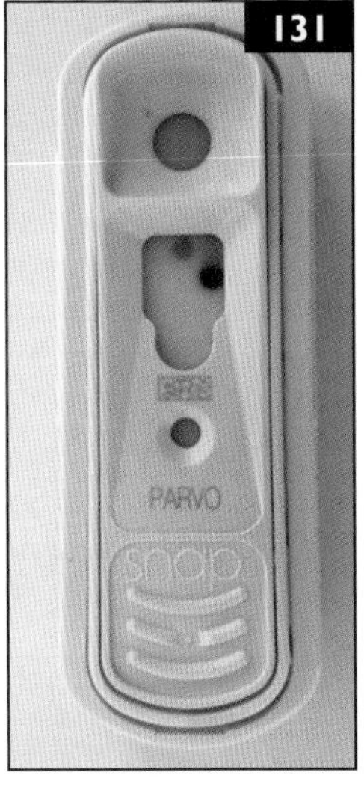

1 What supportive treatment is appropriate in a dog with parvovirosis?
2 Which antibiotics should be used?

CASE 132 Case 132 is the same dog as cases 131 and 130. Although treated intensively, the dog was not improving. Additional treatment options, including recombinant feline interferon-ω (**132**), were considered.

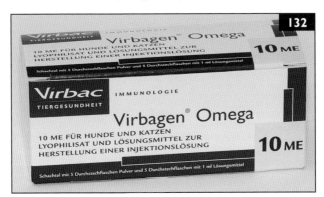

1 Is treatment with recombinant feline interferon-ω useful?
2 Is administration of specific antibodies useful?
3 Are drugs that increase the neutrophil count available and useful?

CASE 133 A 2-year-old male mixed-breed dog, originating from Santa Maria, Brazil, was evaluated because over the last 5 days he had shown lethargy, anorexia, hematochezia, vomiting, weight loss, dark yellow colored urine, and bleeding at the ear pinnal margins. The dog had been regularly vaccinated, but had not received any parasite control within the last year.

Physical examination revealed a poor body condition (BCS 3/9), pale and icteric mucous membranes, peripheral generalized lymphadenomegaly, splenomegaly, hepatomegaly, intermittent fever, and extensive subcutaneous hemorrhage (**133a**). Ticks were found around the dog's ears and feet. A CBC, biochemistry panel, and urinalysis were performed (for significant findings see below). On the blood smear, polychromasia, normoblastemia, spherocytosis, anisocytosis, and Howell–Jolly bodies (**133b**) were noted. There was agglutination of red blood cells on the tube wall.

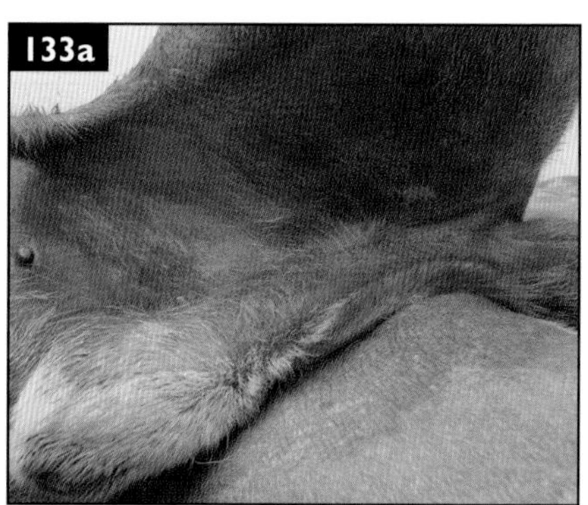
133a

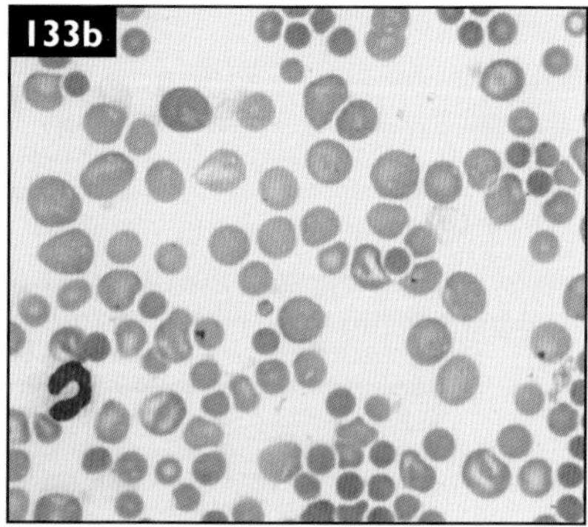
133b

Complete blood count	Results	Reference interval
Hematocrit	0.17 l/l	0.35–0.58
MCV	105 fl	58–72
MCHC	24.7 mmol/l	19–21
Reticulocytes	85 × 10^9/l	0–60
Platelets	61 × 10^9/l	150–500
White blood cells	24.5 × 10^9/l	5–16
Mature neutrophils	19.3 × 10^9/l	3–9
Monocytes	1.8 × 10^9/l	0.04–0.5

Biochemistry panel	Results	Reference interval
ALT	36 U/l	18–110
ALP	45 U/l	13–152
Total protein	64 g/l	55.5–77.6
Albumin	32 g/l	31–43
Bilirubin	10.2 μmol/l	0–5.3

Urinalysis	Results
Color, appearance	Dark yellow
Bilirubin	3+
Hemoglobin	Negative

1 How is the anemia in this dog classified, and what are the main differential diagnoses?
2 What diagnostic tests should be performed next?

CASE 134 Case 134 is the same dog as case 133. Tests for serum antibodies against *Borrelia burgdorferi*, *Ehrlichia canis*, *Ehrlichia ewingii*, *Anaplasma* spp., and *Leishmania* spp., as well as for antigens of *Dirofilaria immitis*, were negative. Cytologic examination of a fine needle aspirate of the left popliteal lymph node was performed (**134**).

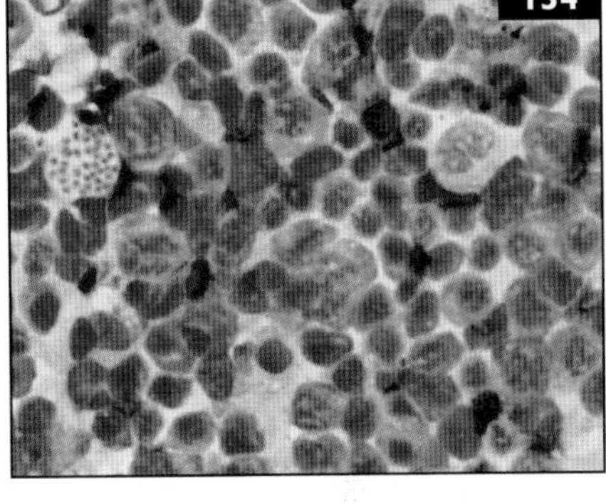
134

1 What are the cytologic findings in the lymph node aspirate?
2 Can a definitive diagnosis be made?

CASE 135 Case 135 is the same dog as cases 133 and 134. The dog was hospitalized for treatment. The hemorrhagic diarrhea and vomiting ceased, and the dog started to eat and drink after 3 days of hospitalization. After 2 weeks, the dog's clinical condition improved, and the icterus resolved (**135**). The dog was discharged from the hospital, and treatment was continued at home.

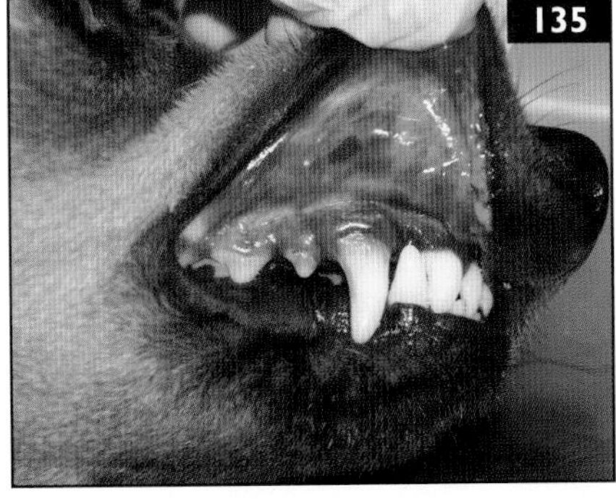
135

1 What is the recommended treatment for this patient?
2 The owner has two other dogs. What preventive measures should be recommended?

CASE 136 A 3-year-old neutered female Doberman Pinscher was evaluated for acute cough and respiratory distress that the owner had first noticed 3 days previously. Before this episode, the dog was in good condition, and there was no previous history of illness. The dog lived in the San Francisco Bay area, California, USA, and had never traveled outside of this region. She was regularly vaccinated and received preventive treatments for endoparasites and ectoparasites on a regular basis.

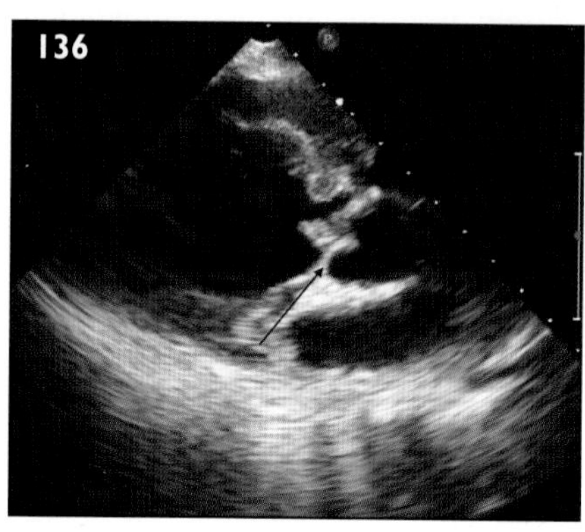

On physical examination, the dog was listless. She had tachypnea with crackles on auscultation of the thorax, and a respiratory rate of approximately 70 bpm. The pulse rate was 160–210 bpm. A grade III/VI left-sided apical heart murmur was detected, with hyperkinetic but synchronous femoral pulses. The BCS was 5/9. Thoracic radiographs showed a severe interstitial to alveolar pattern in the caudodorsal lung lobes and mild left atrial enlargement. An echocardiogram showed moderate left atrial enlargement. A hyperechoic, oscillating lesion was seen on the aortic valve cusps (**136, arrow**). Severe aortic insufficiency was also present.

1 What is your main differential diagnosis for the lesion on the aortic valve, including infectious agents potentially involved, and which pathogen seems most likely based on the clinical findings?
2 What additional diagnostic tests would you recommend?
3 How should this dog be treated pending the results of those diagnostic tests?

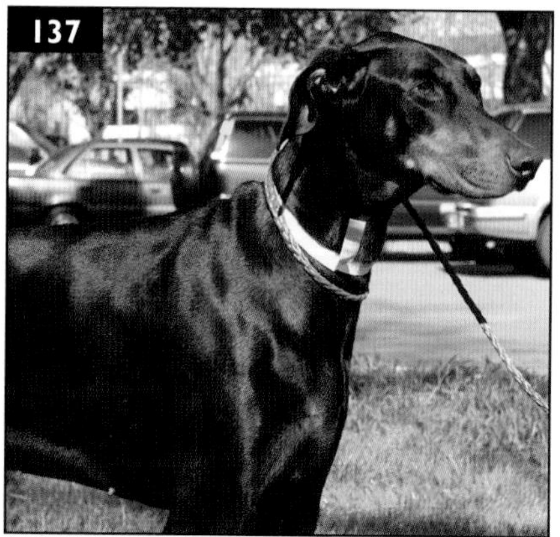

CASE 137 Case 137 is the same dog as case 136 (**137**). The CBC showed a mild non-regenerative anemia (hematocrit 0.32 l/l, RI 0.35–0.58 l/l) with a mild mature neutrophilia (14.227×10^9 cells/l, RI $3–115 \times 10^9$/l). The biochemistry panel revealed hyponatremia (142 mmol/l, RI 145–154 mmol/l), hypochloremia (96 mmol/l, RI 105–116 mmol/l), hyperglycemia (7.6 mmol/l, RI 3.9–6.5 mmol/l), increased serum urea nitrogen concentration (14.6 mmol/l, RI 2.9–11.1 mmol/l), and increased

activities of serum ALP (210 U/l, RI 15–127 U/l) and serum ALT (73 U/l, RI 19–67 U/l). Urinalysis showed a specific gravity of 1.012 and a benign sediment. Blood cultures were negative. A *Bartonella vinsonii* subsp. *berkhoffii* antibody test was positive at 1:256, a *Bartonella henselae* antibody test was positive at 1:64, and a *Bartonella clarridgeiae* antibody test was negative.

1 Do the antibody test results prove that *Bartonella* spp. infection is the cause of endocarditis in this dog, and would it rule out *Bartonella* spp. infection as a cause of disease if the test results had been negative?
2 What is the prognosis for recovery?
3 What is the zoonotic potential of *Bartonella* spp.?

CASE 138 A young puppy of about 3 months of age was adopted 3 days previously from a rescue shelter in Munich, Germany, where it had been boarded for at least 14 days after living as a stray. The dog was vaccinated once on entry into the shelter with an attenuated live canine distemper, adenovirus, and parvovirus vaccine. The new owner noticed a cough, mucopurulent nasal discharge, and diarrhea 1 day after adoption. On contacting the shelter, the owner was informed that several other dogs had developed similar signs and two puppies had died with seizures. On physical examination the puppy appeared weak and lethargic. Rectal temperature was elevated (40.2°C [104.7°F]) and the dog had a mucopurulent nasal discharge and conjunctivitis (**138a**). There were harsh lung sounds on auscultation. Hyperkeratosis was noted on examination of the footpads (**138b**). A CBC revealed mild lymphopenia but a normal neutrophil count.

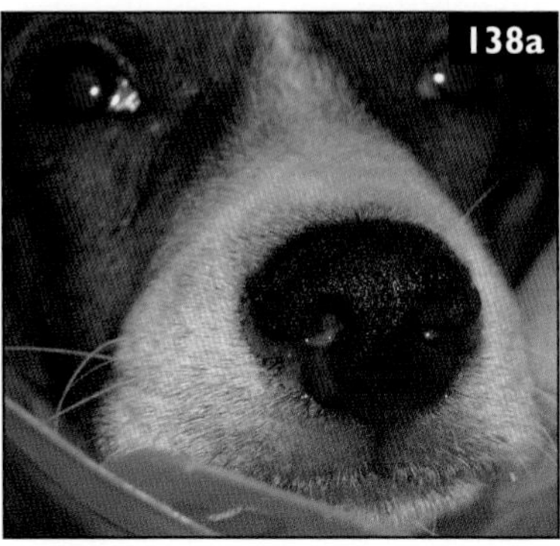
138a

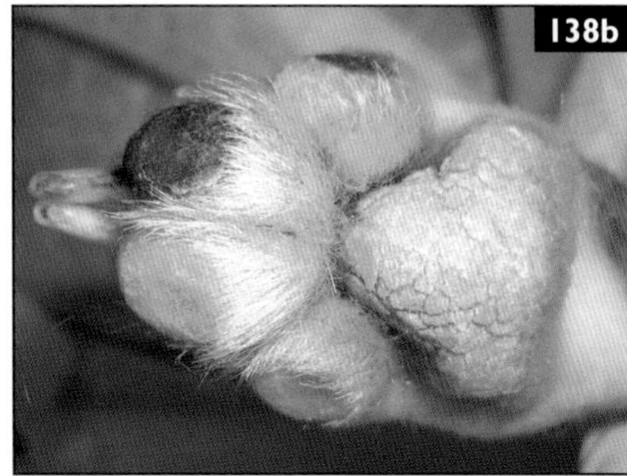
138b

1 What is the main differential diagnosis?
2 What diagnostic tests should be considered?
3 What treatment is recommended, and what is the prognosis?

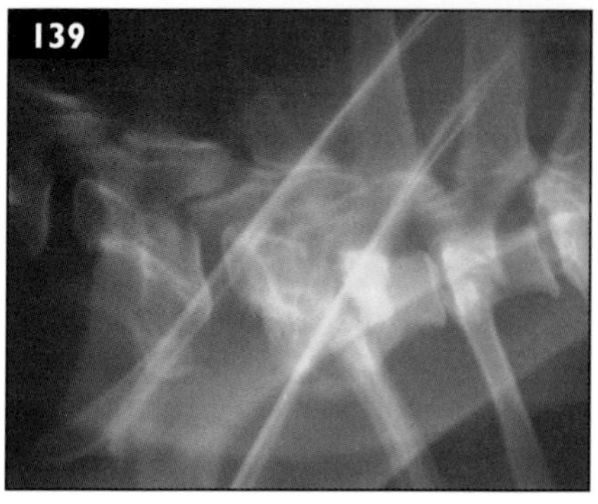

CASE 139 A 3-year-old intact female Doberman Pinscher was evaluated for a 2-day history of lethargy, anorexia, and reluctance to ambulate. The dog lived in Palermo, Italy. It had received complete vaccinations against distemper, adenovirus, parvovirus, *Leptospira*, and rabies, and was on regular heartworm prophylaxis.

On physical examination, abnormal clinical findings included elevated temperature (39.9°C [103.8°F]), cervical pain, and a stiff neck. The remainder of the physical examination, including a detailed neurologic examination, was unremarkable. A radiograph of the cervical region was obtained (**139**).

1 What would be your differential diagnoses for the clinical presentation in this dog (before radiographs were obtained)?
2 What is your interpretation of the radiograph?
3 What diagnostic tests should also be performed?

CASE 140 Case 140 is the same dog as case 139. *Staphylococcus pseudintermedius* bacteriuria was documented by urinalysis and culture, and was associated with urinary cystoliths (**140a, 140b**). The same bacterial species was isolated from two out of three blood cultures. Susceptibility testing showed that all isolates were broadly susceptible, including to all beta-lactam drugs tested. Thus, the source of the organism causing the discospondylitis was suspected to be the urinary tract.

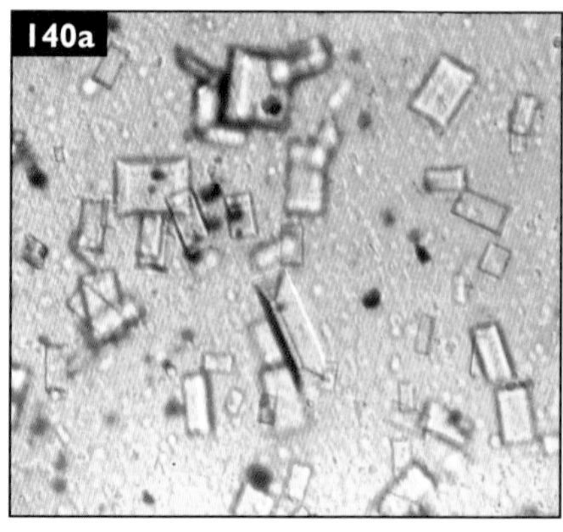

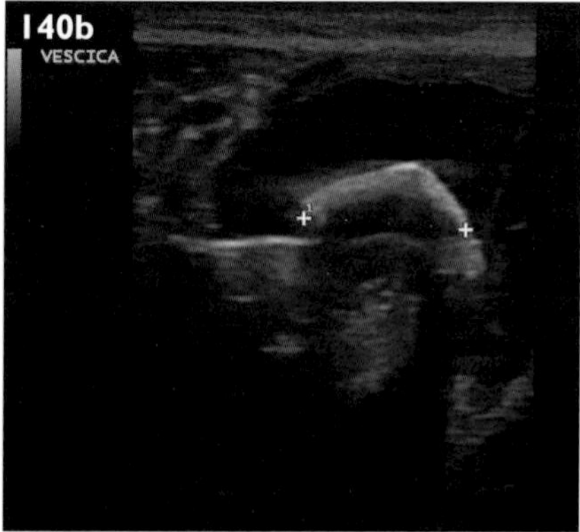

1 What other common sources of infection can be associated with discospondylitis?
2 What are the most common infectious agents associated with discospondylitis?
3 What treatment should be recommended?
4 What is the likely composition of the urolith?

CASE 141 A 3-year-old neutered male American Pitbull Terrier from Tulsa, Oklahoma, USA, was evaluated for lethargy, inappetence, and a stiff gait of 2 days' duration. The dog was up to date on core vaccines and had received heartworm and flea preventatives monthly. The owner took the dog for hikes at weekends, and had found an attached tick 1 week previously. No history of trauma, travel, access to toxins, or previous illnesses was reported.

Physical examination revealed approximately 5% dehydration, a rectal temperature of 40.1°C (104.2°F), petechiation of mucous membranes (**141**), moderate bilateral prescapular lymphadenomegaly, and splenomegaly. The dog seemed painful during the examination, but the pain could not be localized to a specific area. No swelling or joint effusion was present. Neurologic examination was within normal limits. The only abnormalities found on bloodwork were thrombocytopenia (130×10^9 platelets/l, RI $150–400 \times 10^9$/l) and slight hypoalbuminemia (25 g/l, RI 28–40 g/l). An in-clinic ELISA (4Dx SNAP Plus, IDEXX Laboratories) was negative for antibodies to *Anaplasma* spp., *Borrelia burgdorferi*, *Ehrlichia canis* (and *Ehrlichia ewingii*), and antigens of *Dirofilaria immitis*. A PCR panel for detection of *Anaplasma* spp., *Ehrlichia* spp., *Babesia* spp., and *Bartonella* spp. DNA was also negative.

1 What are your primary differential diagnoses?
2 What would be the next diagnostic step?
3 How should this dog be treated?

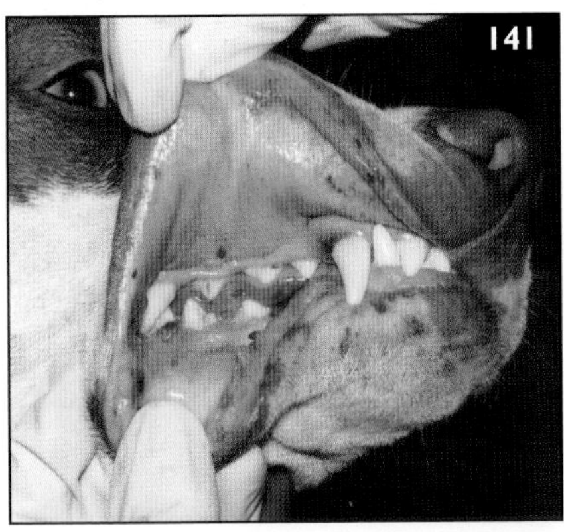
141

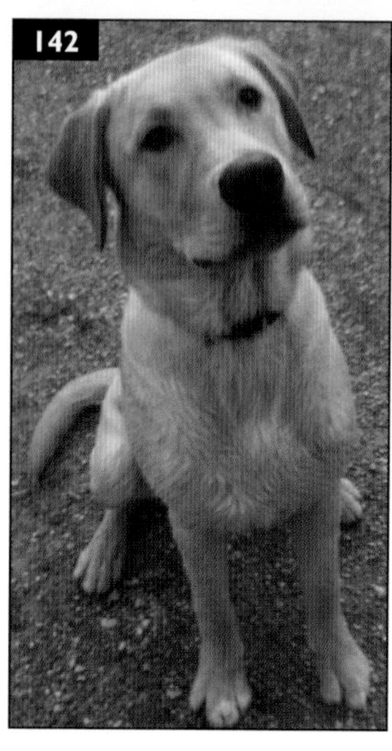

CASE 142 A 6-month-old intact male Labrador Retriever was evaluated for acute diarrhea and lethargy (**142**). Anorexia, refusal to walk, and diarrhea had started 24 hours before evaluation, and the diarrhea progressed in frequency. For the 3 hours before evaluation, the dog had watery diarrhea every 30 minutes. The dog lived in Munich, Germany, and had never been outside the country. He had received a full basic vaccination series, had been treated with endoparasiticides several times, and was on a regular ectoparasite control program. The dog had been fed a raw meat diet over the last 3 months.

On physical examination, the dog showed signs of shock. He was mentally obtunded. Mucous membranes were pink, but tacky. Pulse quality was good. Capillary refill time was 1 second. Heart rate and respiratory rate were 140 bpm and 36 breaths/min, respectively, without abnormal findings on auscultation. On palpation, the abdomen was tense. Rectal body temperature was 40.7°C (105.3°F). The remainder of the physical examination was unremarkable.

1 What are the two clinical phases of shock, and what phase was present in this dog?
2 What are the five pathophysiologic types of shock?
3 How would you characterize the pathophysiologic type of shock in this dog?

CASE 143 143 is the same dog as case 142. On ultrasound, the small intestine appeared partly corrugated (**143**). A 15-cm segment of the jejunal wall was

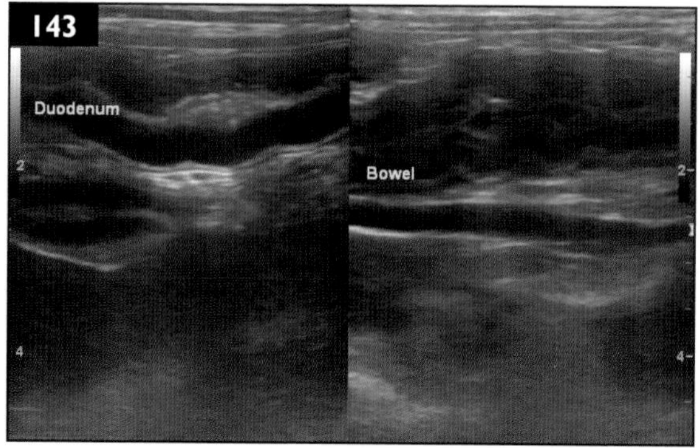

thickened when compared with other parts of the small intestine, with a lack of normal intestinal wall layering. In addition, a mesenteric lymph node in the mid-abdomen was moderately enlarged (diameter 1.5–2 cm; length 4–5 cm) and of heterogeneous echogenicity. A CBC was performed.

Complete blood count	Results	Reference interval
Red blood cells	5.56×10^{12}/l	5.5–9.3
Hemoglobin	7.73 mmol/l	7.45–12.5
Hematocrit	0.37 l/l	0.35–0.58
Platelets	211×10^{9}/l	150–500
White blood cells	9.28×10^{9}/l	5–16
Mature neutrophils	3.29×10^{9}/l	3–9
Band neutrophils	2.37×10^{9}/l	0–0.5
Eosinophils	0×10^{9}/l	0–1.0
Basophils	0×10^{9}/l	0–0.04
Lymphocytes	3.21×10^{9}/l	1–3.6
Monocytes	0.41×10^{9}/l	0.04–0.5

1 Which bacterial species are considered to be enteropathogenic?
2 What are limitations of a fecal culture?
3 How might you make a diagnosis of an enteropathogenic bacterial infection in this case?

CASE 144 Case 144 is the same dog as cases 142 and 143. The enlarged lymph node was aspirated with a fine needle, and the aspirated fluid was transferred into a transport medium and submitted for culture. In addition, two separate blood culture specimens of 10 ml were taken at a 30-minute interval from two different sites after aseptic preparation of the skin. Blood specimens were immediately inoculated into a blood culture system using a fresh needle. The bottles were submitted for aerobic and anaerobic bacterial culture.

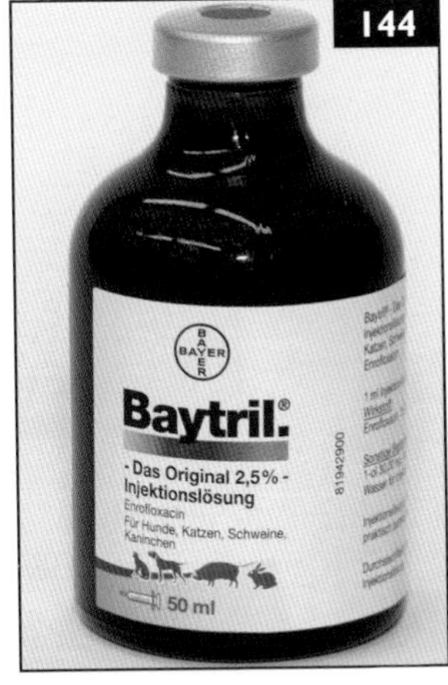

144

After taking specimens for bacterial culture, antibiotic treatment was started with enrofloxacin (**144**). With fluid therapy and antibiotics, the dog improved clinically. On the second day after treatment, the dog showed normal vital parameters and was afebrile. After 3 days of treatment, the diarrhea had resolved and the dog was discharged on oral enrofloxacin and a low fat, highly digestible diet.

Blood cultures were negative, but *Salmonella* spp. were isolated from the lymph node aspirates. Susceptibility testing revealed that the isolate was susceptible to enrofloxacin. A diagnosis of acute intestinal *Salmonella* spp. infection with bacterial translocation and sepsis was made.

1 Should antibiotics be administered to every patient with acute diarrhea and suspicion of an enteric bacterial infection?
2 Do you think antibiotics were indicated in this case?
3 Is there a potential zoonotic risk?
4 What would your recommendations be to the owner?

CASE 145 A 5-month-old intact male American Pitbull Terrier was referred with a 5-day history of progressive illness. For the first 2 days of illness, the dog's clinical signs consisted of lethargy and mild inappetence. On the following day, the owner noticed that the dog had a stiff gait, anorexia, and difficulty opening his mouth. Subsequently, the owner noticed "muscle spasms", which progressed over 24 hours despite treatment with flumethasone, antibiotics, and intravenous fluids at a local veterinary clinic. On admission, the dog was in lateral recumbency with spastic hyperextension of all limbs, extension of the tail, and generalized muscular spastic rigidity (**145**). Rectal temperature was 41.1°C (106.0°F), heart rate 186 bpm, and respiratory rate 54 breaths/min. Hypersensitivity to external stimuli was present, which resulted in profound muscular spasms.

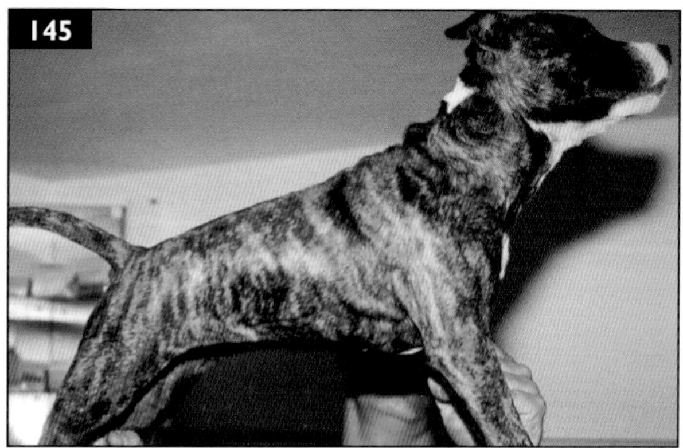
145

1 What is the most likely diagnosis?
2 What are potential differential diagnoses?
3 How is the diagnosis confirmed?
4 What is the prognosis?
5 What are the most common complications of this disease?

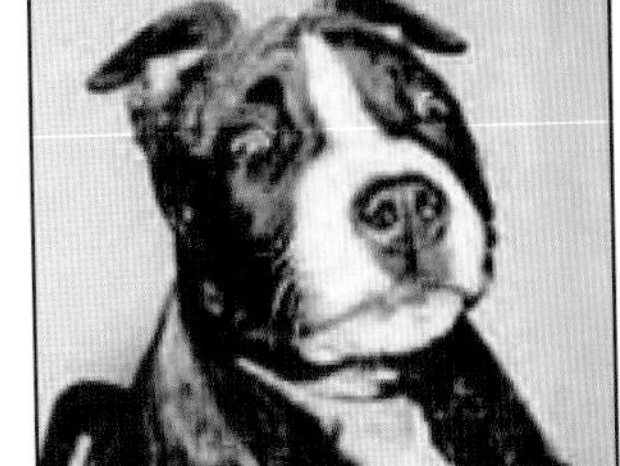

CASE 146 Case 146 is the same dog as case 145. The most common early signs of generalized tetanus are ocular and facial muscular abnormalities (risus sardonicus) (**146**), progressing to rigidity of other muscles. Localized tetanus, which involves only one portion of the body adjacent to the wound, is less common but has a better prognosis.

1 How is *Clostridium tetani* transmitted?
2 What could be the source of infection in this dog?
3 What treatment would be recommended?

CASE 147 A 3-year-old neutered male Golden Retriever was evaluated for a 3-week history of progressive cough, decreased appetite, and weight loss. The dog lived in Minneapolis, Minnesota, USA, and had no history of traveling. He was regularly vaccinated and received regular antiparasitic treatment.

Physical examination revealed a quiet but alert and responsive dog in thin body condition (BCS 3/9). The dog's rectal temperature was 39.7°C (103.5°F), the respiratory rate was 40 breaths/min, and pulse rate was 100 beats/min. There were no other physical examination findings apart from two firm, non-ulcerated cutaneous nodules, one on the trunk (1 cm in diameter) and one on the left distal pelvic limb (0.5 cm in diameter). The left popliteal lymph node was also slightly enlarged and firm. A fundic examination was normal. Thoracic radiographs showed hilar lymphadenomegaly and multifocal pulmonary nodules, as well as some patchy alveolar infiltrates. Cytologic examination of a fine needle aspirate of the left popliteal lymph node revealed yeast organisms consistent with *Blastomyces* spp. (**147**)

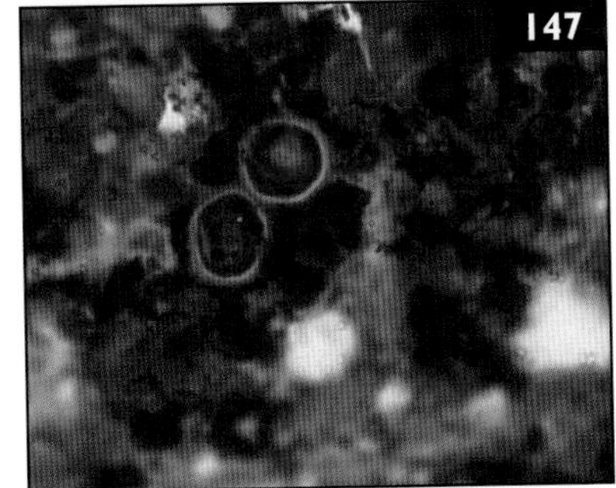

1 What is the geographic distribution of *Blastomyces* spp.?
2 What are other anatomic sites of predilection of this organism?
3 Had the cutaneous lesions not been identified, what other diagnostic tests could have been used to obtain the diagnosis, and what are the limitations of these tests?
4 What treatment should be recommended?

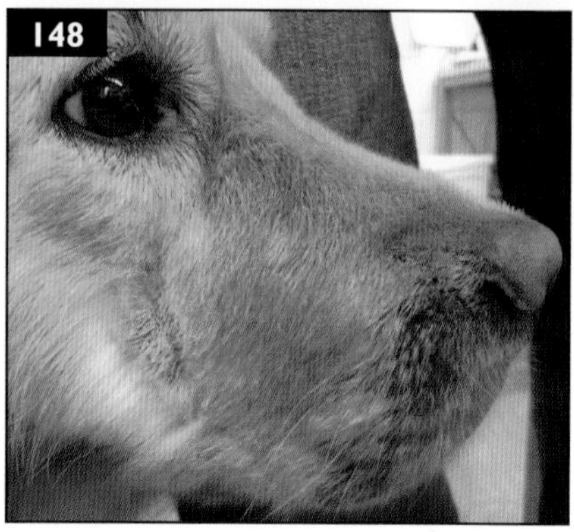

CASE 148 A 6-month-old intact female Golden Retriever was evaluated for two focal regions of hypotrichosis on the muzzle (**148**) of several weeks' duration. The dog was otherwise well, had a good appetite, and was not pruritic. The dog had been regularly vaccinated with core vaccines and was regularly treated for endoparasites. She lived in Munich, Germany, and had never been outside the country.

On physical examination, the only pathologic findings were the lesions described. The affected skin was not erythematous, but was slightly thicker than in adjacent areas and hyperpigmented.

1 What are your differential diagnoses?
2 What tests would you propose?

CASE 149 Case 149 is the same dog as case 148. Cytology revealed keratinocytes and occasional cocci. A deep skin scraping showed mites (**149**).

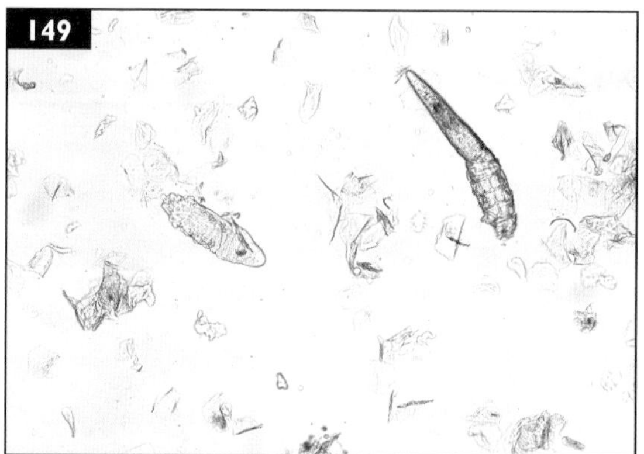

1 What is the prognosis for the disease in this dog?
2 How would you treat this dog?

CASE 150 A 2-year-old mixed-breed dog from Munich, Germany, was evaluated for acute cough of 3 days' duration. The cough began while the dog was boarded in a kennel for 7 days. The owners reported that the dog seemed slightly lethargic and showed a decreased appetite. The dog was up to date on vaccinations (distemper, adenovirus, parvovirus, parainfluenza, *Bordetella*, *Leptospira*, and rabies) and was receiving monthly milbemycin for parasites.

On physical examination, the dog was febrile (rectal temperature 40.3°C [104.5°F]), had a bilateral nasal discharge (**150a**), and harsh inspiratory and expiratory lung sounds on auscultation. Bloodwork was performed and revealed a neutrophilia with a left shift. Radiography was also performed (**150b, 150c**).

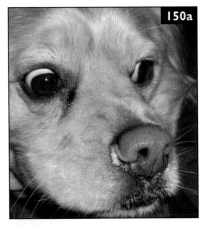
150a

1 What is the most likely diagnosis in this dog, based on the history and clinical signs?
2 How would you interpret the radiographs?
3 What treatment would you recommend?

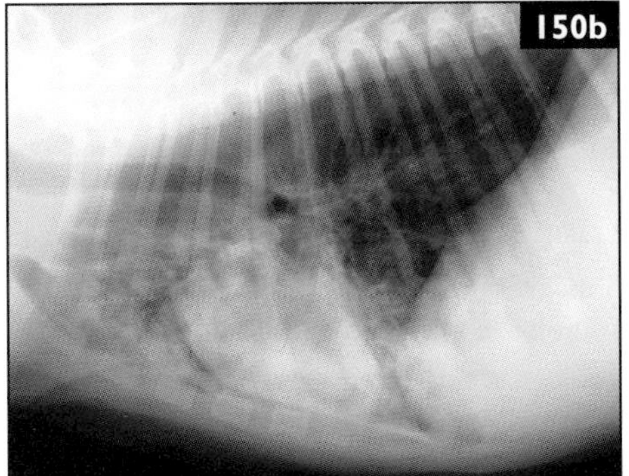
150b

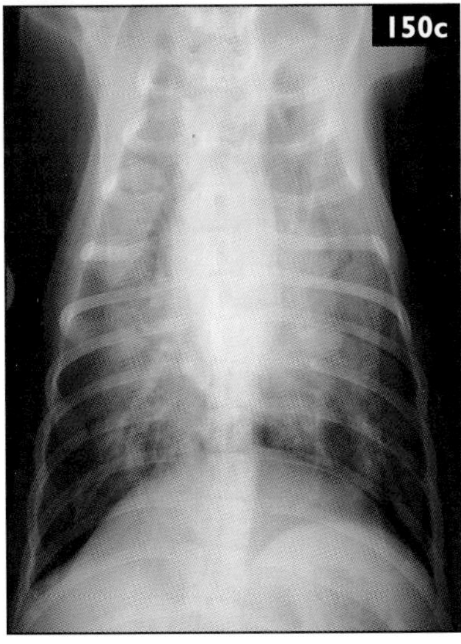
150c

CASE 151 A 4-year-old intact male Dachshund Terrier (**151**) was referred because of a 6-week history of elevated serum liver enzyme activities. Six weeks previously, the dog had an episode of vomiting and lethargy that lasted 2 days. The dog had been evaluated by a veterinarian at that time who had treated the dog with antiemetics and oral antibiotics (amoxicillin–clavulanic acid). The dog improved and appeared healthy thereafter, but elevated ALT and ALP enzyme activities were noted on several rechecks. The dog lived in Ingolstadt, Germany, and had never traveled. The owner worked as a forest ranger and the dog was used as a hunting dog. The dog was up to date on vaccinations, was treated about twice a year for endoparasites, and received ectoparasite control. No previous health problems were known.

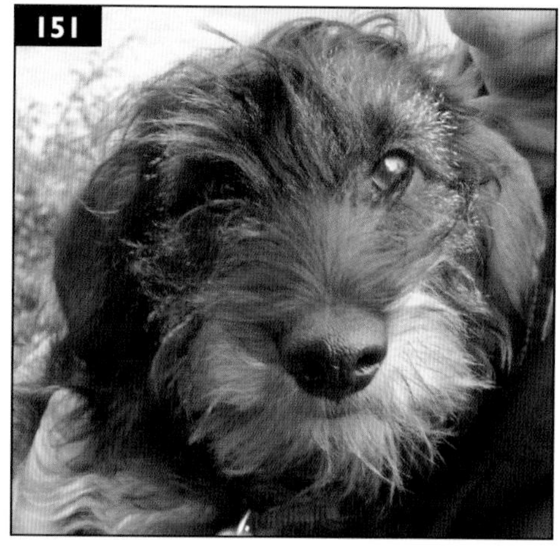

On physical examination, the dog was bright, alert, and responsive, and in good body condition (BCS 4.5/9). On palpation, the abdomen appeared tense, but was not painful. The remainder of the physical examination was unremarkable.

1 What drugs can result in increased serum liver enzyme activity without liver damage?
2 Which extrahepatic diseases can result in increased serum liver enzyme activity?
3 What is the half-life of serum ALT and ALP in dogs?
4 Can a single insult to hepatocytes result in elevated liver enzymes for a period of 6 weeks?
5 Which non-invasive diagnostic tests should be performed to assess the significance of a chronic increase in liver enzyme activities?

CASE 152 Case 152 is the same dog as case 151. An abdominal ultrasound examination was performed. The liver was moderately enlarged and only small parts of the liver showed a normal architecture. Much of the liver parenchyma appeared heterogeneous with increased echogenicity (**152**). The remainder of the liver had a normal appearance.

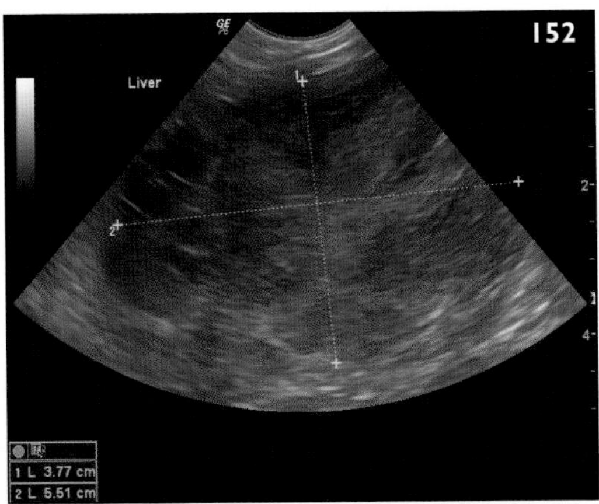

1 What is the most likely differential diagnosis based on the ultrasound examination findings?
2 What would be your next diagnostic step?

CASE 153 Case 153 is the same dog as cases 151 and 152. Several abnormal structures were identified on cytologic examination of fine needle aspirates of the liver (**153**).

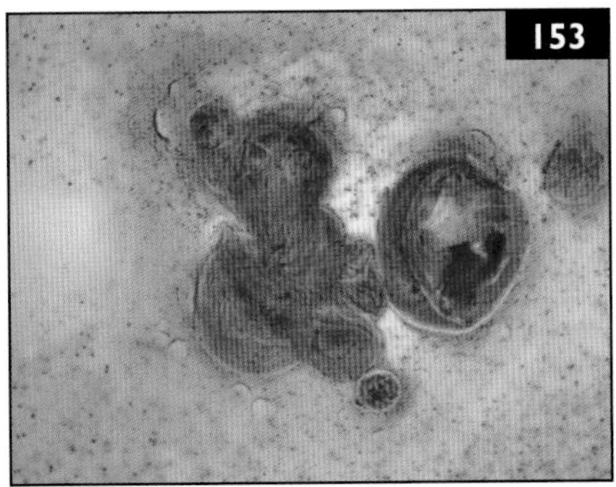

1 What is the diagnosis in this dog, and what forms of this disease are known?
2 Is cytologic identification sufficient to define the species involved, and what tests would be superior?
3 What is the life cycle of this agent and the required hosts?
4 How did the dog in this case fit into the life cycle?
5 What treatment is indicated?

CASE 154 A 1-year-old intact female Poodle living close to Pelotas, Brazil, was evaluated for lethargy, inappetence, and weight loss for several weeks. No vomiting or diarrhea was noted, but the owner reported dark feces and "skin rashes" (**154a, 154b**), which had been observed over the last 3 days. The owner also reported frequent tick infestations, which were treated with amitraz. The dog was up to date on core vaccines and was regularly treated for endoparasites. No access to toxins or plants and no history of trauma, medications, or travel was reported.

Physical examination revealed lethargy, a rectal temperature of 39.5°C [103.1°F], pale mucous membranes, moderately enlarged peripheral lymph nodes, splenomegaly, mucosal petechiation, and skin ecchymoses.

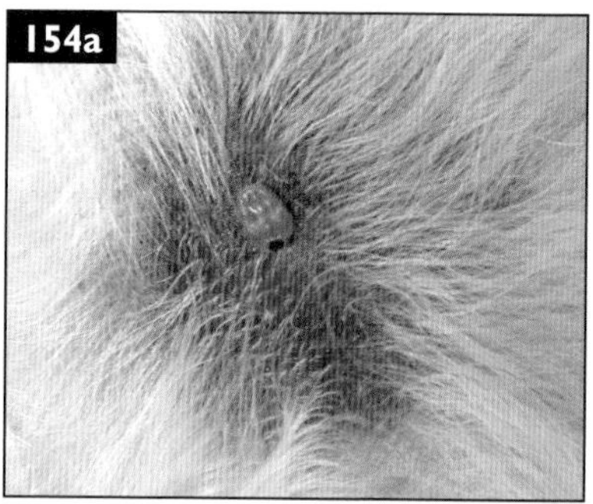
154a

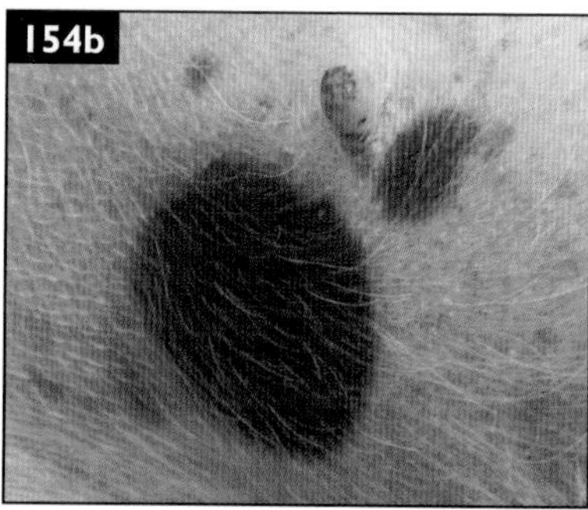
154b

1 What are the differential diagnoses for the petechiation and ecchymoses?
2 What diagnotic tests should be recommended?

CASE 155 Case 155 is the same dog as case 154. A CBC and serum biochemistry panel were performed (for significant results see the boxes). A blood smear was also evaluated (**155a, 155b**). Collection of a free catch urine sample was not possible and cystocentesis was not performed because of the bleeding disorder.

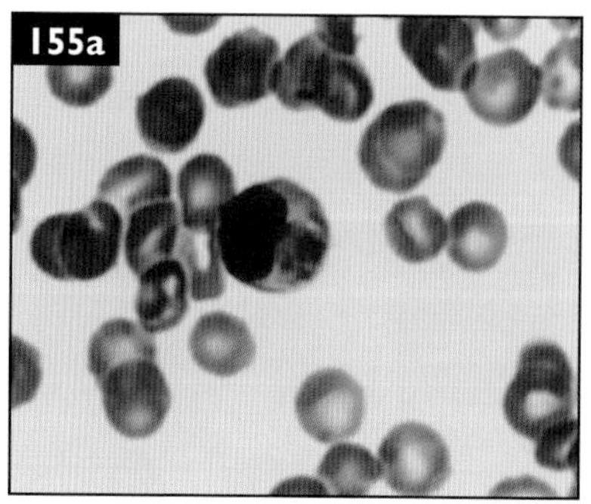
155a

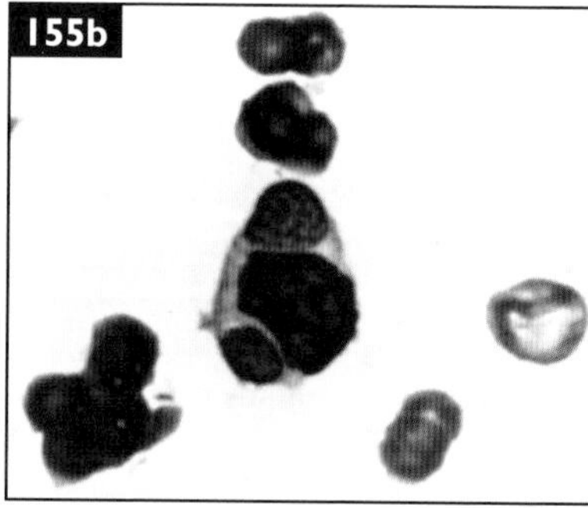
155b

Complete blood count	Results	Reference interval
Hematocrit	0.15 l/l	0.35–0.58
Reticulocytes	0 × 10^9/l	0–60
Neutrophil count	0.8 × 10^9/l	3–9
Monocyte count	0.01 × 10^9/l	0.04–0.5
Platelets	8 × 10^9/l	150–500

Biochemistry panel	Results	Reference interval
ALT	145 U/l	18–110
ALP	180 U/l	13–152
Total protein	94 g/l	56–78
Albumin	25 g/l	31–43
Globulins	69 g/l	24–35

1 What conclusions can you make based on the laboratory test results?
2 What initial treatment is required in this case?

CASE 156 Case 156 is the same dog as cases 154 and 155. During physical examination on the second day of hospitalization, an irregular cardiac rhythm was auscultated, with asynchronous femoral pulses. An ECG was performed (**156**). In addition, blood pressure measurement was performed. The blood pressure was 140 mmHg (systolic). Also, free catch urine could now be obtained and submitted for analysis.

Urinalysis	Results
Specific gravity	1.020
pH	7.2
Protein	3+
Glucose	Negative
Bilirubin	Negative

The urine sediment was benign and the UPCR was 10.2 (RI <0.5).

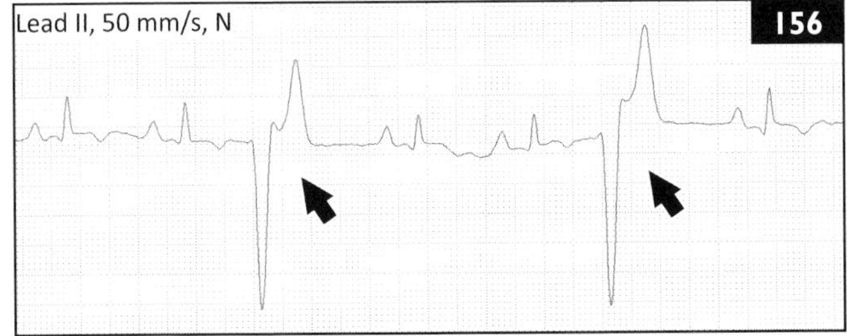

1 What are the important findings from the ECG and urinalysis?
2 Is specific therapy required for these findings?
3 What is the prognosis in this dog?

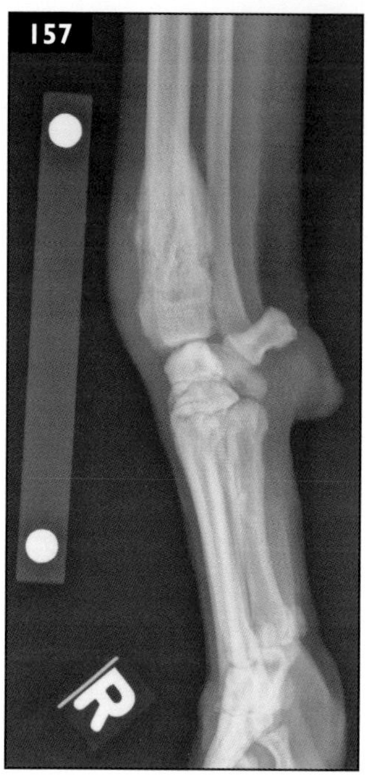

CASE 157 A 1.5-year-old neutered female Boxer dog was evaluated for right thoracic limb lameness and swelling of the carpus of 3 weeks' duration. There had been no response to non-steroidal anti-inflammatory drugs (deracoxib 1.5 mg/kg PO q12h) prescribed by her veterinarian when the lameness first began. The owner also reported that, over the last month, the dog had four episodes of inappetence that resolved within 24 hours. She was currently eating well. There had been no cough, sneezing, vomiting or diarrhea, or increased thirst and urination. There was no history of exposure to trauma. The dog lived in Sacramento, California, USA. Travel history consisted of several visits to Arizona over the last year, with the last visit being 3 months previously. She was up to date on routine vaccinations and was the only pet in the household.

Physical examination was normal apart from moderate weight-bearing lameness of the right thoracic limb and a firm swelling over the right carpus and distal antebrachium that was painful on palpation. Funduscopic examination was normal. Radiographs of the right carpus revealed moth-eaten osteolysis throughout the distal radius, with cortical bone destruction along the cranial aspect of the distal radial diaphysis. There was solid periosteal new bone circumferentially surrounding the distal radius, which was most pronounced along the caudomedial cortices. There was also moderate soft tissue swelling surrounding the distal right antebrachium (**157**).

1 What are the main differential diagnoses, including specific infectious agents that might be involved?
2 What other diagnostic tests should be recommended for this dog?

CASE 158 Case 158 is the same dog as case 157 (**158**). Further diagnostic work-up was performed. The CBC and urinalysis were normal and a biochemistry panel revealed moderate hyperglobulinemia (43 g/l, RI 17–31 g/l) and mild hypoalbuminemia (32 g/l, RI 34–43 g/l). Thoracic radiographs were unremarkable. Fine needle aspirates of the lesion showed moderate mixed inflammation that was characterized by a mixture of non-degenerate neutrophils, histiocytes, reactive lymphocytes, and occasional multinucleated osteoclasts. A *Coccidioides* spp. antibody titer was positive at 1:64.

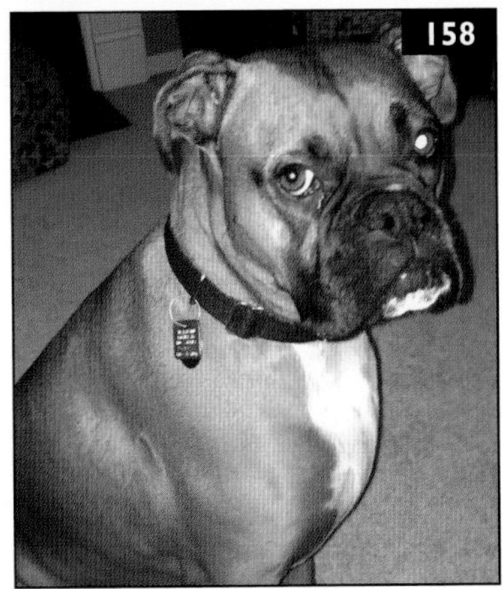
158

1 What is the significance of the positive *Coccidioides* spp. antibody test?
2 Are any additional diagnostic tests indicated?
3 What is the recommended treatment for this patient, and what are the possible adverse effects of therapy?

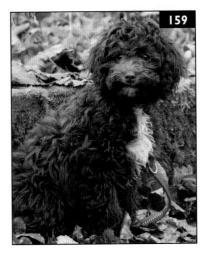
159

CASE 159 A 5-month-old intact female Australian Labradoodle (**159**) was evaluated for several episodes of soft feces within the last 3 months. The dog belonged to a veterinarian who had performed centrifugal zinc sulfate flotation and the test was positive. The dog had been treated several times with fenbendazole and metronidazole, but the *Giardia* spp. test remained positive at three consecutive testings, and the fecal consistency did not improve. Tests for other endoparasites had been negative. The dog was on a commercial puppy diet, was eating well, and had no vomiting. The dog had been born in Australia and was imported into Germany at the age of 10 weeks. Since then, the dog had lived in Munich and had not traveled outside Germany. She had contact with many dogs, because she was attending puppy school and was allowed to run free in parks and around the veterinary hospital. She had received a complete basic vaccination series and was on monthly endo- and ectoparasite treatment.

Physical examination was unremarkable, and the dog was alert and responsive. The BCS was 4/9.

1 What are likely reasons that the *Giardia* spp. test remained positive?
2 How should the dog be treated?

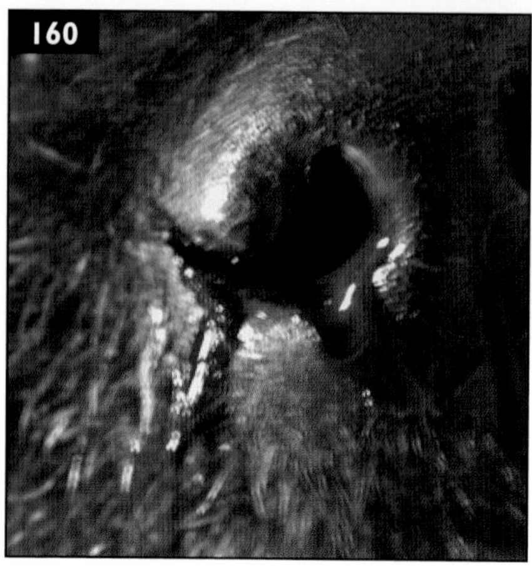

CASE 160 An 8-year-old neutered female German Shepherd Dog mix was referred for evaluation of reverse sneezing followed by epistaxis from the right nostril (**160**). Signs were first noted 3 months ago and had become progressively worse. The referring veterinarian had used an otoscope to search for a foreign body but none was found. A dental procedure was performed under anesthesia to investigate tooth root disease as a cause of the epistaxis but signs continued. The dog lived in a rural area close to Davis, California, USA, had no travel history, and was regularly vaccinated and on heartworm prophylaxis.

On presentation, the dog was mildly obtunded with a rectal temperature of 38.4°C (101.1°F), pulse of 100 bpm, and respiratory rate of 32 breaths/min. Mild intermittent blepharospasm was noted bilaterally, along with a brown serous to crusted ocular discharge. Nasal airflow was present bilaterally; however, the dog resisted full examination of the head and oral cavity. The right mandibular lymph node was enlarged (2 cm).

1 What are the most likely differential diagnoses for the problems of unilateral epistaxis and ipsilateral lymphadenopathy?
2 If only one diagnostic test was allowed in this patient, what would you perform?
3 If the owner agreed to a full work-up, what would you recommend?

CASE 161 Case 161 is the same dog as case 160. A test for *Aspergillus* spp. antibodies was negative. Cytologic examination of a lymph node aspirate (**161a**) and CT of the nasal cavity (**161b, c**) were performed.

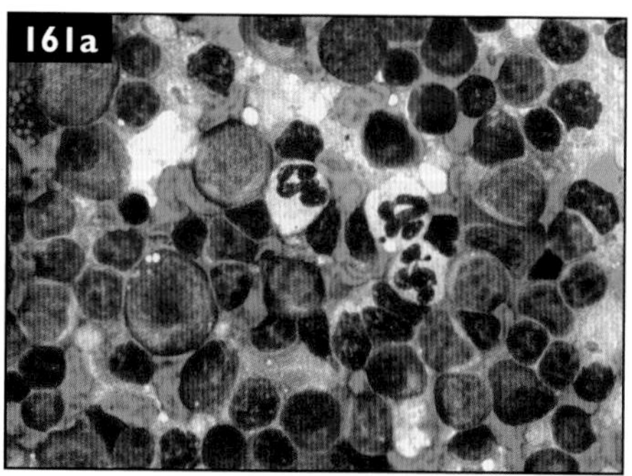

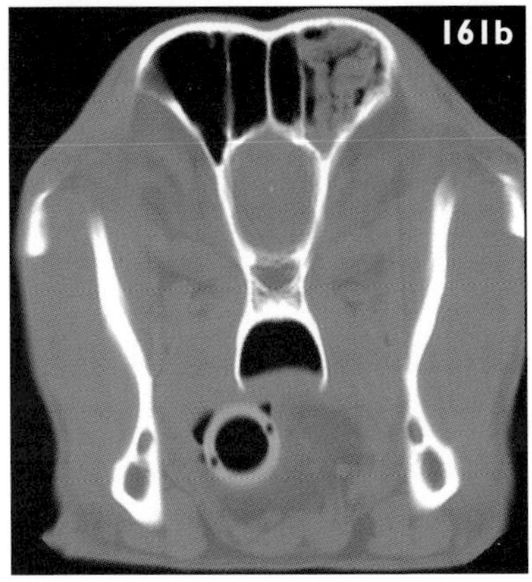

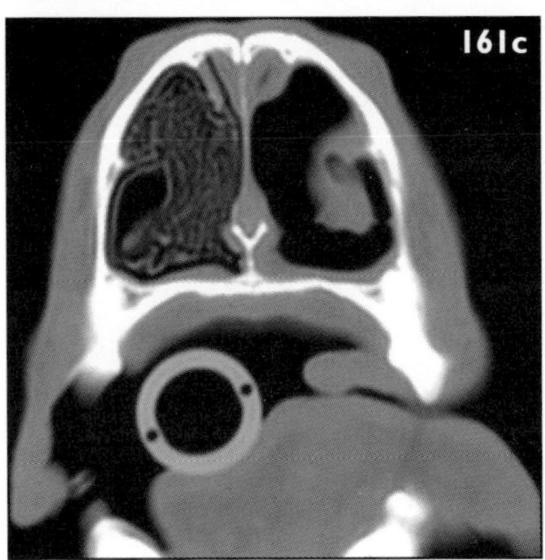

1 What is your interpretation of the lymph node cytology?
2 What is your interpretation of the CT images?

CASE 162 A 7-year-old intact male Jack Russell Terrier was evaluated for a single skin lesion on the lateral thorax that the owner had discovered 3 days ago (**162**). The dog was a bright and alert hunting dog and had no other known illnesses besides the skin lesion. The lesion was moderately pruritic. The dog lived in Regensburg, Germany, and had never been outside the country. He received regular core vaccinations and preventive treatment for endoparasites and ectoparasites.

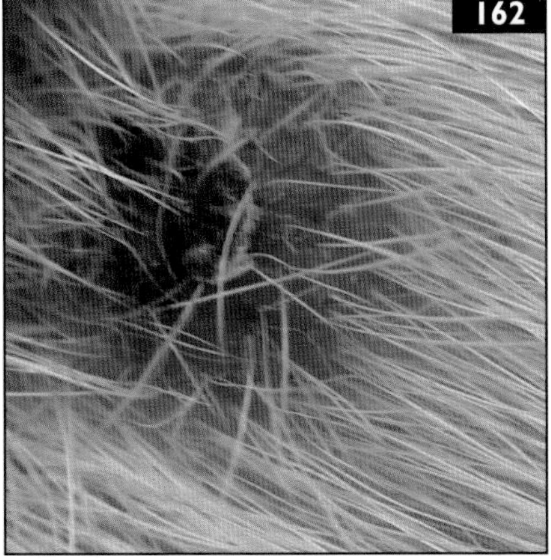

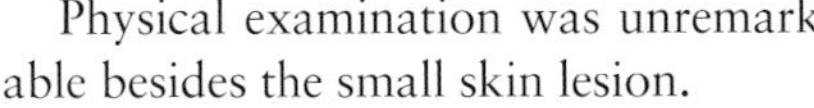

Physical examination was unremarkable besides the small skin lesion.

1 What are the main differential diagnoses?
2 What would you recommend as the minimal diagnostic approach for this case?
3 What is the most complete diagnostic approach to this case?

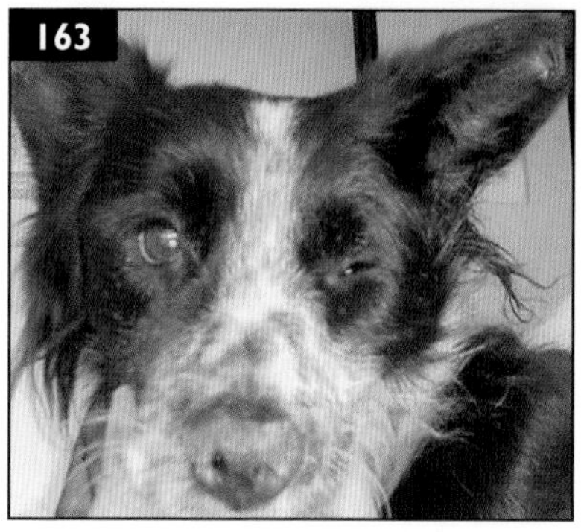

CASE 163 A 4-year-old intact male mixed-breed dog was evaluated because of a 4-day history of left-sided head tilt and uncoordinated gait that had become progressively worse over that time. The dog lived in Messina, Italy. He was regularly vaccinated with core vaccines and received prophylaxis for endoparasites and ectoparasites.

On physical examination, abnormal findings included a left-sided head tilt, circling and falling, Horner's syndrome, facial nerve paralysis (**163**), and positional strabismus on the left side. Neurologic examination revealed no abnormalities in mentation, placing reaction abnormalities, limb paresis/paralysis, or involvement of other cranial nerves.

1 What differential diagnoses should be considered?
2 What is your initial diagnostic plan?

CASE 164 Case 164 is the same dog as case 163. Otoscopic evaluation was performed under sedation and revealed exudate in the left horizontal ear canal (**164**). The tympanic membranes could not be examined because of severe ear canal stenosis. Open-mouth anterior–posterior radiographs of the skull revealed a bilateral thickening of the bullae that was more severe on the left side.

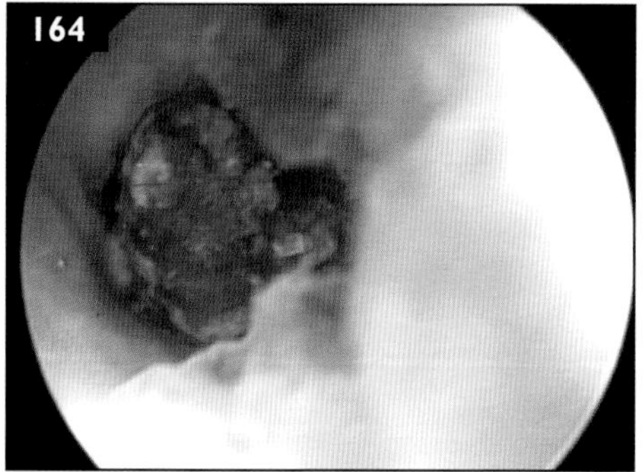

1 What is your diagnosis?
2 What additional diagnostic tests might be useful to better understand the condition?
3 What treatment is indicated?

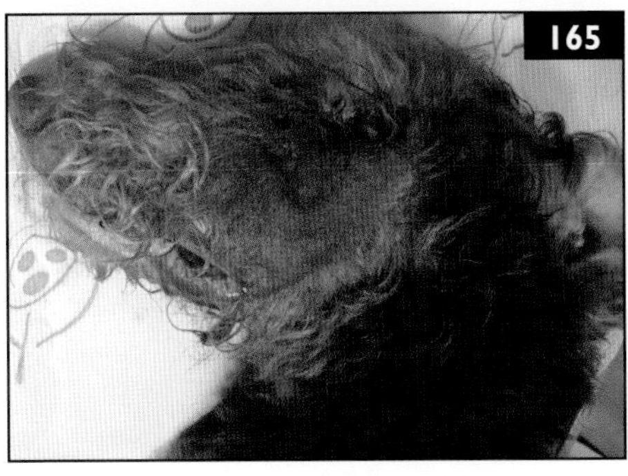

CASE 165 A 2-year-old intact male Wirehair mix dog was evaluated by an emergency clinic for a 2-day history of anorexia, vomiting, and agitation. Over the last day, the owner noted that the dog had developed severe pruritis, especially involving the head. The dog lived in a village about 30 km from Krakow, Poland, and was used as a hunting dog. Four days before the onset of clinical signs, the dog had been in contact with, and possibly consumed, a wild boar carcass. The dog was vaccinated against rabies, but not against any other infectious diseases and had not been treated with any antiparasitic drugs.

On physical examination, the dog was obtunded, vocalizing, and in lateral recumbency. Tachycardia, tachypnea, fever (40.6°C [105.1°F]), and hypersalivation were noted. In addition, tremor, strabismus, and anisocoria were identified. Around the mouth, on the lips, and in the temporal area, asymmetric excoriations due to self-mutilation were apparent (**165**).

1 What is the most likely diagnosis?
2 What other differential diagnoses are there for the neurologic signs combined with fever?
3 What is the prognosis?

CASE 166 Case 166 is the same dog as case 165. The dog died within a few hours. Lesions noted at necropsy, due to self-mutilation, were also found on the gingiva, tongue, and buccal mucosa (**166**).

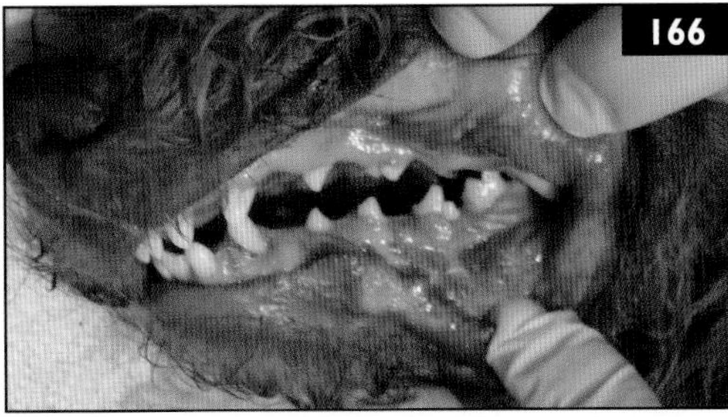

1 How is a diagnosis of Aujeszky's disease confirmed?
2 What was the likely source of this infection in this case?
3 Can a dog with Aujeszky's disease infect other animals?
4 Is Aujeszky's disease a zoonosis?

CASE 167 A 2-year-old neutered female Labrador Retriever was referred for cutaneous lesions that had been present for 10 days. The dog had been treated with oral marbofloxacin for the past week. The dog had lived in the countryside close to Athens, Georgia, USA, for her entire life. The owners had a lakefront property, and the dog spent up to 2 hours per day in the lake. The dog had been regularly vaccinated and received regular prophylactic treatment for ecto- and endoparasites.

On physical examination, non-pruritic ulcerative nodular cutaneous lesions on the right carpus and left tarsus were seen (**167**). The masses were 4–6 cm long and 2 cm wide, with overlying erythematous, alopecic, and ulcerated skin. Popliteal and prescapular lymph nodes of the respective limbs were enlarged and firm. The remainder of the physical examination was unremarkable.

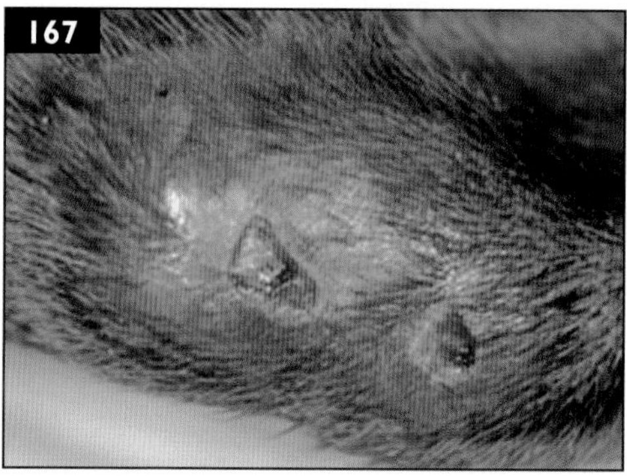

1 What are the differential diagnoses for nodular ulcerative skin lesions?
2 What would be the diagnostic plan to evaluate the skin lesions?

CASE 168 Case 168 is the same dog as case 167. Fine needle aspirate cytology, examined with a modified Wright's stain, showed granulomatous and eosinophilic inflammation; however, organisms were not observed. Radiographic findings revealed only mild periosteal proliferation on bones of the affected carpal joint.

Histopathology of a biopsy sample showed severe, multifocal, eosinophilic to pyogranulomatous deep dermatitis with fibroplasia and neovascularization. Intralesional filamentous structures were observed. They did not stain with periodic acid–Schiff stain. With Gomori's methenamine silver stain, wide (5–10 μm) bulbous, irregularly septate branching hyphae were observed (**168**). Aseptically obtained skin biopsy specimens were cultured on blood agar, MacConkey agar, Sabouraud dextrose agar, and Mycosel agar plates. All cultures were negative. However, tests for anti-*Pythium insidiosum* antibodies were positive. PCR was performed on tissue specimens taken from the biopsy and confirmed the presence of *Pythium* spp. in the lesions.

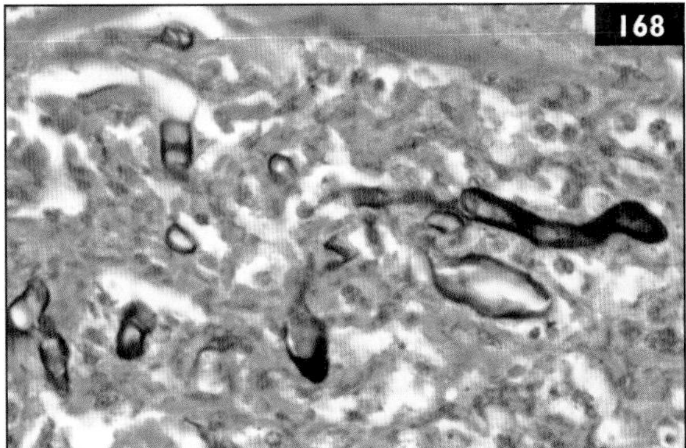

1 What are the treatment options for *Pythium insidiosum* infection?
2 What other genera of bacteria or fungi can cause ulcerated (with or without drainage) nodular granulomatous or pyogranulomatous skin lesions in dogs?

CASE 169 A 6-month-old female Dachshund (**169**) was presented for a consultation. The dog had lived together with one of her male siblings at the owner's house for the last 3 months. The male sibling had mild diarrhea since he was introduced into the household, but the female puppy had normal feces. A fecal PCR panel for infectious agents was performed on the feces of both dogs and was unremarkable in the diarrheic male dog, but coronavirus RNA was detected in the feces of the the female dog. The owner was seeking advice concerning coronavirus infection. The dog lived in Munich, Germany, and had no travel history. The dog had received a full basic vaccination series and been treated for endoparasites five times within the last 3 months. She had also received ectoparasite treatment once a month. Physical examination was unremarkable.

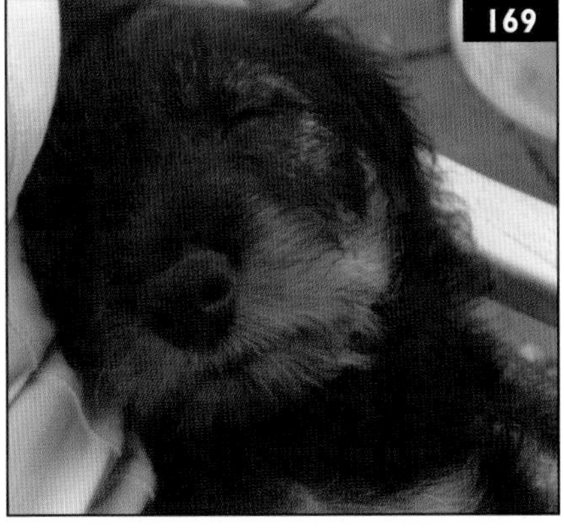

1 What coronaviruses are known to infect dogs, and what is their role as pathogenic agents?
2 Is it necessary to treat this dog for coronavirus infection?

CASE 170 A 5-year-old intact male German Shepherd Dog was evaluated because of "red eyes" and sudden loss of vision. The dog was kept entirely outdoors in Bari, Italy. He was only vaccinated against rabies and had not been regularly treated for endoparasites or ectoparasites.

Physical examination revealed pale mucous membranes and enlargement of peripheral lymph nodes and the spleen. On ophthalmic examination, severe bilateral hyphema (**170a**) was identified. A CBC, biochemistry panel, coagulation tests, and urinalysis, as well as cytology of a fine needle aspirate of the enlarged lymph nodes, were performed. The relevant abnormalities were moderate non-regenerative anemia (0.21 l/l, RI 0.37–0.55 l/l), moderate neutropenia (1.2×10^9 cells/l, RI 3–115 $\times 10^9$/l), severe thrombocytopenia (5×10^9 platelets/l, RI 150–400 $\times 10^9$/l), hyperglobulinemia (70 g/l, RI 24–35 g/l), hypoalbuminemia (21 g/l, RI 29–37 g/l), proteinuria with a UPCR of 2.5, slightly prolonged PT and aPTT, as well as severely prolonged buccal mucosal bleeding time. Plasmacytosis was identified in the lymph node cytology (**170b**).

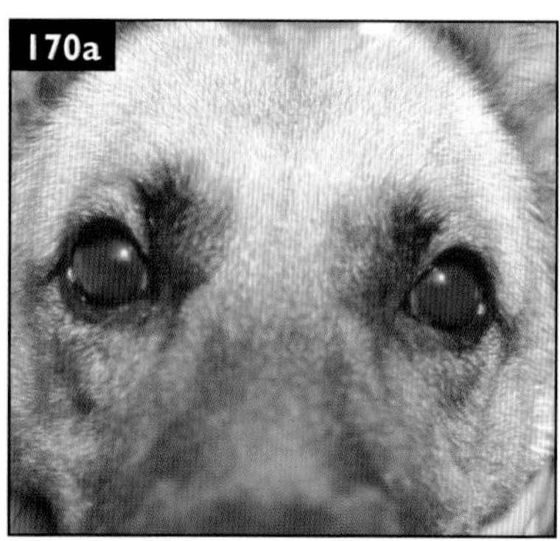
170a

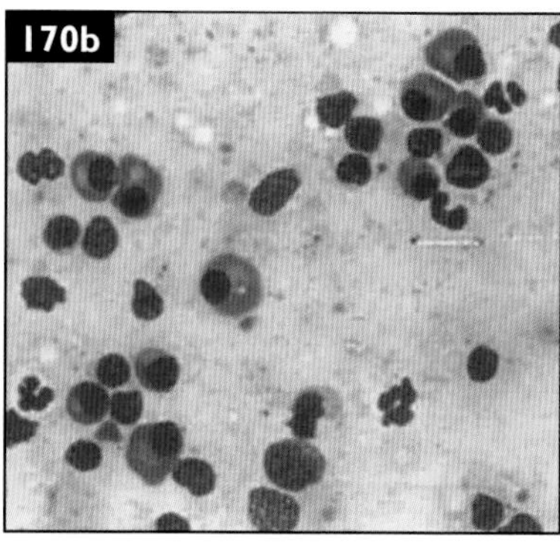
170b

1 What are the main problems in this dog, and what are the most important differential diagnoses?
2 What diagnostic procedures should be performed next?

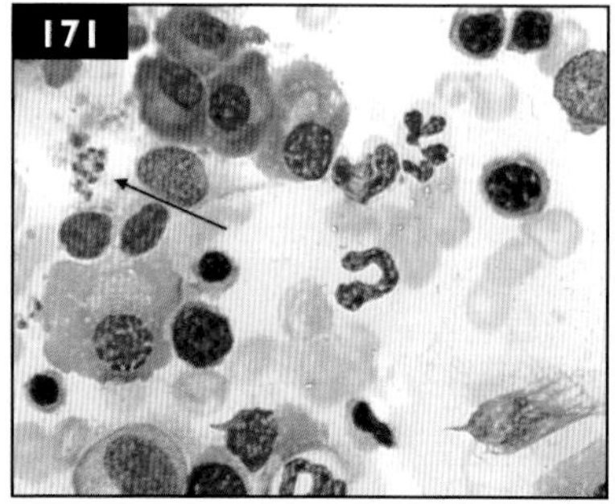
171

CASE 171 Case 171 is the same dog as case 170. High antibody titers were present for both *Ehrlichia canis* (1:12,800) and *Leishmania infantum* (1:128). Bone marrow cytology confirmed severe plasmacytosis and hypoplasia of all other cell lineages. In addition, *L. infantum* amastigotes were found in the bone marrow (**171**, arrow). PCR of a lymph node aspirate was positive for *E. canis*. Therefore, both infectious diseases, ehrlichiosis and leishmaniosis, associated with bone marrow suppression and possible glomerulonephritis were diagnosed.

1 What are possible complications in this dog secondary to the abnormalities identified?
2 What treatment should be given and what is the prognosis?

CASE 172 An 8-year-old neutered male Chihuahua was evaluated for a 2-day history of anorexia and lethargy. The dog had shifting-leg lameness and was reluctant to walk (**172**). The dog lived in a rural area close to Bemidji, Minnesota, USA, mostly indoors but with supervised access to the woods. Ticks had been found on the dog at least twice in the previous 6 months, despite regular treatment with fipronil. The dog had received regular core vaccinations, but had not been treated for endoparasites for the last 5 years.

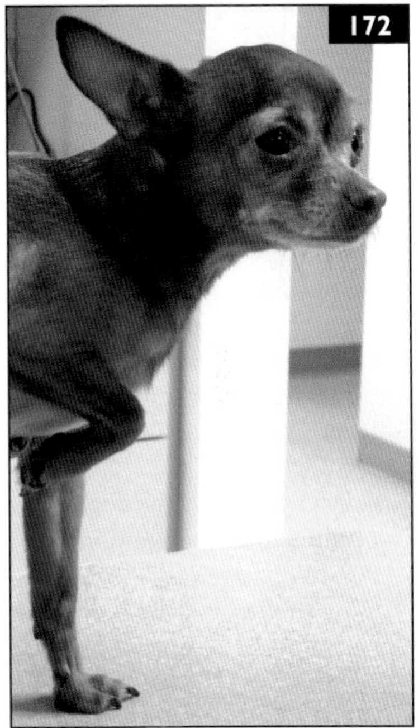

Physical examination revealed a temperature of 39.9°C (103.8°F), stiffness, and joint pain, which was most evident in the carpal joints. A CBC revealed mild thrombocytopenia (125×10^9 platelets/l, RI $150–400 \times 10^9$/l). The biochemistry panel was within normal limits, but urinalysis revealed 1+ proteinuria with a specific gravity of 1.045 and a benign sediment. Synovial fluid analysis showed 15,872 WBC/μl (normal <3,000 cells/μl), with 90% non-degenerate neutrophils (normal <5%), 35 g/l protein (normal <25 g/l), and absence of bacteria. An in-house ELISA (SNAP 4Dx Plus, IDEXX Laboratories) was positive for antibodies to the C6 peptide of *Borrelia burgdorferi*.

1 How should the ELISA result be interpreted in this case?
2 What other diagnostic tests should be considered?
3 What treatment should be recommended?
4 What is the prognosis?

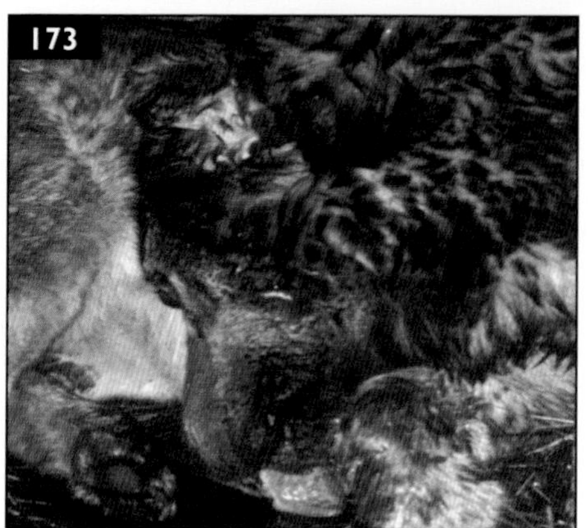

CASE 173 A 7-year-old intact female Caucasian Shepherd Dog, used as a watchdog on a sheep farm in Przemysl, Poland (close to the Ukrainian border), was evaluated for sudden onset of lameness, inappetence, and lethargy. The owner had not noticed any trauma recently. The vaccination and antiparasitic treatment history was unclear, because the dog was brought to the veterinarian by the owner's son, who had little knowledge about the dog's history.

On physical examination, the dog appeared disorientated and had ataxia due to pelvic limb paresis. Pyrexia was present (39.9°C [103.8°F]). The dog had anisocoria, reduced pupillary light responses, and an inability to swallow water (which ran back out of the dog's mouth). A CBC revealed neutrophilia and mild lymphopenia. Additional diagnostics were declined by the owners. Treatment with IV fluid therapy and antimicrobial drugs was initiated.

On day 2 of hospitalization, the dog showed generalized incoordination, seizures, and hypersalivation due to a "dropped jaw". This progressed to torticollis, coma, and death on the same day (**173**). At that time the owner recalled that the dog had been in a fight with a fox about 2 months previously, in a region where rabies was endemic in red foxes. The dog had never received any vaccination against rabies.

1 Considering that the dog did not show aggression, could this still be rabies?
2 Could detection of antibodies have been helpful to confirm or rule out rabies in this dog?
3 How should dogs be protected from rabies?

CASE 174 A 1-year-old intact male mixed-breed dog was evaluated for a 4-day history of lethargy, inappetence, reluctance to move, vomiting, and diarrhea, which had recently progressed to hematochezia. The dog lived in a suburban area near Krakow, Poland, and was frequently walked in the forest on a leash. The dog had never been vaccinated or treated for parasites.

Physical examination revealed fever (40.0°C [104.0°F]), tachypnea, tachycardia, mild dehydration, tonsillar enlargement, and pharyngeal hyperemia. An in-house test for fecal canine parvovirus antigen was negative (**174**). The dog was started on intravenous fluid therapy and amoxicillin–clavulanic acid. There was no clinical improvement over the following 24 hours and the dog's rectal temperature remained at 40.1°C. During physical examination on day 2 of hospitalization, cranial abdominal pain was noted. A CBC revealed neutrophilia, thrombocytopenia, hyperbilirubinemia, hypoalbuminemia, and severely increased activities of serum ALT and ALP.

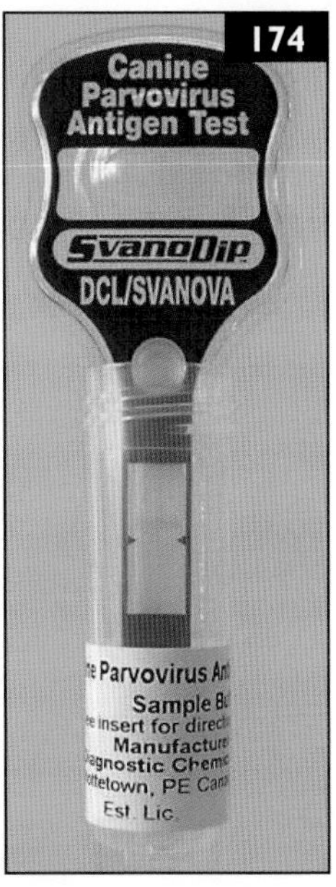

1 What are the main differential diagnoses for the vomiting and diarrhea before the laboratory results are available?
2 What are the main differential diagnoses after the laboratory results become available?
3 What other diagnostic tests should be performed?

CASE 175 Case 175 is the same dog as 174. Abdominal ultrasound showed that the liver was diffusely hyperechoic and enlarged with rounded lobar edges. Changes consistent with gallbladder edema were visible. Mesenteric lymph nodes were enlarged and a small amount of free peritoneal fluid was noted. The dog's blood tested positive by PCR for canine adenovirus 1 (CAV-1).

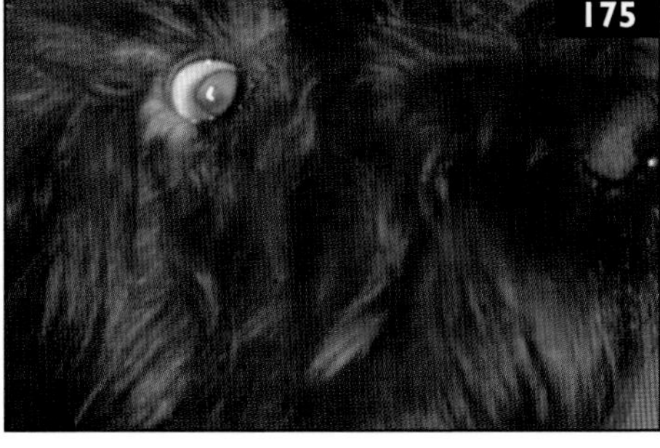

The dog improved gradually with supportive treatment, and within a few days started to eat again. During this convalescent phase (about 10 days after onset of the disease), the owner noted opacity of the right cornea (**175**). The other eye was unaffected and the dog was clinically otherwise apparently healthy.

1 What is the pathogenesis of the ocular changes?
2 What is the prognosis for this dog?
3 How should the ocular disease be treated?
4 What could have been the source of CAV-1 infection in this dog?

CASE 176 A 1-year-old neutered female Poodle was evaluated for a 6-month history of intermittent cough and gagging episodes that did not coincide with eating, drinking, or exercise. These episodes persisted for weeks at a time and were sometimes accompanied by lethargy and inappetence. The dog lived in Sacramento, California, USA, had received her basic vaccination series, and was on heartworm prophylaxis; she had been neutered at around 6 months of age. A local veterinarian had examined the dog and a lateral thoracic radiograph had been obtained (**176**). The dog had been treated with one course of 7 days of amoxicillin–clavulanic acid but the cough had not improved.

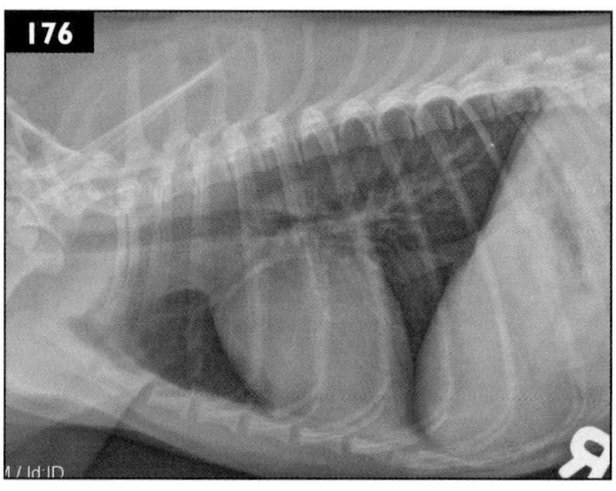

On physical examination, the temperature was 39.1°C (102.4°F), pulse 124 bpm, respiratory rate 32 breaths/min, and spontaneous coughing occurred throughout the examination. Normal bronchovesicular lung sounds were present in all lung fields and a cough was easily elicited on tracheal palpation. The remainder of the physical examination was normal.

1 What is your interpretation of the radiograph?
2 What differential diagnoses should you consider?
3 What additional diagnostic tests should be performed?

CASE 177 Case 177 is the same dog as case 176. The owners elected to have bronchoscopy performed (**177a**). Based on the bronchoscopic findings, bronchoscopic-guided brush biopsies and cytology of impression smears of the brushings were performed (**177b**).

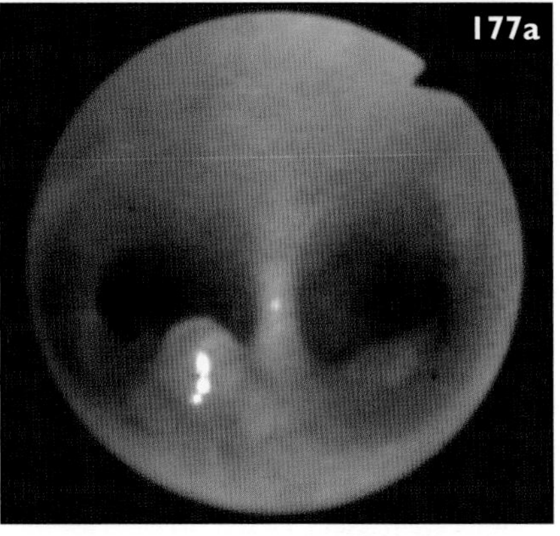

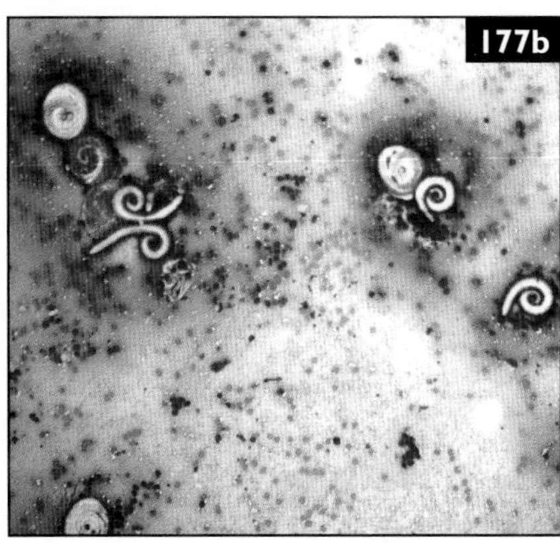

1 With what disease process are the bronchoscopic image and the histopathology most consistent?
2 Is there an additional diagnostic test that could have provided the diagnosis prior to bronchoscopy?

CASE 178 A 6-month-old intact female Wire-haired Dachshund (**178**) was evaluated at a wellness visit that included advice regarding a planned trip to Italy. The owner reported that the dog was apparently healthy and eating well. However, the owner's husband currently had influenza and the dog used to sleep in their bed. The owner was worried that the dog could contract influenza from her husband and wanted to know whether the husband should sleep in a separate room.

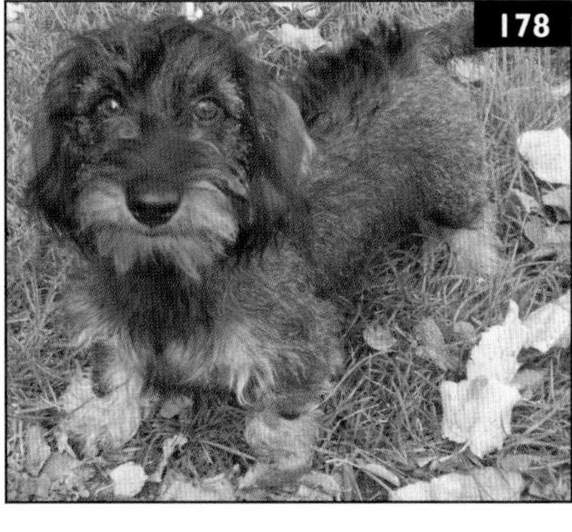

The dog lived in Munich, Germany, and had never been outside the country. The dog had received a basic vaccination series at 8 weeks, 12 weeks, and 16 weeks of age, and was treated for endoparasites and ectoparasites regularly. Physical examination was unremarkable.

1 What influenza viruses can infect dogs?
2 Are dogs with influenza virus infection a zoonotic risk?
3 What is the risk of the husband transmitting infection to the dog?

CASE 179 A 3-year-old neutered male Chow/Golden Retriever mix was evaluated for a 3-month history of progressive large bowel diarrhea with hematochezia. There had been no improvement with metronidazole, a combination of amoxicillin–clavulanic acid and enrofloxacin, or a low fat diet. One month after the signs began, the dog was treated with prednisone (0.5 mg/kg PO q12h) with initial improvement, but when the dose was tapered 1 week later, the diarrhea recurred and did not resolve when the dose was increased again. Over the last month, the frequency of diarrhea with hematochezia had increased to eight times/day. Vomiting began a week before presentation and was occurring every other day, containing bile or food. The dog was eating a normal amount of food, but was slower to eat than normal. The dog had been rescued 2 years previously and had an unknown travel history before that time. He now lived in Sacramento, California, USA. Since then, travel had been limited to the San Francisco Bay area. The dog was up to date on routine vaccinations (distemper, adenovirus, parvovirus, rabies) and was on regular ecto- and endoparasite control.

Physical examination revealed a bright, alert, and well-hydrated dog with normal vital signs and a BCS of 3/9. The only abnormal finding was pain on rectal examination, and soft to liquid brown diarrhea on the glove, with frank blood. A CBC was unremarkable apart from thrombocytopenia (72 × 10^9 platelets/l, RI 150–400 × 10^9 l/l). A biochemistry panel showed hyperglobulinemia (42 g/l, RI 17–31 g/l) and mild hypoalbuminemia (28 g/l, RI 34–43 g/l). Urinalysis was unremarkable. A centrifugal zinc sulfate fecal flotation was negative. Abdominal ultrasound showed an enlarged and hyperechoic liver. The spleen was mildly enlarged and had a diffuse hypoechoic mottling. The mesenteric, colic, and sublumbar lymph nodes were mildly enlarged and hypoechoic. There was multifocal bowel wall thickening with associated loss of wall layering within the duodenum, jejunum, ileum, and colon. Cytologic examination of a fine needle aspirate of one of the abdominal lymph nodes revealed intracellular yeast organisms consistent with *Histoplasma capsulatum* (**179**).

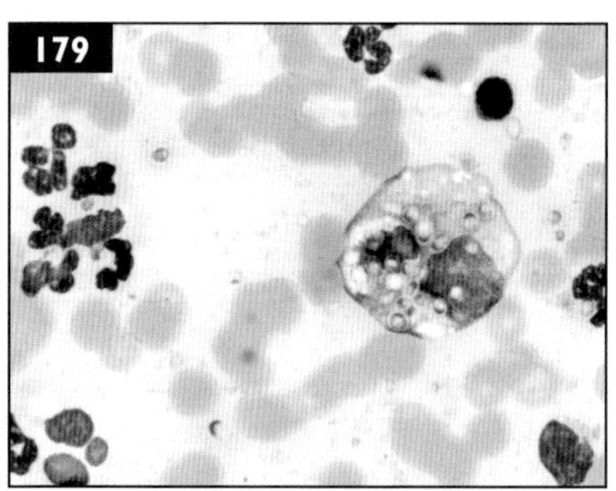

1 What other differential diagnoses should have been considered in this dog before the results of cytology were available?
2 What is the normal geographic distribution of *Histoplasma capsulatum*?
3 What are the anatomic sites of predilection of *Histoplasma capsulatum* in dogs?
4 How could the success of antifungal drug therapy be monitored in this dog?

CASE 180 A 2-year-old recently neutered female Sighthound was evaluated for a several-month history of lethargy and difficulty walking up stairs. The dog had been adopted by the owners 1 year ago from an animal shelter in Romania and now lived in Munich, Germany. Since that time, the dog had not travelled outside of Germany. She had received a vaccination series at the time of adoption and received tick and flea preventives regularly.

General physical examination revealed an elevated rectal body temperature (39.2°C [102.6°F]), but was otherwise unremarkable. Neurologic examination showed kyphosis, low carriage of the neck, and pelvic limb proprioceptive deficits. The dog exhibited pain when the neck was manipulated and pain was also evident on palpation of multiple regions of the lumbar and thoracic vertebrae.

Radiographs of the cervical and thoracolumbar spine were obtained (**180a, 180b**).

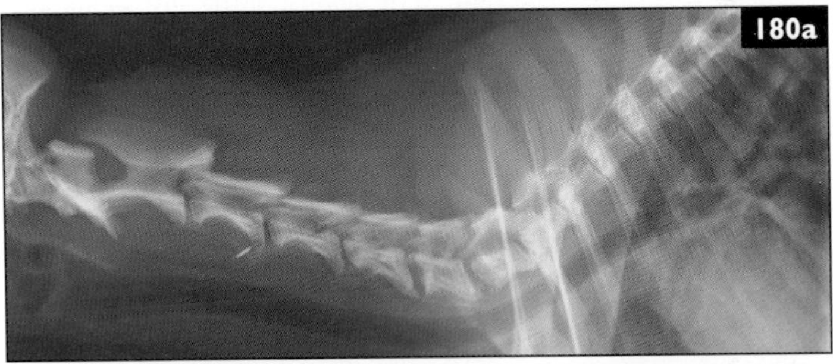
180a

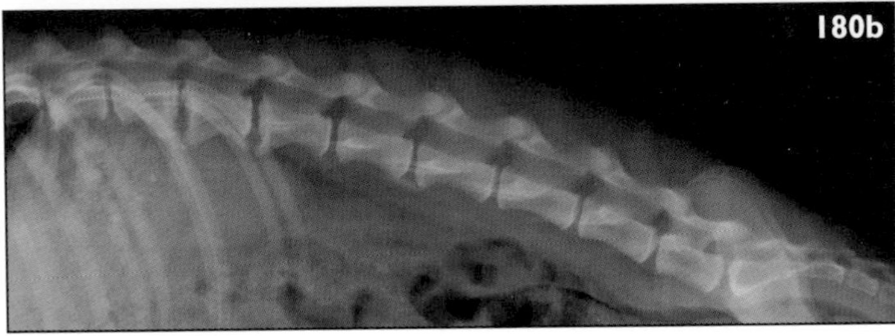
180b

1 What are the main differential diagnoses for this dog's neurologic abnormalities based on the physical and neurologic examination findings?
2 How would you interpret the radiographs?
3 What are the next diagnostic steps?
4 What treatment would you recommend?

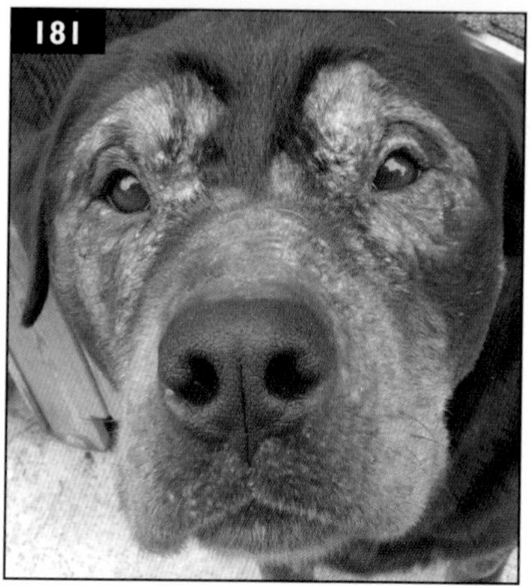

CASE 181 A 4-year-old intact male Rottweiler was evaluated because of multifocal alopecia and mild pruritus. The dog had been treated with an immunosuppressive dose of prednisone and azathioprine for the last 6 months because of severe inflammatory bowel disease. The skin problems had begun about 3 weeks previously on the dog's face and were progressively worsening. The dog lived in a rural area near Taormina, Italy. He had been vaccinated against rabies but not against other infections and the last time a parasiticide was administered was about 2 years previously.

Physical examination revealed a multifocal alopecic dermatitis with well-defined margins, scaling, and some crusting (**181**). Otherwise the physical examination was unremarkable.

1 What are the main differential diagnoses for the skin changes in this dog?
2 What diagnostic tests should be performed?

CASE 182 Case 182 is the same dog as case 181. Deep skin scrapings were negative and a few extracellular cocci were found in impression cytology of the crusts. *Leishmania* spp. antibody testing was negative. A Wood's lamp evaluation and trichogram were also negative. Dermatophytes grew on Sabouraud agar, and the geophilic fungus *Microsporum gypseum* was identified (**182a, 182b**).

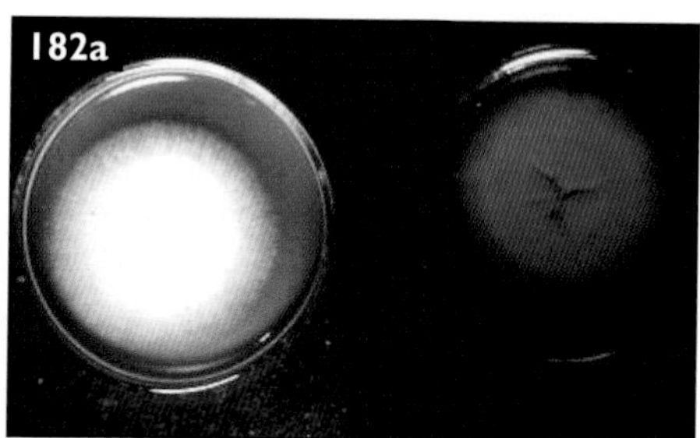

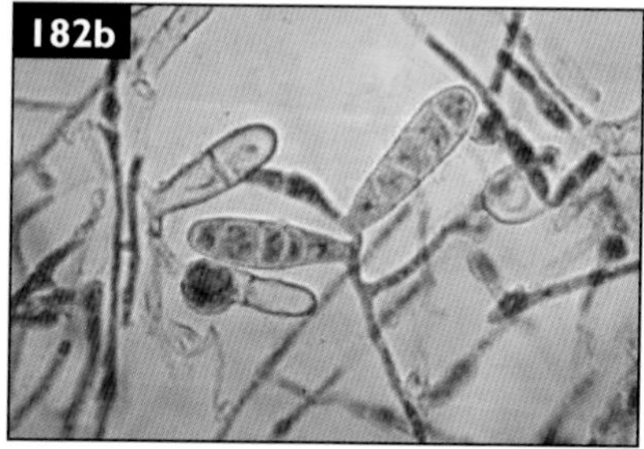

1 What are the therapeutic options?
2 What should be done to reduce contamination of the environment?

CASE 183 A 5-year-old intact male Belgian Shepherd from San Diego, California, USA, was evaluated for progressive lethargy, inappetence, vomiting, and diarrhea for 5 days. The owner reported two generalized seizures on the day of the presentation. The dog had not been vaccinated for several years and did not receive ectoparasite or heartworm preventives.

Physical examination revealed stuporous mentation, a rectal temperature of 40.5°C (104.9°F), severe dehydration, a capillary refill time of 3 seconds, white mucous membranes with petechiation, tachycardia, tachypnea, and tick infestation. Despite appropriate emergency therapy, the dog developed acute respiratory distress and ventricular tachycardia and died. Initial bloodwork revealed a hematocrit of 0.9 l/l (RI 0.40–0.55 l/l%), total protein of 50 g/l (RI 55–75 g/l), 0.14×10^9 WBC/l (RI $6–17 \times 10^9$/l), and 5.96×10^9 platelets/l (RI $150–400 \times 10^9$/l). Necropsy and histopathology were performed. The results of necropsy and histopathology (hematoxylin and eosin stain) of the heart are shown (**183a, 183b, 183c**).

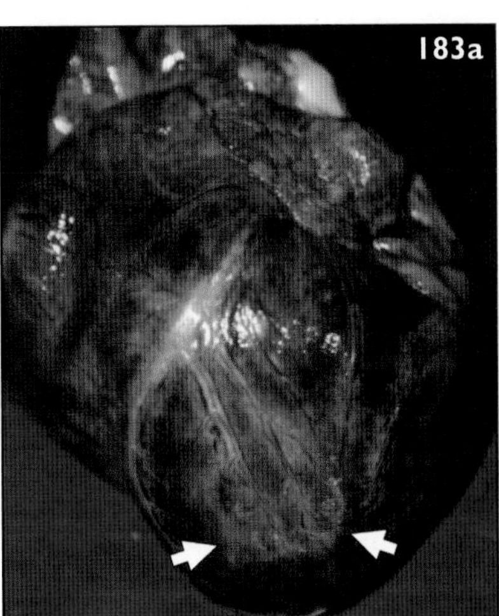
183a

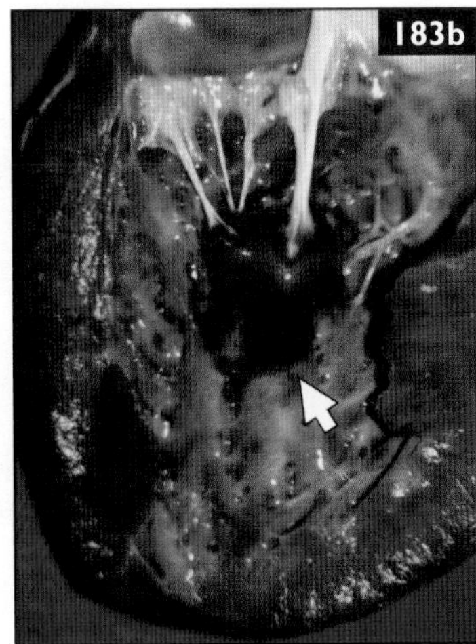
183b

1 What are the most important findings of the necropsy and histopathology of the heart?
2 What are the differential diagnoses for these abnormalities in this case?

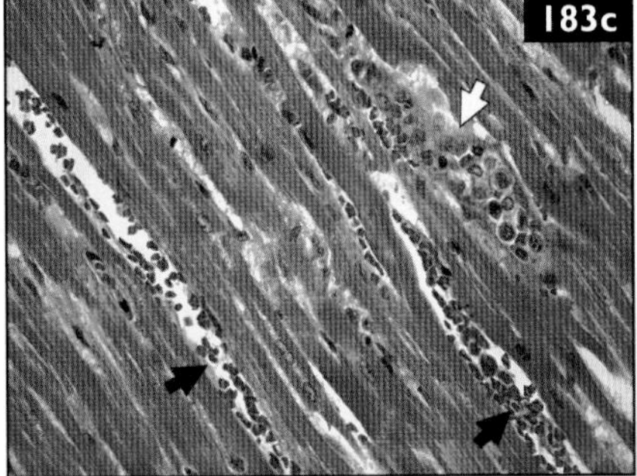
183c

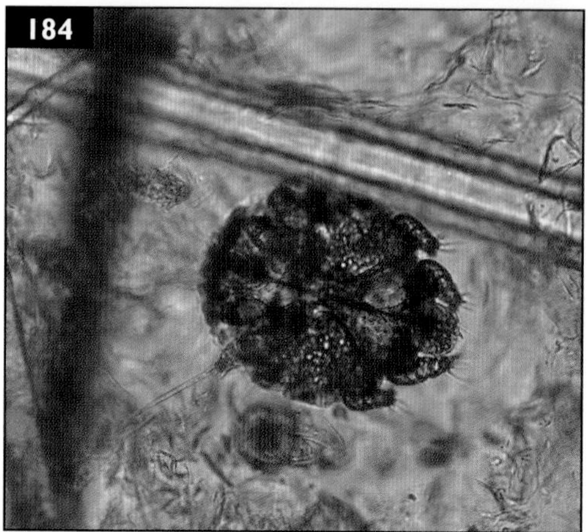

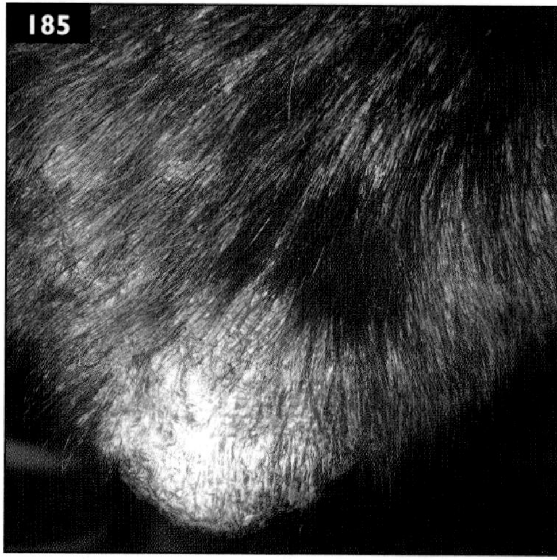

CASE 184 A 6-month-old Poodle was evaluated for severe acute pruritus for the last 2 weeks. The dog had severe crusting and erythema on the pinnae, face, elbows, tarsi, and ventrum. During the last week, the owner had also developed pruritus. The dog lived in Munich, Germany, and had received its initial vaccination series. He had been treated for endoparasites several times.

Physical examination was otherwise unremarkable. Superficial skin scrapings from several large areas of the dog's body revealed scabies mites (**184**).

1 How would you treat the dog?
2 How would you treat the owner?
3 How would you treat the environment?

CASE 185 A 6-year-old neutered male Labrador Retriever had been rescued in Spain 2 years ago. A history prior to the rescue was not available. Since that time, the dog had never left Germany (it now lived in Munich), and was appropriately vaccinated and treated regularly for ectoparasites and endoparasites. The dog had not had any known health problems until 8 weeks previously, when alopecia and scaling developed on both ear tips without any evidence of pruritus (**185**).

At the time of evaluation, the physical examination was normal besides the skin lesions and being slightly thin (BCS 3/9). A CBC, serum biochemistry panel, and urinalysis were all normal.

1 What are your differential diagnoses for the skin lesions?
2 What tests are indicated in this dog?
3 What is the prognosis for each of the major differential diagnoses?

CASE 186 A 4-year-old neutered male mixed-breed dog was referred for treatment of acute kidney injury due to leptospirosis. The dog had been anorexic for the last 5 days, but had no vomiting. He had been treated with maropitant, a metoclopramide continuous rate infusion, and famotidine at adequate doses. The dog lived in Ingolstadt, Germany, and had not traveled outside the country. He had only been vaccinated as a puppy and had not received any parasite prevention or treatment within the last 2 years.

On physical examination, the dog was obtunded. Ulceration and necrosis of the tongue were present (**186a, 186b**). The dog exhibited signs of pain when the kidneys were palpated. The rest of the physical examination was unremarkable.

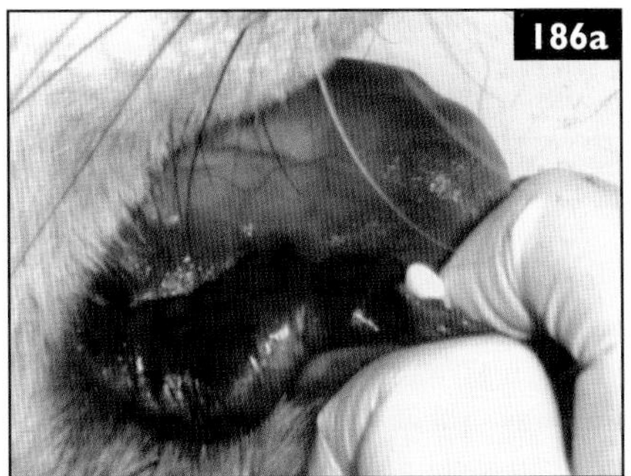
186a

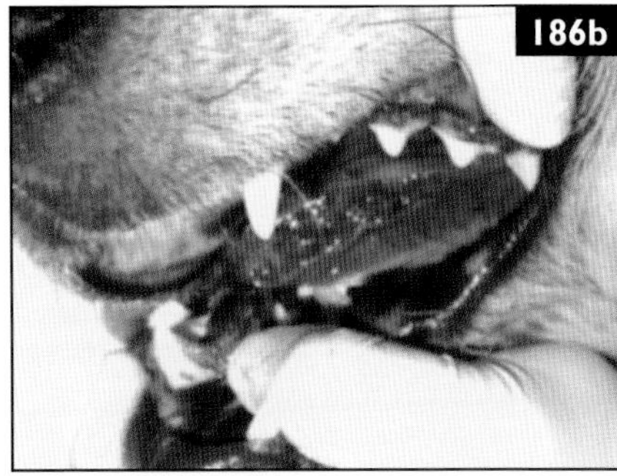
186b

1 What would be an adequate analgesia protocol for painful oral ulceration?
2 What would be appropriate routes for food administration in this dog?

CASE 187 A 2-year-old intact male Smooth-coated Fox Terrier was evaluated for a 3-day history of hematuria. The dog lived in Napoli, Italy, and was owned by a breeder. The dog had been mated with bitches from several European countries. He had been vaccinated on a regular basis (distemper, adenovirus, parvovirus, *Leptospira*, and rabies) and was on heartworm prophylaxis.

Physical examination revealed a BCS of 3/9 and a mild enlargement of the popliteal lymph nodes. Examination of the prepuce and penile mucosa showed a congested proliferative lesion around the urethral orifice (**187**).

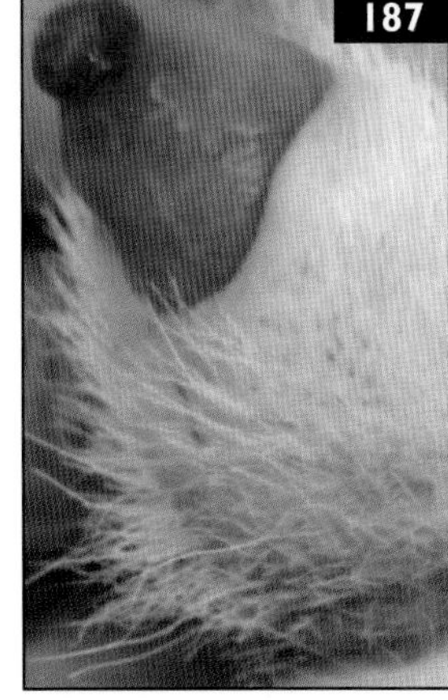
187

1 What are the main differential diagnoses for the genital lesion?
2 What diagnostic tests should be performed?

CASE 188 A 3-year-old intact male Labrador Retriever mix was presented for booster vaccination. The dog lived in Warsaw, Poland. He had been treated for endoparasites 1 week before presentation. The dog's vaccination history was as follows (see below).

Age	Vaccination
6 weeks	Attenuated live canine distemper virus (CDV) and canine parvovirus (CPV)
9 weeks	Attenuated live CDV, CPV, and canine adenovirus 2 (CAV-2); *Leptospira* bacterins (Canicola and Icterohaemorrhagiae)
13 weeks	Attenuated live CDV, CPV, and CAV-2; *Leptospira* bacterins (Canicola and Icterohaemorrhagiae), inactivated rabies virus
1 year	Attenuated live CDV, CPV, and CAV-2; *Leptospira* bacterins (Canicola and Icterohaemorrhagiae), inactivated rabies virus
2 years	Attenuated live CDV, CPV, and CAV-2; *Leptospira* bacterins (Canicola and Icterohaemorrhagiae), inactivated rabies virus

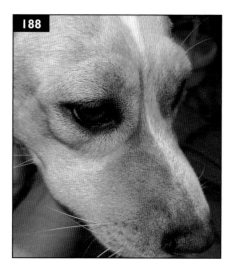
188

At evaluation, the dog appeared clinically healthy. The same combination of vaccine antigens given at the 2-year visit was administered. About 25 minutes after vaccination, the owner noticed swelling around the dog's eyes and returned to the veterinarian.

On physical examination, non-painful periocular edema was evident (**188**). There were no signs of upper or lower respiratory involvement. The dog's temperature, heart rate, and capillary refill time were normal, and there was no evidence of abdominal pain or signs of anaphylactic shock. Thus, a diagnosis of angioedema secondary to vaccination was made.

1 How should the dog be treated?
2 Is this dog at higher risk for allergic reactions after future vaccinations?
3 How should this dog be vaccinated in the future?

CASE 189 A 6-year-old intact male Pointer mix was evaluated for a 4-week history of progressive cloudiness in the right eye. Additionally, the dog had exfoliative skin lesions around his head and ear pinnae, and had appeared to be debilitated with decreased activity levels for about 4 weeks prior to the onset of the ocular and skin signs. The owner lived in a suburb of London, UK, and travelled with the dog to Spain during the summer months, where they spent several weeks in the coastal area of Malaga.

On physical examination, in addition to the skin lesions, the right mandibular lymph node was slightly enlarged. Otherwise, physical examination was unremarkable. On ophthalmic examination of the right eye (**189**), the conjunctiva was very hyperemic with markedly injected episcleral vessels. There was increased tearing and mucoid discharge. The lower eyelid appeared slightly swollen and mildly hyperemic. There was an absent menace response. Slit lamp examination revealed diffuse and deep corneal edema; no details of the anterior chamber could be visualized. The fluorescein test was negative in this eye. The left eye had very mild perilimbal corneal edema in the dorsal aspect, but was otherwise normal.

Ophthalmic examination	Right eye (OD)	Left eye (OS)
Menace response	Absent	Present
Dazzle reflex	Present	Present
Pupillary light reflex	No visibility of pupil	Direct and indirect present
Schirmer tear test	15 mm/min	15 mm/min
Intraocular pressure	10 mmHg	15 mmHg

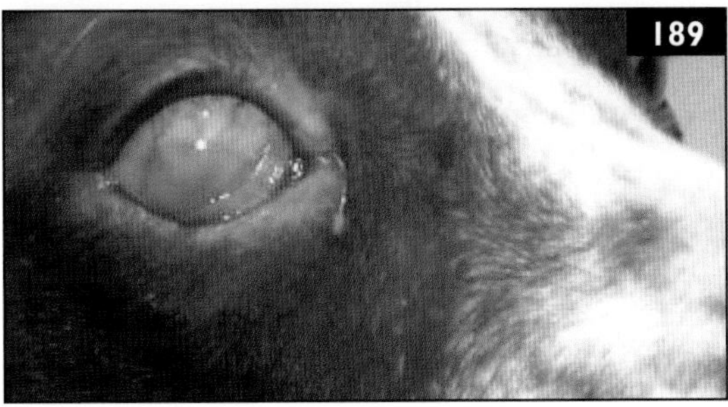
189

1 What is the ocular diagnosis based on the clinical presentation and ocular examination?
2 Which underlying disease would you suspect based on the clinical findings and history?
3 What further diagnostic tests do you suggest?
4 What is your ocular and systemic treatment plan for this dog?

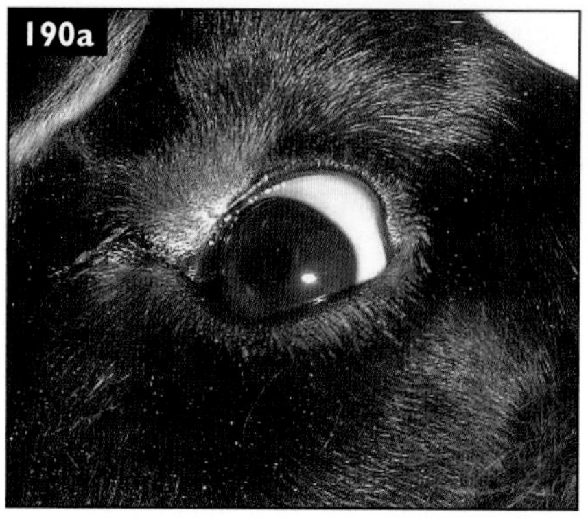

CASE 190 A 2-year-old intact male Border Collie mix was evaluated for lethargy, anorexia, and weakness that had lasted a week. The owners had noticed a yellow tinge to the dog's sclera over the last 3 days (**190a**). The dog had three episodes of vomiting over the 2 days before presentation. The vomit was described as yellow and watery. No diarrhea, polyuria, polydipsia, cough or neurologic signs were reported. The dog had no previous disease history and no travel history. It lived in Salvador, Brazil. The dog had unsupervised outdoor access. Ticks and fleas were infrequently found on the dog, after which the owners applied topical fipronil. The dog was up to date on vaccinations against rabies, parvovirus, and distemper.

Physical examination revealed 5–7% dehydration, icterus (**190b, 190c**), a rectal temperature of 39.8°C (103.6°F), splenomegaly, and abdominal pain.

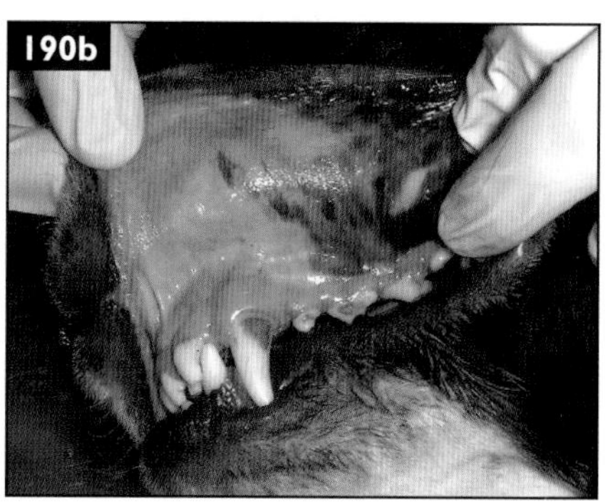

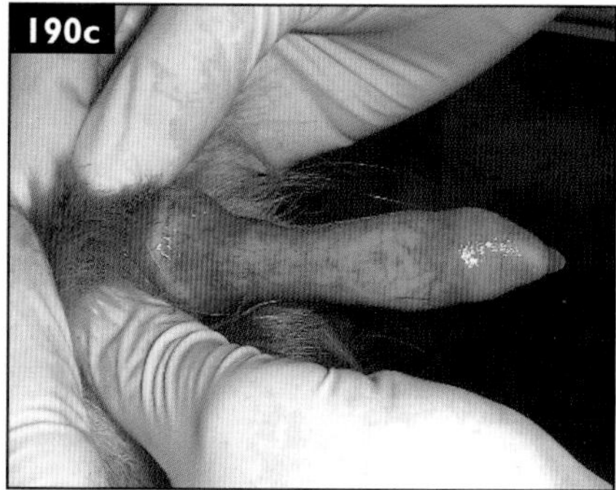

1 What are the differential diagnoses for the main problem in this dog?
2 What are the next diagnostic steps?
3 Does this patient represent a risk for transmission of infection to other dogs and to humans?

CASE 191 Case 191 is the same dog as case 190. Laboratory tests showed regenerative anemia (hematocrit: 0.28 l/l, RI 0.40–0.55 l/l), thrombocytopenia (63.3 × 10^9 platelets/l, RI 150–400 × 10^9/l), normal WBC count, hyperbilirubinemia (total bilirubin 29.1 µmol/l, RI 0–13.7 µmol/l), normal activity of serum liver enzymes, and a positive Coombs test. A blood smear was evaluated (**191**). Antibodies against

Leptospira spp. serovars Autumnalis, Bratislava, Canicola, Grippotyphosa, Icterohaemorrhagiae, and Pomona were undetectable, as was a *Leptospira* PCR on blood and urine specimens.

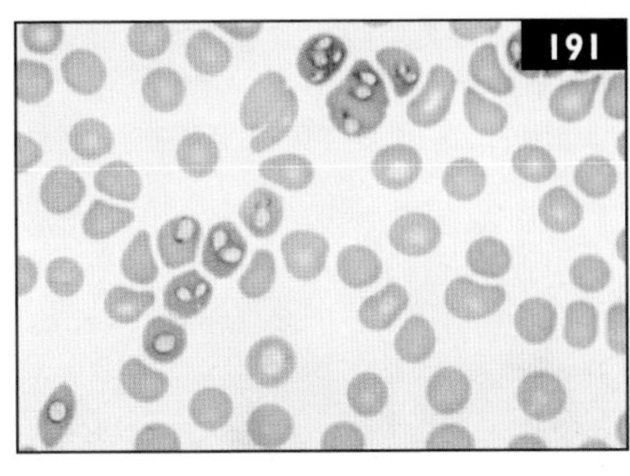

1 What are the abnormalities seen on the blood smear?
2 How did this dog become infected with these organisms?
3 How should this disease be treated?
4 What is the prognosis?

CASE 192 A healthy 4-year-old neutered male mixed-breed dog (**192**) was evaluated for lameness. The owner was a hobby hunter and had recently been diagnosed with Lyme disease. Four weeks previously, the dog had an episode of mild lameness in the left pelvic limb, after a 10-hour mountain hiking tour in the German Alps, that lasted for 10 days and then resolved without treatment. During this episode, the dog was eating well and did not show any other signs of illness. The owner was now concerned that the dog also could have Lyme disease. The dog lived in Munich, Germany, and frequently went hiking with the owner in the German or Austrian Alps, but he had never been to Southern or Eastern European countries. The owner also took the dog frequently on hunting trips. The dog had only been vaccinated regularly against rabies and was not on any ecto- or endoparasite control. The owner reported that he removed a tick from the dog about once a month during the summer months.

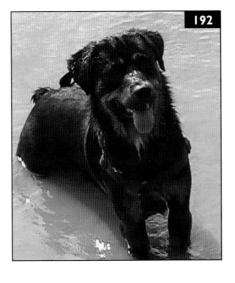

Physical examination revealed no abnormalities.

1 What is Lyme disease, and how is it transmitted?
2 How common are clinical signs in dogs?
3 Is it possible that the infection was transmitted from the dog to the owner?
4 How could you quickly rule out a diagnosis of Lyme disease in this dog?

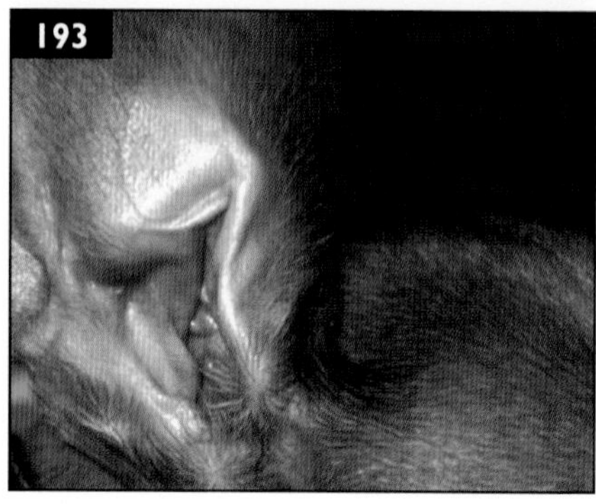

CASE 193 A 1.5-year-old intact female Dachshund was evaluated for a 3-day history of lethargy, anorexia, and diarrhea. On the day of evaluation the owner had also noted yellow coloration of the skin (**193**). The dog lived with three other Dachshunds in a suburban area close to Prague, Czech Republic, near a waste recycling facility, where the dog was known to catch and eat rodents. The dog had been vaccinated as a puppy twice for distemper, parvovirus, and adenovirus hepatitis, and later against rabies. She had not been treated with antiparasitic drugs on a regular basis.

On physical examination, dehydration, icterus, and petechial hemorrhages on mucous membranes were noted. The cranial abdomen was painful on palpation. Laboratory findings were consistent with renal failure. In addition, thrombocytopenia and increased liver enzymes were noted. Antibody titers against *Leptospira* serogroups Canicola, Icterohaemorrhagiae, Grippotyphosa, and Australis were determined by the microscopic agglutination test (MAT). The titer to Icterohaemorrhagiae was high at 1:6,400, with low (1:100) or negative titers to other serovars. A urine PCR for *Leptospira* spp. was positive.

1 What treatment is indicated for leptospirosis?
2 Are other dogs in this household at risk of infection?
3 Could handling this dog represent a risk for humans?

CASE 194 A 2-year-old intact male Labrador Retriever was evaluated for a very cloudy left eye, which the owner had first noticed about 3–4 days previously. The dog lived with one other dog and two cats in the countryside near London, UK, and there was no travel history. The dog was regularly vaccinated, treated for endoparasites, and received preventives for ectoparasites. There was no history of previous ocular disease or other illnesses.

Physical examination was unremarkable besides the ocular changes. On ocular examination of the left eye, there was diffuse, subtle corneal edema, diffuse conjunctival hyperemia, mild chemosis, and mild to moderate mucoid discharge (**194**). Slit lamp examination of the anterior chamber revealed aqueous flare ++/++++ (positive Tyndall effect) and traces of hyphema. The iris was diffusely swollen and hyperemic (rubeosis iridis), with the pupil being miotic. The lens was clear. Examination of the posterior segment was limited because of the aqueous flare and miotic pupil, but no gross lesions were detected. However, the tapetum appeared to have multifocal "dull looking" (hyporeflective) areas in the dorsal aspect.

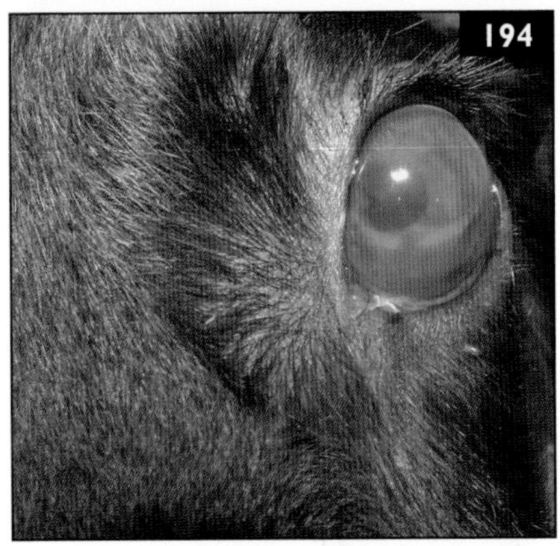
194

Ophthalmic examination	Right eye (OD)	Left eye (OS)
Menace response	Present	Decreased
Dazzle reflex	Present	Present
Pupillary light reflex	Normal	Pupil miotic
Schirmer tear test	15 mm/min	15 mm/min
Intraocular pressure	17 mmHg	5 mmHg

1 Based on the ophthalmic findings in the left eye, what is your ocular diagnosis?
2 What ocular treatment would you suggest?
3 What further diagnostic tests would you perform to identify the underlying etiology?

CASE 195 A 2-year-old Labrador Retriever was evaluated for numerous skin lesions (**195**). The dog was pruritic predominantly on the ventrum, inguinal area, flanks, thighs, and dorsal trunk. Otherwise, the dog was bright and alert. The dog lived in Munich, Germany, and was regularly vaccinated and treated for endoparasites, but was not on any ectoparasite control.

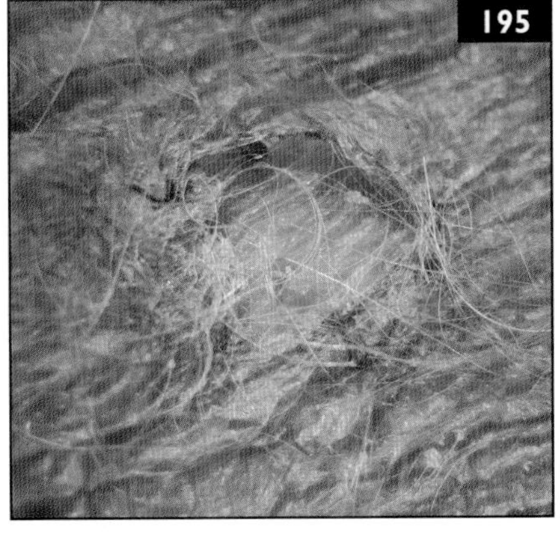
195

On physical examination, the dog showed no other clinical abnormalities besides the pruritus and skin lesions. An impression smear revealed numerous cocci and occasional neutrophils with engulfed bacteria.

1 What is the most likely underlying cause for the pyoderma?
2 How would you treat this dog?
3 Does the treatment have consequences for any tests used to identify underlying disease?

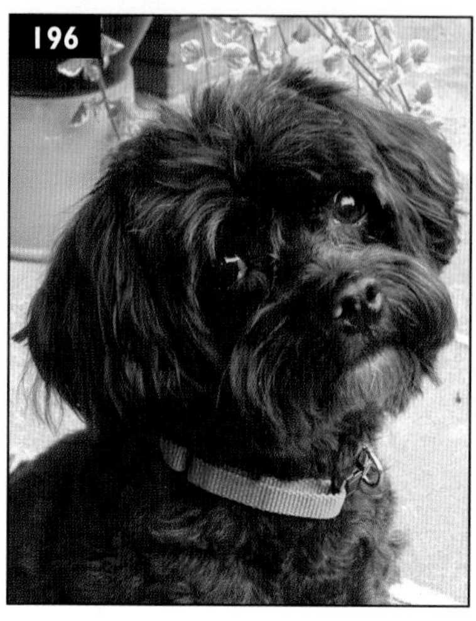

CASE 196 A 4-year-old intact female mixed-breed dog (**196**) was evaluated at a wellness visit. The dog had been diagnosed with immune-mediated thrombocytopenia at the age of 2 years. The disease was well controlled with treatment and the dog was currently receiving a low dose of prednisolone and azathioprine. The dog lived in downtown Munich, Germany, and had never been outside the country. The dog was never allowed to run free and had not much contact with other dogs. The owner's neighbor (from an apartment on the same floor of the apartment building) had recently purchased a puppy from the internet, and the puppy had died of parvovirosis 1 week previously. The owner was concerned that the dog could also get parvovirosis and asked for advice on whether to vaccinate the dog or not. The dog had been vaccinated against parvovirus infection at the age of 8 weeks, 12 weeks, and 16 weeks, and 12 months later, but never since. The dog had not received preventive treatment for endoparasites or ectoparasites within the last 2 years.

Physical examination was unremarkable. A CBC revealed no abnormalities, and the platelets were in the RI.

1 What would be your assessment of the vaccination history of this dog?
2 Could vaccination against parvovirus infection present an increased risk of adverse effects for this dog?
3 What would you recommend as an alternative to vaccination?

CASE 197 A 6-year-old neutered female German Shepherd Dog from Sacramento, California, USA was evaluated for inappetence, weight loss, and lethargy. Five months previously, the owner had noted pelvic limb lameness that did not respond to carprofen. Subsequently the dog developed inappetence and transient small bowel diarrhea, and began to lose weight. Water consumption and urination were normal to slightly decreased. There was no history of trauma, toxin exposure, or ticks. The dog had no travel history, was last vaccinated 4 years ago, and had not received any preventive treatments for parasites for at least 1 year.

On physical examination, the dog was quiet, dull, mildly dehydrated, and thin (BCS 2/9). Although ambulatory, the dog had a stilted gait and appeared mildly ataxic. A neurologic examination showed placing deficits in both pelvic limbs.

The dog exhibited pain when her tail was raised and also on palpation of the lumbosacral region and mid-thoracic spine. All other physical examination findings were normal. A CBC was unremarkable. A chemistry panel showed severe azotemia (creatinine 760.3 µmol/l [RI 50–119 µmol/l], BUN 58.2 mmol/l [2.6–9.9 mmol/l]) and hyperglobulinemia (47 g/l). Urinalysis showed a specific gravity of 1.011, 0.75 g/l of protein, pH 6, and >100 WBC and >100 RBC/hpf. Urine culture revealed large numbers of *Aspergillus terreus* (**197**).

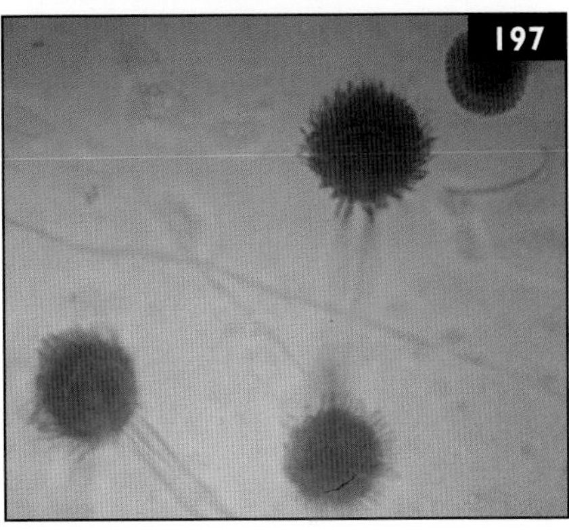
197

1 What is the significance of finding *Aspergillus terreus* in this dog's urine?
2 What is the likely cause of the pelvic limb paresis?
3 Had the urine culture been negative, what additional test could have been performed to make a diagnosis?
4 What treatment would be recommended, and what is the prognosis?

CASE 198 An 8-month-old intact female American Pitbull Terrier was evaluated for acute anorexia, severe lethargy, and high fever (temperature 40.2°C [104.4°F]). The owners lived in Rome, Italy, but had recently been on a trip to Croatia with the dog. The dog was up to date on core vaccinations (distemper, adenovirus, parvovirus, rabies, *Leptospira*), but had not received prophylaxis for internal or external parasites.

On physical examination, the dog had very pale mucous membranes, icteric sclera, and a weak pulse, and an arrhythmia was detected on auscultation of the heart. A CBC and biochemistry profile showed severe anemia (0.12 l/l, RI 0.37–0.55 l/l), autoagglutination, and mild thrombocytopenia (100×10^9 platelets/l, RI $150–400 \times 10^9$/l). Blood smears were obtained (**198**).

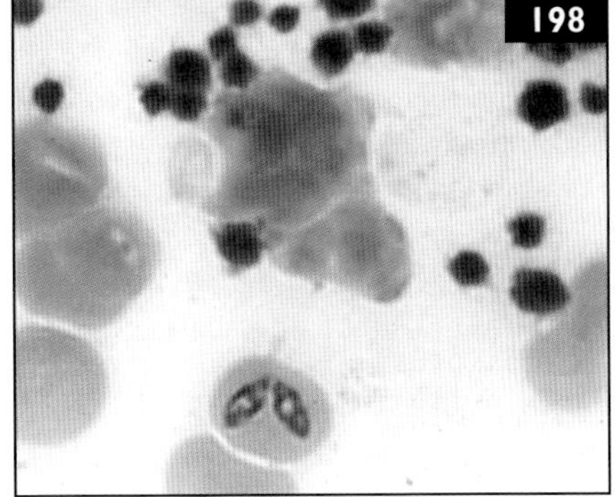
198

1 What is the diagnosis?
2 What is the prognosis?
3 How should the dog be treated?

CASE 199 An adult intact male mixed-breed dog was rescued from the streets in San Diego, California, USA, and taken to a local humane society, where he was found to have severe tick infestation (**199a**) and blindness.

Physical examination revealed a BCS of 2/9, normal vital signs, pale mucous membranes, lymphadenopathy, and splenomegaly. There was no menace response or dazzle reflex bilaterally. Pupillary light reflex was also absent, and both pupils were fixed and dilated (**199b**). Scleral injection was present in both eyes, and was most severe in the left eye. Palpebral and corneal reflexes were normal bilaterally, and a Schirmer tear test was normal in both eyes. Intraocular pressure (IOP) was 9 mmHg in the right eye and 10 mmHg in the left eye (RI 12–25 mmHg).

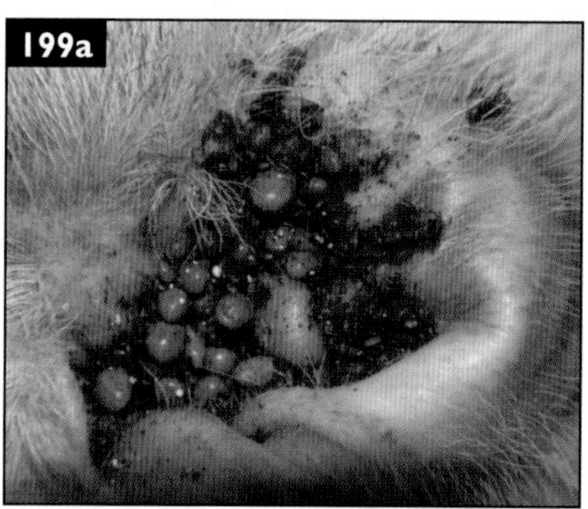
199a

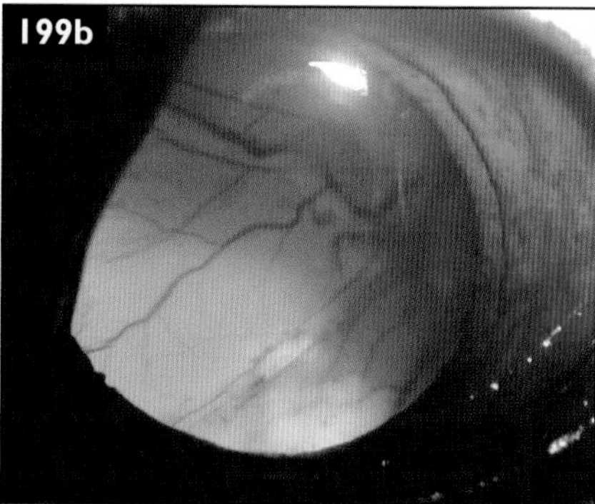
199b

1 What are the clinically relevant findings from the ophthalmic examination?
2 What are the most likely diseases causing these problems?
3 What is the prognosis for this dog?

CASE 200 A 2.5-month-old intact male Polish Tatra Sheepdog was presented for its first vaccination. The puppy had been recently treated for endoparasites. It had come from a breeder in Warsaw, Poland, and now lived in a rural area close to Warsaw. On physical examination the puppy appeared healthy. A vaccine containing live attenuated canine distemper virus, canine parvovirus 2, canine adenovirus, and two inactivated *Leptospira* serovars (Canicola and Icterohaemorrhagiae) was administered subcutaneously.

Within 15 minutes after administration of the vaccine, the puppy developed edema on the nose and around the eyes (**200**) and ptyalism, followed almost immediately afterwards by an episode of vomiting, marked abdominal pain, diarrhea with hematochezia, urination, tachypnea, bradycardia, and cyanotic mucous membranes. These clinical signs were suggestive of anaphylactic shock.

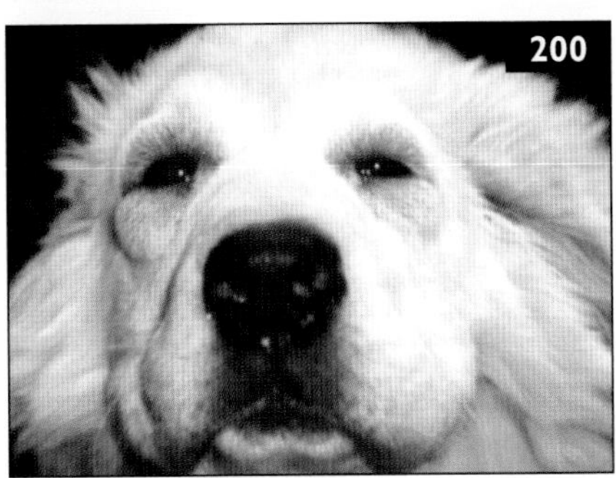

1 Given that this puppy has never been vaccinated before, could the vaccine be the cause of the anaphylactic shock?
2 How common is postvaccinal anaphylaxis in dogs?
3 How would you treat this dog?

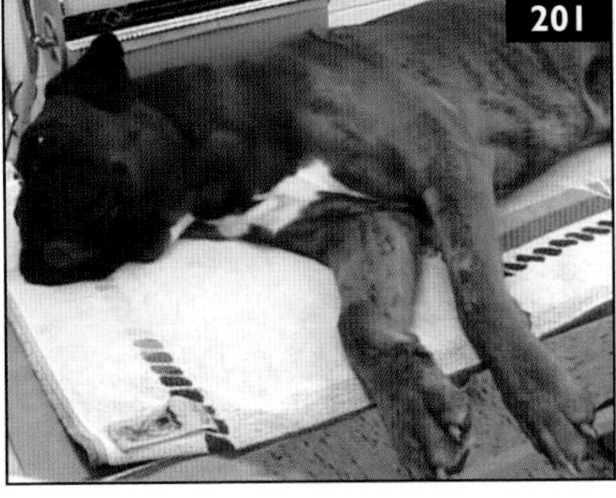

CASE 201 A 3-year-old intact male Boxer dog (**201**) was referred for progressive neurologic abnormalities. The dog had been ataxic over the last 7 days, and 5 days previously circling had been observed. Over the past 4 days, the dog had been non-ambulatory. A veterinarian had treated the dog with prednisolone, chloramphenicol, and diazepam, but this did not lead to any improvement. The dog lived in Freiburg, Germany, and had not traveled outside the country. He had only been vaccinated in his first year of life, and had only received endoparasite and ectoparasite treatment as a puppy. The owner reported that the dog had frequent tick infestations, but he always removed the ticks immediately because the dog had a short hair coat.

On physical examination, the dog presented in lateral recumbency and was unable to stand or walk; he had a reduced menace response bilaterally. Voluntary movement of the thoracic limbs was present, but this was absent in the pelvic limbs. The dog also had bilateral mydriasis.

A CSF analysis revealed a high WBC count and a moderate CSF protein concentration. The CSF was positive for tick-borne encephalitis virus by PCR.

1 What is tick-borne encephalitis?
2 What are the typical clinical signs?
3 What is the prognosis?

CASE 1

1 How would you interpret the findings in this dog? This dog has renal failure, based on the presence of increased serum urea and creatinine and the low specific gravity of the urine. Glucosuria with normoglycemia suggests renal tubular injury. The history of acute onset and the good BCS together with the slightly enlarged kidneys suggest acute kidney injury rather than chronic kidney disease. Although a low hematocrit is commonly associated with chronic kidney disease, in one study, 55% of dogs with acute kidney injury had a hematocrit below the RI. Thrombocytopenia is likely associated with the underlying disease causing the acute kidney injury. The dog's acute kidney injury would be non-oliguric grade III according to the grading system suggested by the International Renal Interest Society (IRIS).

2 What are the differential diagnoses for this dog? Causes of acute kidney injury include ischemic events secondary to hypovolemia, infections (e.g. leptospirosis or pyelonephritis), renal neoplasia (especially lymphoma), and toxins (such as ethylene glycol or non-steroidal anti-inflammatory drugs). Based on the clinical findings (thrombocytopenia, azotemia, glucosuria), leptospirosis is a likely underlying cause. More than half of dogs with leptospirosis are thrombocytopenic, and glucosuria is also a common finding in this disease.

CASE 2

1 How would you make a specific diagnosis of leptospirosis? Antibody testing for diagnosis of leptospirosis is usually done by the microscopic agglutination test (MAT). The MAT can be negative in the first week of illness. Therefore, convalescent titers 1–2 weeks after the acute titer are recommended, and a 4-fold (2 titer steps) increase indicates recent infection. Single high titers >1:800 against non-vaccinal serovars have been used for the diagnosis of leptospirosis. However, given the widespread availability of new four-serovar vaccines and the inaccuracies of the MAT, use of a single titer for diagnosis is no longer recommended, and a 4-fold titer increase must be demonstrated to confirm the diagnosis. PCR assays for use on whole blood and urine are also available. PCR is considered very specific, but false-negative results are common, especially in dogs that have already received antimicrobial drugs. In-clinic ELISA antibody tests are also available, but these may be negative early in the course of infection and positive results can occur as a result of recent vaccination or subclinical exposure.

2 How would you treat this dog? The dog should be treated aggressively for acute kidney injury with intravenous fluids and other supportive treatments while awaiting the results of further diagnostics. Oral doxycycline is recommended for the treatment of leptospirosis in dogs. However, vomiting in this dog precludes oral medications and administration of intravenous ampicillin or amoxicillin is

recommended until vomiting subsides. Once vomiting subsides, treatment with doxycycline for 2 weeks is recommended to eliminate leptospires from the kidneys.
3 Is there a risk of human infection when handling the dog? Leptospirosis is a zoonosis and veterinary staff should take precautions when handling dogs with this disease. Contact with urine should be minimized, because the spirochete is shed in urine and can penetrate intact mucous membranes and abrasions in the skin. Gloves and a gown should be worn, and pregnant women should not be in contact with dogs suspected to have the disease. These precautions should remain in place until dogs have received at least 2–3 days of appropriate antimicrobial drug therapy.

CASE 3

1 What are the most likely differential diagnoses for this dog based on your assessment of the history and image provided? In a young dog from this region with crusty skin disease, infectious diseases are top of the differential diagnosis list, particularly demodicosis, dermatophytosis, and bacterial pyoderma. However, this could also be puppy strangles, although clinical signs are mild for the long duration of disease.
2 What diagnostic tests should be done immediately? An impression smear and deep skin scrapings are the first tests to be conducted, because they assist with the diagnosis of bacterial pyoderma and demodicosis. If neutrophils and macrophages predominate on cytology, bacteria are sparse or absent, and the scrapings are negative, a dermatophyte culture, PCR, or multiple skin biopsies are the next diagnostic tests to consider. If multiple biopsies are collected, the first biopsy is taken under aseptic conditions; the top part of the biopsy specimen is removed with a sterile scalpel blade, and the bottom part is submitted for bacterial culture. The other specimens are placed in formalin and submitted for histopathologic evaluation. A dermatophyte culture is indicated if historical information favors that diagnosis (or if other animals or humans in the household are affected). A combination of those two tests can also be considered.
3 Could this dog have a transmissible infectious disease? Of the four differential diagnoses only dermatophytosis is contagious. All the other diseases are caused by an insufficient or exaggerated immune response of the host and are not transmitted to humans or other animals. Demodicosis was diagnosed in this dog by deep skin scrapings.

CASE 4

1 What are the differential diagnoses for draining skin lesions? Pyogranulomatous or purulent infections caused by foreign bodies, certain bacteria, or fungi are the main differential diagnoses for draining skin lesions.

2 What diagnostic plan should be considered for the skin lesions? The initial diagnostic plan should involve cytologic examination of stained specimens of the discharge material. Sometimes, material for microscopic examination can be obtained by fine needle aspiration or flushing of the drainage site. Radiographs should be taken to determine whether there are any underlying bony lesions responsible for, or associated with, the drainage. Ultrasound of local soft tissues can sometimes lead to detection of a foreign body and sinus tract. If biopsy or surgical examination is needed, further procedures could be a CBC, biochemical profile, and urinalysis. Biopsies should be taken under anesthesia, and the lesion should be carefully explored. With surgical intervention, culture specimens can be obtained in an aseptic manner. Antibody or PCR testing can be performed to help determine whether pathogenic agents are associated with these lesions.

CASE 5

1 What is the source of the organism isolated in this infection? *Basiobolus ranarum* belongs to the filamentous fungi, phylum Zygomycota, which is most commonly found in soil, decaying organic matter, and the gastrointestinal tracts of amphibians, reptiles, fish, and bats. *Basiobolus ranarum* is the causative agent of zygomycosis, which is a chronic inflammatory or granulomatous disease in humans and animals. Subcutaneous, gastrointestinal, respiratory, and systemic infections have been reported in dogs.

2 What treatment is indicated? Surgical drainage and resection of inflamed tissues is the first management consideration. Drugs most active against filamentous fungi should be used when antifungal susceptibility testing is not available. Amphotericin B has to be given parenterally and is potentially nephrotoxic. Azoles, specifically itraconazole, voriconazole, or posaconazole, can be given orally. Iodides and trimethoprim/sulfonamide combinations have been used in human infections; however, efficacy has not been shown in any of the canine cases reported.

CASE 6

1 What is the differential diagnosis for icterus? Icterus is the description for yellowish pigmentation of skin and mucous membranes caused by hyperbilirubinemia. Hyperbilirubinemia can be classified into one of three categories of underlying etiologies: prehepatic (increased red blood cell destruction); hepatic (liver cell dysfunction); and posthepatic (a cholestatic disorder).

2 What non-invasive tests would you perform first to investigate this problem? First, a CBC should be performed. Moderate to severe regenerative anemia is most typical with prehepatic hyperbilirubinemia. A mild to moderate normocytic, normochromic, nonregenerative anemia is often present in chronic intra- and posthepatic inflammatory diseases (anemia of inflammatory disease) and should be discriminated from prehepatic hemolytic anemia. Changes in erythrocyte morphology consistent with increased erythrocyte destruction (e.g. spherocytes, schistocytes) are helpful to differentiate prehepatic from hepatic and posthepatic causes of anemia. Prehepatic hyperbilirubinemia is unlikely when the hematocrit is within the RI, without evidence of regeneration. A serum chemistry panel and urinalysis should be performed to determine whether there are liver function abnormalities (e.g. low cholesterol, albumin, glucose) that can indicate hepatic hyperbilirubinemia, or findings supportive of cholestatic disease (e.g. increased serum cholesterol concentration). The magnitude of serum liver enzyme activities can be influenced by a number of different factors, so these are more difficult to interpret. For example, both prehepatic (oxygen deficiency in hemolytic anemia) and posthepatic (e.g. bile duct obstruction due to pancreatitis) factors can cause secondary hepatocellular damage. An abdominal ultrasound is also recommended to aid differentiation of hepatic and posthepatic causes of hyperbilirubinemia. Posthepatic hyperbilirubinemia is unlikely when the gallbladder size, gallbladder wall thickness, diameter of the extrahepatic bile duct, and pancreas appear normal.

CASE 7

1 What form of icterus can be ruled out based on the results of the CBC? Prehepatic icterus is unlikely, based on the high hematocrit. With normal liver function, massive numbers of erythrocytes must be destroyed for icterus to develop. Therefore, anemia is generally observed in icterus due to hemolysis.

2 What is your assessment of the neutrophilia observed in this dog? Neutrophilia can be due to glucocorticoids or stress, inflammation, or, in rare cases, leukemia. A significant inflammatory response due to a bacterial infection is most likely in this case given the magnitude of neutrophilia and the left shift. In contrast, a mild to moderate elevation of mature neutrophils often characterizes a stress leukogram, typically in association with a reduction in the eosinophil and lymphocyte counts. Granulocytic leukemia is a rare disorder and can be suspected when there is a very high number of neutrophils ($50–100 \times 10^9$/l) without a significant left shift.

3 What are reasons for distension of the common bile duct? Two reasons for distension of the common bile duct are obstruction and inflammation.

4 Which reason is more likely in this case, and what test would you perform to confirm your suspicion? A complete obstruction of the common bile duct would cause distension of the intra- and extrahepatic biliary system upstream of the obstruction, as well as enlargement of the gallbladder. In this case, the gallbladder and intrahepatic biliary ducts were not distended. This imaging finding, together with the elevated rectal temperature and the significant left shift, makes an inflammatory cause of the bile duct distension more likely and should increase suspicion for bacterial cholangitis. To confirm a bacterial cholangitis, aspiration of bile for cytologic examination and aerobic and anaerobic bacterial culture is indicated.

CASE 8

1 **What are the most common bacterial species involved in bacterial cholangitis and, therefore, what antimicrobial would you choose empirically while the results of culture and susceptibility are pending?** A study of 190 dogs with a positive culture of bile, gallbladder, or liver showed that *Escherichia coli*, *Enterococcus* spp., *Bacteroides* spp., *Streptococcus* spp., and *Clostridium* spp. were the most common bacteria isolated. More than 80% of Enterobacteriaceae were susceptible to ciprofloxacin or aminoglycosides, whereas only 30–67% were susceptible to first-generation aminopenicillins and cephalosporins. In this dog, intravenous antibiotics are indicated. Fluoroquinolones are a reasonable first choice, because Enterobacteriaceae susceptible to this group of antibiotics are most frequently isolated. Anaerobic bacteria might also be involved, and thus fluoroquinolones should be combined with metronidazole, clindamycin, and/or a beta-lactam/beta-lactamase inhibitor combination such as ampicillin/sulbactam.

2 **Are bacterial infections of the hepatobiliary system common in dogs?** In contrast to cats, in which neutrophilic cholangitis is common, bacterial cholangitis is uncommon in dogs.

3 **What predisposing factors contribute to ascending bacterial cholangitis?** Predisposing factors in dogs include biliary stones, inflammatory bowel disease (causing sphincter odi incompetence), pancreatitis, vomiting, and immunosuppression. In this dog, a foreign body was suspected on the basis of the results of an upper gastrointestinal tract contrast study (**8b**), and was confirmed using ultrasound. The foreign body was surgically removed (**8c**).

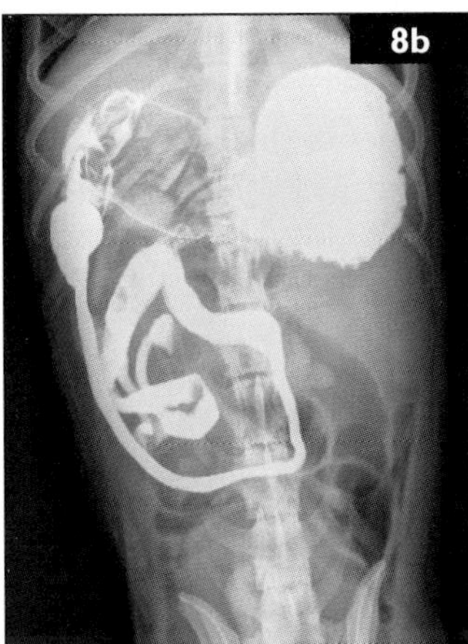
8b

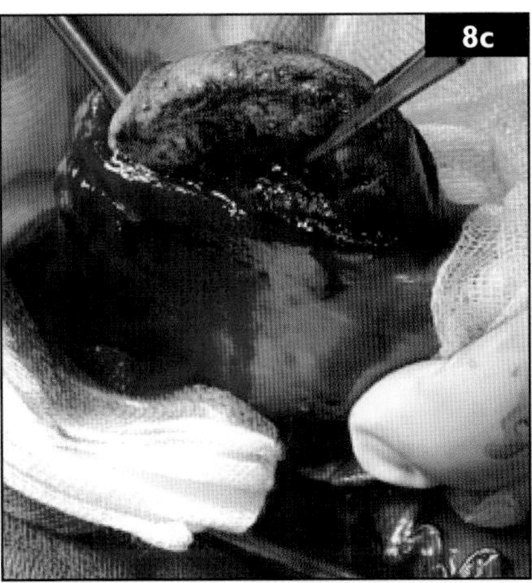
8c

4 For how long would you continue antimicrobial treatment? Based on reports of successful treatment of bacterial cholangitis with long-term follow-up, antibiotics should be continued for 2–4 weeks. The dog recovered uneventfully with pradofloxacin selected as the outpatient antibiotic in this case (pradofloxacin is a new fluoroquinolone that is licensed for use in dogs, but so far only in Europe).

CASE 9

1 Which infectious agents can be transmitted by *Rhipicephalus sanguineus*? Tick-borne infections transmitted by *R. sanguineus* that are endemic in Brazil include *Anaplasma platys*, *Ehrlichia canis*, *Babesia vogeli*, and *Hepatozoon canis*. *R. sanguineus* is also suspected as a vector of *Rangelia vitalii* and possibly also *Mycoplasma haemocanis*. Co-infections with more than one of these organisms commonly occur.

In the United States, *R. sanguineus* can also transmit *Rickettsia rickettsii*.

2 What are the two most striking abnormalities in the CBC, and which tick-borne diseases can cause these abnormalities? The two major findings in the CBC are a severe thrombocytopenia (which explains the hemorrhage in this dog) and a marked neutrophilia. An acute *E. canis* infection could explain the severe thrombocytopenia in this dog. The massive neutrophilia is suggestive of infection by *H. canis*.

3 What diagnostic tests should be performed to diagnose these infections? Blood smear evaluation is a simple test that might show *Ehrlichia* spp. morulae and *Hepatozoon* spp. intracellular inclusions. Both infections can be detected by PCR, and antibody tests could also be performed. Both antibody testing and PCR are required for acute *E. canis* infections; acute and convalescent antibody testing might be required to confirm the diagnosis.

CASE 10

1 Which clinical signs and laboratory abnormalities in this dog are caused by *Hepatozoon canis* and which are more likely to be caused by *Ehrlichia canis*? Anorexia, lethargy, weight loss, pale mucous membranes, lymphadenomegaly, splenomegaly, and fever could be attributed to both infections. The bleeding is likely the result of the severe thrombocytopenia, which probably results primarily from infection by *E. canis*. The extreme neutrophilia is caused by the *H. canis* infection. Hyperproteinemia, hypoalbuminenia, and hyperglobulinemia can be caused by both infections.

2 What are the differences between the modes of transmission of *Hepatozoon canis* and *Ehrlichia canis*? *E. canis* is transmitted by an infected *Rhipicephalus* tick that feeds on a non-infected dog. After inoculation, the organisms multiply in the macrophages of the mononuclear phagocyte system and disseminate throughout the body. *H. canis* can only be transmitted by ingestion of a tick that contains mature oocysts. Once within the canine gastrointestinal tract, sporozoites penetrate the intestinal wall and are transported through the blood to hemolymphatic tissues, including the spleen, bone marrow, and lymph nodes, where meronts are formed. Merozoites released from meronts invade neutrophils or monocytes, in which they form gamonts in the peripheral blood.

3 What treatments are indicated for the two infections? For *E. canis* infection, treatment with doxycycline (10 mg/kg PO q24h or 5 mg/kg PO q12h for 21–28 days) is recommended. The recommended treatment for *H. canis* infections is imidocarb dipropionate (6 mg/kg SC) every 14 days until gamonts are no longer present in the blood smear. Although some dogs require only one or two treatments, at least 8 weeks of treatment is usually required for dogs with heavy infections.

CASE 11

1 What is your assessment of this case, and how would you proceed? The history and clinical signs in this dog are suggestive of infection with one or more pathogens that belong to the canine infectious respiratory disease complex. If only viral pathogens are present, clinical signs are often mild and self-limiting. In this dog, clinical signs increased in severity within the first week and the dog had a left shift on the hemogram, suggesting a primary or secondary bacterial infection. Infection with *Bordetella bronchiseptica* has been associated with young age (<1 year), fever, and more severe clinical signs, so this dog seems to be at risk of bordetellosis. To confirm the diagnosis and to guide antimicrobial therapy, a bronchoalveolar lavage (BAL) or transtracheal wash is indicated.

2 How would you interpret the cytology of bronchoalveolar lavage fluid in this patient? The BAL fluid cytology revealed predominantly degenerate neutrophils with intracellular rod-shaped bacteria, indicating bacterial infection.

3 What treatment would you recommend? Several factors should be considered when selecting an appropriate antimicrobial for this dog. Bacterial culture and susceptibility testing should be performed, because some gram-negative pathogens including *B. bronchiseptica* have shown multiple drug resistance in some studies. The chosen antibiotic should have a good distribution into the respiratory tract. Doxycycline is a reasonable first choice and it also has activity against mycoplasmas. An alternative would be a beta-lactam antibiotic, such as amoxicillin, although this would not be effective against mycoplasmas. A fluoroquinolone, such as enrofloxacin, would also be an appropriate choice.

CASE 12

1 What is the neuroanatomic localization of the problem? The lack of a menace response (cranial nerve II) together with the lumbosacral pain and the history of neurologic signs are suggestive of multifocal CNS disease.

2 What are your differential diagnoses for this dog's problem, and what infectious agents might be involved? The most likely differential diagnoses, given the concurrent presence of ocular signs, are neoplasia (such as lymphoma) or infectious disease. Possible infectious causes in California include protozoal diseases (especially neosporosis), fungal diseases (coccidioidomycosis, cryptococcosis, or other less common pathogens, such as hyalohyphomycetes or phaeohyphomycetes), or protothecosis. *Toxoplasma gondii* infection is less common in this region.

3 What is your plan for further work-up of this dog's problem? The work-up should ideally include a CBC, biochemistry profile, and urinalysis, as well as thoracic radiographs, spinal radiographs, and abdominal ultrasound to determine whether there are other abnormalities that could be accessible for specimen collection, and possibly an MRI and CSF tap with CSF analysis. Depending on those results, serum antibody testing for *Coccidioides* spp. should be considered, and testing for *Cryptococcus* spp. should be performed using the latex agglutination cryptococcal antigen test. If a CSF tap is performed and the serum *Cryptococcus* antigen test is negative, fungal culture and *Cryptococcus* antigen testing of the CSF could also be performed. In one study, only 15 of 18 dogs with cryptococcosis from northern California had positive serum antigen tests, and in some of those dogs, antigen testing in the CSF was positive. The sensitivity of serum antigen testing in cats is much higher (>95%).

CASE 13

1 What species of *Cryptococcus* cause infections in dogs, and are there differences in their ecologic niches and clinical presentations? Cryptococcosis in dogs can be caused by *Cryptococcus neoformans* and *Cryptococcus gattii*. The recognized ecologic niche for *C. neoformans* is pigeon guano, whereas *C. gattii* has been found in association with a variety of tree species depending on region and molecular type. For example, in Australia, *C. gattii* has been found in association with Eucalyptus tree species, whereas in British Columbia and the Pacific Northwest of the United States, *C. gattii* has been found in association with Douglas fir trees and a variety of other hardwood tree species. It has also been found in water, soil, and air samples in the region. In the United States, dogs infected with *C. neoformans* tend to have widely disseminated infections that commonly involve the CNS and a variety of other tissues, including the gastrointestinal tract, which was probably involved in this dog. In contrast, dogs infected with *C. gattii* often have localized mass lesions, commonly of the nasal cavity with associated destruction of the cribriform plate. Most affected dogs are infected with *C. neoformans*. Factors that predispose dogs to cryptococcosis are unknown, but genetic susceptibility is suspected for disseminated infections with *C. neoformans*.

2 What is the recommended treatment for this dog? Treatment should optimally include intravenous amphotericin B (ideally lipid-complexed amphotericin B, dosed at 3 mg/kg). This is administered on a Monday–Wednesday–Friday basis for 12 treatments. This could be combined with fluconazole, an azole that has excellent penetration of the CNS. For CNS infections, a high dose of fluconazole, 10 mg/kg PO q12h, is recommended.

3 What are possible adverse effects of drug therapy and how should response to treatment be monitored? Possible adverse effects of drug therapy include renal failure in dogs treated with amphotericin B, and gastrointestinal adverse effects, such as diarrhea and inappetence, in dogs treated with fluconazole at higher doses. Hepatopathy is also possible in dogs treated with fluconazole, but is uncommon. Kidney values should be monitored before each treatment with amphotericin B, and if creatinine increases above the RI, treatment should be withheld until azotemia resolves. Liver enzymes should be monitored monthly, and the serum cryptococcal antigen titer should be monitored every 1–3 months initially. Treatment can be discontinued once the cryptococcal antigen test becomes negative and the dog is clinically normal.

CASE 14

1 What is the primary problem in this dog and the most likely underlying disease? The primary problem is acute kidney injury. The two most common causes of acute kidney injury in previously healthy dogs are leptospirosis and a toxic injury, such as through ethylene glycol ingestion. Leptospirosis is more likely in this case given the neutrophilia with left shift combined with thrombocytopenia.

2 What additional tests would you perform? Additional tests that should be performed are: (1) *Leptospira* urine PCR and/or acute and convalescent antibody measurement 1–2 weeks later for diagnosis of leptospirosis; (2) complete urinalysis; (3) abdominal ultrasound to assess for chronic anatomic renal changes or urethral obstruction; and (4) measurement of blood pressure, because many dogs with acute kidney injury are hypertensive.

3 What treatment would you initiate? Supportive treatment should include: (1) antiemetics (e.g. metoclopramide [care should be taken when metoclopramide is used because increased gastrointestinal motility can predispose to intussusception, especially in young dogs with leptospirosis], maropitant, or ondansetron); (2) gastric protectants (e.g. famotidine or omeprazole); (3) diuresis to address overhydration and hyperkalemia if present (e.g. mannitol [reduces interstitial swelling of the kidneys and flushes cellular debris from the tubules] or furosemide [can additionally reduce hyperkalemia]), although no diuretic is proven to improve outcome; (4) analgesic drugs (e.g. buprenorphine); (5) careful fluid therapy to address losses and dehydration; (6) hemodialysis to remove uremic toxins and to address overhydration and hyperkalemia if the dog does not respond to treatment within 12–24 hours.

Specific treatment for leptospirosis initially involves intravenous administration of penicillin derivatives (e.g. ampicillin [20 mg/kg q8h]). Once gastrointestinal signs have resolved, doxycycline should be administered (10 mg/kg q12h PO for 2 weeks) to eliminate leptospires from the kidney.

CASE 15

1 What should be the monitoring plan for this dog? The monitoring plan for this dog should include: (1) regular physical examination, including mentation, heart rate, mucous membrane color, capillary refill time, pulse quality, respiratory rate and effort every 4 hours; (2) rectal body temperature and body weight every 8–12 hours; (3) blood pressure every 8–12 hours (if hypertensive or hypotensive, more frequent monitoring might be needed); (4) continuous ECG in case of arrhythmias or bradycardia; (5) urine output and 'ins and outs' every 4–8 hours; (6) venous blood gas analysis every 12–24 hours to monitor for acidosis; (7) electrolyte status every 8–12 hours to monitor serum potassium concentration; (8) serum glucose concentration every 12–24 hours; (9) serum total protein and albumin concentration every 24 hours; (10) serum creatinine and urea concentration every 24 hours; (11) food intake, and presence of vomiting, diarrhea, and other abnormalities if present.

2 What are the next diagnostic and therapeutic considerations in regards to the respiratory distress? Respiratory distress could be caused by leptospiral pulmonary hemorrhage syndrome, aspiration pneumonia, or pulmonary edema due to cardiac failure or overhydration in this dog. Thoracic radiographs should be taken for identification of these disorders. Cardiac failure could be further excluded on the basis of physical examination and, if necessary, echocardiography. To determine the degree of hypoxemia, arterial blood gas analysis is recommended. Pulse oximetry could also be used, but is less reliable. Diuretics could be considered if overhydration (and, less likely, cardiac failure) is present, but might not be useful in an anuric patient. Alternatively, overhydration could be addressed using hemodialysis if available. If arterial oxygen partial pressure falls below 70–80 mmHg or oxygen saturation gets below 92–95%, oxygen supplementation should be introduced. If arterial partial pressure of oxygen does not increase to over 60 mmHg with oxygen supplementation, intubation and mechanical ventilation should be considered.

CASE 16

1 Would you proceed with the dental cleaning procedure? Despite the fact that this dog is apparently healthy, elective surgical procedures should not be performed because of the thrombocytopenia, which can predispose to severe bleeding. Generally, when platelets are below 30–60 × 10^9/l, spontaneous bleeding can occur (epistaxis, gum bleeding, petechiation, melena, etc.), although in some dogs with severe thrombocytopenia bleeding does not occur.

2 What are the most likely differential diagnoses for the thrombocytopenia? Differential diagnoses for thrombocytopenia include decreased production, increased destruction, increased sequestration, and consumption. Typical causes of decreased production are infection (e.g. with *Rickettsia* spp.), neoplasia, or drugs that affect the bone marrow. Increased destruction can result from primary or secondary immune-mediated disease. Infectious causes such as *Ehrlichia* spp., *Anaplasma* spp., and *Babesia* spp. should be excluded as secondary causes of immune-mediated thrombocytopenia, because immunosuppressive therapy can exacerbate disease severity if caused by infection. Splenomegaly can result in sequestration of platelets. Hemorrhage, vasculitis, neoplasia, bone marrow disease, and DIC are less likely in this case on the basis of history, physical examination, and CBC findings.

CASE 17

1 Describe the blood smear findings. The blood smears show morulae within platelets, compatible with *Anaplasma platys*. Other organisms from the Anaplasmataceae family target different blood cells, such as monocytes or granulocytes. Confirmatory tests are recommended because stain precipitates can be mistaken for organisms within platelets.

2 What tests could be performed to confirm the diagnosis? Antibody tests are available for *A. platys*, but dogs with recent infection can be antibody negative, because antibody production occurs 1–2 weeks post infection. Antibodies against *A. platys* cross-react with *Anaplasma phagocytophilum* antigens, so positive antibodies should be reported as those to *Anaplasma* spp. PCR testing is highly sensitive and specific, and can determine the *Anaplasma* spp. involved. However, PCR can be negative if bacteremia is very low at the time of sample collection, because of the cyclic nature of *A. platys* parasitism. Over half of dogs infected with *A. platys* are co-infected with other tick-borne diseases; therefore, testing for other organisms can be considered. Some pathogens, such as *Bartonella* spp. or *Babesia* spp., require specific therapy if detected.

3 Does this dog need specific therapy for this problem? Doxycycline (10 mg/kg PO q24h) for 3–4 weeks is recommended for this dog, even though the optimum duration of the treatment is still unknown. Tick and flea preventives are generally recommended year-round.

CASE 18

1 How would you interpret the gastroscopy picture? Gastroscopy shows an edematous and erythematous gastric mucosa consistent with gastritis.

2 What would be your diagnostic plan? Multiple gastric biopsies should be obtained from the gastric fundus, body, and antrum, as well as from the duodenum and jejunum. Impression smears of the biopsies can allow detection of gastric *Helicobacter*-like organisms (GHLOs), although it can be hard to make an association with disease given that many healthy dogs are colonized by GHLOs. Histopathology, culture of biopsy specimens, and rapid urease testing have also been used to identify the presence of GHLOs. Some species of *Helicobacter* are very fastidious and difficult or impossible to culture.

CASE 19

1 How would you interpret the results? The diagnosis is chronic gastritis associated with GHLOs. In most cases, mixed *Helicobacter* spp. infections are detected and species identification can only be obtained by a combination of electron microscopy, culture, and PCR, which is usually only done on a research basis. GHLOs can be found in many healthy animals and it is unclear under which circumstances they cause disease. The *Helicobacter* species, the amount of bacteria, or the presence of underlying disease might play a role in the development of clinical signs. When severe gastritis is identified on histopathology together with GHLOs, and other treatments have not been successful (e.g. elimination diet for dietary hypersensitivity), specific treatment for helicobacteriosis can be attempted.

2 How should this dog be treated? Protocols used to treat helicobacteriosis in dogs are derived from those used in humans with *Helicobacter pylori* gastritis. Triple-therapy consists of two oral antibiotics (e.g. metronidazole 20 mg/kg PO q12h and amoxicillin 20 mg/kg PO q12h) together with an antacid (such as omeprazole) or bismuth salicylate for 2 weeks. Improvement of the gastritis should ideally be confirmed by repeating endoscopically obtained gastric biopsies, but typically monitoring is done on the basis of clinical signs.

CASE 20

1 What are the most likely differential diagnoses for this dog? In a dog with follicular papules and pustules (indicated by the lesion with the hair shaft emerging from the center), demodicosis, dermatophytosis, and bacterial pyoderma are the most important differential diagnoses.

2 What diagnostic tests should be done immediately? An impression smear and deep skin scrapings are the first tests to be conducted to assess for bacterial pyoderma and demodicosis. If bacteria are sparse or absent on cytology and numerous macrophages are present, and scrapings are negative, a dermatophyte culture or PCR (if available) are the next steps. If humans or other animals in the household are affected, a fungal culture should always be recommended.

CASE 21

1 What questions should the owner be asked before performing further diagnostic tests? A macrophage and many segmented neutrophils with intra- and extracellular cocci are seen on cytology. This is diagnostic for bacterial pyoderma and there typically is an underlying disease that needs to be diagnosed and treated. As the dog is older, the duration of the disease should be ascertained and the owner should be asked whether there have been previous episodes. If this is the first time the dog has had skin or ear problems, then questions should be asked that might identify the possibility of underlying hypothyroidism (e.g. is the dog heat seeking, exercise intolerant, or gaining weight?), hyperadrenocorticism (e.g. is there polyuria/polydipsia or polyphagia or panting?). If however, the dog has had numerous episodes of skin and/or ear problems over many years, hypersensitivity to environmental, flea, or food allergens could be contributing to the disease. This is particularly likely if the dog was pruritic before it developed the lesions. Which of the hypersensitivities is most likely will depend on the history.

2 How should you proceed based on the possible responses from the owner? If flea control in the household is non-existent or sporadic, and if the skin problems seem to have occurred more in the warmer months in temperate climates, good flea control should be the first recommendation. If gastrointestinal signs, such as occasional vomiting or diarrhea, are reported, and the problems have occurred at any time of the year, then adverse food reaction is possible and an elimination diet should be tried for 8 weeks using a previously unfed protein and carbohydrate source. If both flea control and elimination diet do not improve the clinical signs, then environmental allergy is most likely the underlying cause for the pyoderma.

CASE 22

1 What is the likely etiology of the clinical signs? The dog has tetanus. Typical clinical signs of tetanus consist of focal or generalized spasticity following a wound infection with the ubiquitous anaerobic bacterium *Clostridium tetani*. Infections of the paws often are associated with tetanus in dogs, but any contaminated wound favoring anaerobic bacterial growth can be the underlying cause. Clinical signs reflect the action of tetanus toxin in the CNS. The toxin interferes with the release of the neurotransmitters glycine and gamma-aminobutyric acid (GABA) at inhibitory synapses in the CNS. This results in uninhibited muscle contractions and muscle spasms, which worsen with excitement. The clinical signs of tetanus develop typically within 2 weeks (3 days to 3 weeks) following the infection. The time delay between infection and development of the clinical signs is attributed to the fact that the toxin reaches the CNS after uptake in the peripheral nerve terminal by retrograde axonal transport and transsynaptic migration to its specific site of action. Thus, the time until clinical signs of tetanus develop following the wound infection depends on the distance between the wound and the CNS. In this case, the history of a recent nail bed infection and the characteristic clinical signs, including prolapse of the third eyelid, wrinkling of forehead and facial muscles, drawn-back ears, and trismus, suggested tetanus.

2 How would you describe the different clinical stages of this disease, and what is the prognosis? The two forms of tetanus are the generalized and the localized (focal) forms. Generalized tetanus with involvement of the head musculature and generalized spasticity is more common in dogs than in cats. Generalized tetanus is always associated with spasticity of the facial and masticatory muscles and swallowing difficulties. Focal tetanus rarely occurs in dogs. With focal action of the tetanus toxin, signs are limited to the spinal cord segments next to the injury site and spasticity involves only one or two limbs adjacent to the injury. With generalized tetanus, four severity classes have been defined: Class I – facial involvement alone; Class II – generalized rigidity or dysphagia (dysphagia is often caused by trismus, but pharyngeal muscle spasms can also contribute); Class III – recumbency in addition to Class I or Class II signs, often characterized by rigid extension of all limbs, muscle fasciculations, spasms, opisthotonus, and sometimes seizures; Class IV – rigidity accompanied by autonomic dysregulation of heart rate, respiratory rate, and blood pressure. Clinical signs can progress within the first few days as toxin continues to reach the CNS, and also as long as there is continued release of toxin from the wound infection. Progression from one stage to the next can also occur with excitement, pain, and excessive manipulation of the patient. Prognosis depends on the clinical stage, with the worst prognosis associated with Class IV tetanus. Dogs with Class I signs can be managed at home, if a dark, quiet place is provided and if they can swallow and spasms are controlled with sedation with acepromazine, phenobarbital, and methocarbamol as a centrally acting muscle relaxant. However, owners should be aware that treatment of more severe cases can involve intensive care for up to 3–4 weeks. Numerous complications can arise during treatment of Class III and Class IV tetanus. Trismus and pharyngeal and laryngeal muscle spasms impair food and water intake and increase the risk of aspiration pneumonia. Other complications in severely affected animals are respiratory distress, hyperthermia, gastrointestinal ulceration, and multiple organ failure. Chances for recovery and discharge after 28 days range from 50 to 75%.

CASE 23

1 How would you describe the radiographic findings? There is soft tissue swelling and osteolysis of the distal phalanx of the first toe of the affected paw. No foreign body is seen. Radiographic findings are consistent with osteomyelitis.

2 What are your further treatment recommendations? Because of the osteomyelitis, amputation of the digit was recommended in this case in order to remove the infected site and source of continuing toxin production. As the dog underwent general anesthesia for the surgical procedure, placement of a feeding tube was performed in order to ensure nutrition and minimize the risk of aspiration pneumonia. Management with a gastric tube is preferred to parenteral nutrition because dogs with tetanus can be dysphagic for 2–4 weeks, and enterocyte function is best preserved and gastrointestinal ulceration avoided if nutrients are supplied to the gut. The gastric tube can be placed either surgically or with a minimally invasive endoscopic procedure. Endoscopic placement is usually less painful, which can be a consideration in dogs with tetanus. Increased tetanic muscle contractions can occur in the postoperative period due to pain, and so it is important to provide adequate analgesia.

Muscle spasms can be managed successfully with simultaneous continuous infusions of acepromazine (0.01–0.02 mg/kg/h), methocarbamol (10 mg/kg/h), and/or a medetomidine or dexmedetomidine. Additional drugs that should be considered are phenobarbital (2 mg/kg q8h or 3 mg/kg q12h) to suppress any seizure activity and as a baseline for its GABA-enhancing action, and metronidazole (10–15 mg/kg q8h for a minimum of 10 days). Pain medication should include opioids (e.g. a fentanyl CRI, or morphine or buprenorphine q6h).

Intensive care of tetanus also involves placement of a central venous catheter or two peripheral catheters with multiple venous access ports to ensure application of multiple CRIs at the same time. Intensive monitoring should include fluid and caloric in- and output, body temperature, ECG, blood pressure, and detection of potential development of any signs of aspiration pneumonia, respiratory impairment, seizures, or urinary tract infection.

CASE 24

1 Why is the presence of CNS inflammation likely in this case? Multifocal CNS disease commonly results from CNS inflammatory disorders (e.g. encephalitis, meningitis). Other considerations for the presence of multifocal CNS signs would be metabolic diseases, inherited neurodegenerative disorders, CNS trauma, or hemorrhage. Metabolic disease and inherited neurodegenerative disorders tend to result in bilaterally symmetric neurologic signs and not lateralized signs, as in this dog. CNS trauma or hemorrhage were not suggested by the history. CNS inflammation can be of infectious or non-infectious origin. Non-infectious causes of CNS inflammation are very common in dogs and summarized as "meningoencephalitis of unknown origin". Common infectious causes of CNS inflammation are viral infections (e.g. canine distemper, rabies, Aujeszky's disease, eastern equine encephalitis, and West Nile encephalitis limited to certain geographic endemic regions) and protozoal infections (e.g. neosporosis, toxoplasmosis, and rarely leishmaniosis or infection with *Hepatozoon canis*). Neurotropic bacterial infections are not recognized in dogs, but bacterial infections can originate from local extension (e.g. otitis media or interna, sinusitis, bite wounds) and less frequently from hematogenous spread or thromboembolic disease (e.g. infective endocarditis) or be related to severe systemic chronic infections. Fungal infections (e.g. cryptococcosis) and parasitoses (e.g. angiostrongylosis) need to be considered in certain geographic regions and are usually associated with signs of systemic disease. Unremarkable results of a CBC and a biochemistry panel and absence of fever do not exclude the presence of CNS inflammation.

The presence of mild conjunctivitis, respiratory signs, and gastrointestinal signs prior to the development of neurologic disease should raise a strong suspicion for the presence of an infectious cause and is most characteristic of distemper. Canine distemper virus is an enveloped paramyxovirus of the genus *Morbillivirus*. Despite vaccination, it remains an important cause of encephalitis in dogs worldwide. Respiratory and gastrointestinal signs can be mild or absent in some dogs with distemper, and neurologic signs can be the only clinical sign in affected dogs. Canine distemper virus has a predilection for the cerebellar peduncles and, thus, cerebellar signs (which are often asymmetric) and central vestibular disease are frequently observed. However, seizures, other cranial nerve deficits, paraparesis, or tetraparesis can also occur. In surviving dogs, residual neurologic signs can persist throughout life. A specific manifestation is the development of spinal myoclonus as a consequence of distemper virus infection of the CNS. This type of myoclonus is also classified as constant repetitive myoclonus because it persists even during sleep and throughout life. Affected muscle groups show repetitive contractions that can interfere with the ability to stand, walk, or sleep. Rarely, this type of myoclonus has been reported with other infectious CNS diseases. Hyperkeratosis of the footpads and nasal planum, chorioretinitis, and dental and enamel hypoplasia are also consequences of distemper.

2 What diagnostic tests should be performed? In any dog with suspected distemper, ophthalmic examination including a dilated fundoscopic examination should be performed. Distemper can be associated with chorioretinitis or optic neuritis, as well as conjunctivitis, corneal edema, uveitis, and keratoconjunctivitis sicca. CSF analysis typically shows a mild lymphocytic or monocytic pleocytosis. CSF leukocyte counts are often lower than 50–100 WBC/μl, and protein concentration is in the range of 0.3–0.6 g/l. Magnetic resonance imaging is sometimes performed together with CSF analysis in dogs suspected to have CNS inflammatory disorders. Focal areas of T2 and FLAIR hyperintensities as well as loss of the cerebellar gray and white matter junction can be seen. A specific diagnosis of distemper encephalitis is usually obtained through canine distemper virus PCR on CSF. It can be advantageous to submit multiple specimens to enhance sensitivity (e.g. blood, urine, conjunctival swabs) in addition to CSF.

3 **What are the potential diagnostic pitfalls?** When interpreting PCR results for distemper, the possibility of false-positive and false-negative results should always be considered. Distemper virus is a RNA virus that is prone to degradation during transport to the laboratory. In addition, only small amounts of RNA might be present within CSF lymphocytes, therefore, native CSF rather than the centrifuged supernatant is the preferred sample for PCR. Positive PCR results can occur for several weeks after vaccination because vaccines utilize attenuated live virus that replicates in vaccinated dogs. Currently available PCR assays do not differentiate between field and vaccine strains, although some assays can suggest natural infection based on high viral loads. Another diagnostic pitfall is that CSF analysis can be normal in dogs with distemper encephalitis. Owing to the immunosuppression induced by canine distemper virus infection, co-infections, such as with protozoa (e.g. neosporosis, toxoplasmosis), can occur.

4 **What treatment should be initiated?** To date, there is no effective antiviral treatment for distemper. If neurologic signs are evident, they will often progress. Phenobarbital (2.5–3 mg/kg PO q12h) should be started when seizures occur. However, treatment response can be poor and other anticonvulsants might have to be added. Vitamin C and vitamin A supplementation might be advantageous, based on experimental studies in ferrets and observations in humans with measles, but evidence for efficacy in dogs is still poor. Treatment with a short course of glucocorticoids in anti-inflammatory dosages is recommended by some authors in an attempt to modify demyelination and inflammation in the CNS, but evidence to support this regimen is lacking. Therapeutic trials for amelioration of distemper myoclonus with mexiletine or lidocaine have been unrewarding.

CASE 25

1 **What is your interpretation of the radiographs?** The thoracic radiographs reveal consolidation of the right middle lung lobe, most evident on the dorsoventral view. On the right lateral image, a lobar sign is evident but is silhouetted against the cardiac silhouette. Inclusion of a left lateral view would improve visualization of the consolidated right middle lung lobe by increasing aeration of the right lung.

2 **What differential diagnoses are most likely in this animal?** The primary differential diagnosis in this patient is aspiration pneumonia, although other differential diagnoses should be considered that could lead to bronchial obstruction, including

foreign body inhalation, neoplasia, and lung lobe torsion. Fungal disease should also be considered. The absence of pleural effusion makes lung lobe torsion less likely, and the young age of the patient places neoplasia lower on the differential list. Absence of vomiting or regurgitation in the history does not rule out aspiration pneumonia.

3 What additional tests should be performed? A CBC, biochemistry panel, and urinalysis would be indicated to assess the overall health of the animal. CT of the thorax followed by bronchoscopy with or without exploratory surgery may be necessary to establish a diagnosis and determine appropriate treatment. Given the possibility of aspiration pneumonia, a thorough laryngeal examination should be performed on induction of anesthesia to ensure there are no laryngeal abnormalities such as laryngeal paralysis.

CASE 26

1 What findings can be seen on bronchoscopy and on cytologic examination of the bronchoalveolar lavage fluid? The bronchoscopy image reveals foreign material, likely a grass awn, protruding from a bronchus that appears to be obstructed with mucus. Cytology shows an abundance of degenerate neutrophils. Large numbers of bacteria are found extracellularly. These are composed of a mixed population of small cocci (often in pairs or tetrads) and small, short bacilli. Scattered neutrophils appear to contain intracellular bacteria. This is indicative of bronchopneumonia secondary to a foreign body.

2 What additional tests should be submitted on the bronchoalveolar lavage fluid? Aerobic and anaerobic bacterial culture should be requested on the bronchoalveolar lavage fluid. Fungal culture could be considered but fungal infection is rarely found in such cases.

CASE 27

1 What can be seen in the urinary sediment? On this slide, fungal pseudohyphae of *Candida* spp. are visible.

2 How common are fungal urinary tract infections? Fungal urinary tract infections are rare. The most common species causing infection in the urinary tract is *Candida albicans*, but less than 1% of all urinary tract infections are caused by *Candida* spp.

3 What are risk factors for this infection? Urinary tract infections caused by *Candida* spp. are usually associated with a breach in the normal host defenses. Common underlying disorders are endocrinopathies, especially diabetes mellitus, or lower urinary tract diseases such as neoplasia, urolithiasis, or chronic bacterial infections that have been repeatedly treated with antibacterial drugs. Most animals

diagnosed with *Candida* spp. urinary tract infection have received antibacterial medications within the last month preceding the diagnosis.
4 What treatment should be recommended? Either systemic or local therapies can be used. Treatment with oral fluconazole, which concentrates in the urine, for 4–6 weeks is successful in some cases. If this therapy fails (usually because of the presence of large mats of fungus), bladder lavage followed by intravesical infusion of 1% clotrimazole can be performed under anesthesia.

CASE 28

1 What are the differential diagnoses for the petechial lesions? Petechial hemorrhages can be caused by thrombocytopenia or thrombocytopathy. In this case, the petechial lesions were associated with fever. Therefore, an infectious/inflammatory etiology is most likely in this dog. In this region, *Ehrlichia canis*, *Anaplasma platys*, *Leptospira* spp., and *Rickettsia* spp. infections should be considered.
2 What useful information could be obtained from a CBC? A CBC can confirm thrombocytopenia. The mean platelet volume can be increased in dogs with primary or secondary immune-mediated thrombocytopenia. If thrombocytopenia is accompanied by non-regenerative anemia and neutropenia, bone marrow suppression is likely (such as in chronic *E. canis* infection). Evaluation of blood smears can show inclusion bodies in circulating platelets (*A. platys*) or mononuclear cells (*E. canis*).
3 Antibody testing for which infectious diseases would be indicated, and what are the limitations of these assays for establishing a diagnosis? In the acute stage of disease, a single antibody test detecting only IgG antibodies against these pathogens is commonly not diagnostic, because antibodies are only detectable starting from a few days to up to 2 weeks after the onset of clinical signs. Therefore, immediately collected and also convalescent IgG titers (about 2 weeks apart) are needed; a 4-fold increase in titer documents recent infection. In the early stage of infection, blood PCR is sometimes positive and diagnostic in dogs with acute onset of clinical signs (provided laboratory quality assurance is high and false positives resulting from contamination are not occurring).

CASE 29

1 What is the diagnosis? The diagnosis is acute *Ehrlichia canis* and *Anaplasma platys* co-infection. The presence of both infectious agents was also confirmed by blood PCR. Acute *E. canis* infection typically causes a hemostatic disorder, while *A. platys* usually only induces thrombocytopenia with minimal clinical signs. However, co-infections with both agents can worsen the severity of the disease.

2 How should the dog be treated? Doxycycline (10 mg/kg PO q24h or 5 mg/kg PO q12h) is used for both agents and early treatment is associated with a favorable outcome. Treatment should be for 2–4 weeks based on CBC monitoring.

CASE 30

1 What would be the first step to work-up the problem of pale mucous membranes? The two primary rule outs for pale mucous membranes are anemia and shock. Shock is unlikely because of the normal capillary refill time. In addition, the veterinarian had already diagnosed anemia on a previous CBC. The next step would be to obtain a reticulocyte count to differentiate between regenerative and non-regenerative anemia.

2 What infectious disease are American Pitbull Terriers predisposed to, and what is the likely reason for this breed predisposition? American Pitbull Terriers are predisposed to infection with *Babesia gibsoni*, a blood parasite belonging to the small *Babesia* spp. In the USA, American Pitbull Terriers are used for dog fighting. *B. gibsoni* is transmitted through biting and, thus, dogfights are a major mode of transmission. In addition, intrauterine transmission of *B. gibsoni* is possible. Therefore, breeding of American Pitbull Terriers also leads to spread within the breed.

CASE 31

1 If no parasites can be found on a blood smear, what would be the diagnostic test of choice? Molecular diagnosis using PCR is the most sensitive and specific method of detecting infection with *Babesia gibsoni*. Species identification can be performed by DNA sequencing or by the use of species-specific PCR assays.

2 What is the recommended treatment? Atovaquone (13.3 mg/kg PO q8h) and azithromycin (10 mg/kg PO q8h) combination therapy is the most effective treatment for *B. gibsoni* infection. For initial treatment, the two drugs are given for a period of 10 days. Atovaquone should be administered with a meal to maximize intestinal drug absorption. However, many dogs fail to clear *B. gibsoni* infection and clinical relapses can occur. Therefore, two follow-up PCRs, approximately 60 and 90 days after completing therapy, are recommended. An alternative treatment regimen for dogs that fail to respond to atovaquone and azithromycin involves clindamycin, metronidazole, and doxycycline given for at least 3 months. Monotherapy with clindamycin might also improve clinical signs.

CASE 32

1 What is your initial assessment of this case, and what are your differential diagnoses for the dog's problems? The problem list includes exercise intolerance, cough, a thin body condition, as well as hypoalbuminemia. The combination of exercise intolerance and cough in a large breed dog could be due to a cardiac problem, such as dilated cardiomyopathy. However, no arrhythmia or abnormal heart sounds were noted, the pulse quality was normal, and the dry cough made cardiac disease less likely. Pulmonary hypertension is another common cause of respiratory problems and cough, and can also lead to exercise intolerance. Other primary respiratory problems could also cause exercise intolerance due to decreased arterial oxygen saturation. Hypoalbuminemia is a non-specific finding that could be due to decreased production (liver disease), gastrointestinal or urinary loss, loss into body fluids with pleural effusion or ascites, or reactive due to hypergammaglobulinemia.

2 What diagnostic tests would you perform? The next diagnostic step for the problem cough would be thoracic radiographs. A CBC should be performed to assess for anemia as a cause for the exercise intolerance, determine the number of platelets, and look for signs of inflammation/infection. A biochemistry panel would be useful to verify the hypoalbuminemia and to check parameters of liver and kidney function. A urinalysis is also indicated to assess renal function and whether proteinuria is present.

CASE 33

1 What is your interpretation of the radiographs? The radiographs show severely dilated and tortuous pulmonary arteries. This is indicative of pulmonary hypertension, most likely related to heartworm disease.

2 What is your assessment of the laboratory findings? Eosinophilia can be seen with parasitic infection as well as in eosinophilic disorders (e.g. hypereosinophilic syndrome or eosinophilic leukemia), fungal disease, neoplasia (such as mast cell tumors), and hypoadrenocorticism. Hypoalbuminemia is most likely related to loss through the kidneys given the high UPCR. Proteinuria can be classified as preglomerular, glomerular, or post glomerular. Postglomerular proteinuria is unlikely, because the urine sediment shows no evidence of inflammation and hemorrhage. Preglomerular proteinuria caused by multiple myeloma/plasmacytoma is unlikely given the normal total protein concentration. The high UPCR (>5) indicates glomerular disease, most likely glomerulonephritis, but amyloidosis or glomerular sclerosis would be other considerations. A kidney biopsy would be necessary to differentiate these conditions definitively, and would help to disclose the underlying etiology as well as direct therapy. Given that glomerulonephritis is often a secondary complication of infectious, autoimmune, or neoplastic conditions, a diagnostic work-up should be performed to identify any underlying disease.

CASE 34

1 What is your interpretation of the echocardiographic examination? The volume overloaded right ventricle and tricuspid regurgitation of >2.5 m/s indicate pulmonary hypertension, as pulmonic stenosis can be excluded (1.8 m/s is normal). Therefore, a diagnosis of severe pulmonary hypertension can be made in this dog. Pulmonary hypertension can be primary (rare in dogs) or secondary to heartworm disease, *Angiostrongylus vasorum* infection, pulmonary thromboembolism, lung lobe torsion, or severe pulmonary disease.

2 What further tests would you recommend? Heartworm disease is a likely differential because the disease can also be associated with glomerulonephritis. A heartworm antigen test was performed and was positive. A modified Knott test was also performed and microfilaria were detected.

3 What is the likely underlying pathophysiology for proteinuria in this dog? Antigen–antibody complexes, formed in response to heartworm antigens, can cause glomerulonephritis in heartworm-infected dogs. The result is proteinuria, sometimes ultimately leading to renal tubular failure. The bacterium *Wolbachia* is known to infect *Dirofilaria immitis* worms. *Wolbachia* surface proteins have been identified in the glomeruli and lungs of heartworm-infected dogs, and *Wolbachia* are suspected to contribute to the host's inflammatory reaction to worm death. Therefore, the suspected glomerulonephritis in this dog is most likely related to chronic heartworm disease.

4 What is your treatment plan? Given that the dog was diagnosed with severe heartworm infection with microfilaremia, the dog initially received milbemycin monthly for 3 months to kill the microfilaria, and doxycycline (5 mg/kg PO q12h or 10 mg/kg q24h for 30 days) to kill *Wolbachia*. One month after the initial diagnosis, melarsomine (2.5 mg/kg IM) was injected, followed by two additional injections after 1 month (2.5 mg/kg IM q24h). Strict cage rest was advised for 2 months after the start of the first melarsomine injection. Two months after the first melarsomine injection, tricuspid regurgitation was reduced to 3.2 m/s, indicating a reduction of pulmonary hypertension. Six months after the treatment, another antigen test was performed and was negative. Furthermore, the amount of proteinuria had improved and the UPCR was 1.3.

CASE 35

1 What is the diagnosis? The diagnosis is small bowel diarrhea due to giardiasis. The fecal flotation shows *Giardia* spp. cysts. When evaluating diarrhea, one negative zinc sulfate fecal flotation does not definitively rule out giardiasis. Ideally, three flotations should be performed over 3–5 days because the cysts are shed intermittently.

2 If you are not sure about the microscopic interpretation, what additional test(s) could you perform to confirm the diagnosis? Diagnosis of giardiasis can be made by zinc sulfate fecal flotation, *Giardia* spp. antigen test via ELISA, immunofluorescent assays, or PCR. Most commonly used in-house *Giardia* spp. fecal ELISAs are very sensitive and therefore useful to rule out a *Giardia* spp. infection in case of a negative test result. However, these in-house tests have a poor positive predictive value at common prevalence rates in most clinical settings. Therefore, the combination of direct fecal smear, fecal centrifugal flotation, and *Giardia* spp. antigen assay is currently recommended by the Companion Animal Parasite Council. PCR can also be used to detect *Giardia* spp. DNA in feces. However, PCR is only available in a few reference laboratories.

3 Do you think there is a zoonotic risk for the owners and their children? All dogs with idiopathic acute diarrhea or a definitive diagnosis of *Giardia* spp. infection should be potentially considered contagious. Currently, there is little epidemiologic evidence that strongly supports the risk of zoonotic transmission. However, results of studies suggest that a significant proportion of dogs harbor zoonotic *Giardia* spp. Therefore, all animals with diarrhea that test positive for *Giardia* spp. parasites on fecal flotation or antigen test should be treated.

CASE 36

1 What treatment is recommended? Given that *Giardia* spp. cysts are ubiquitous in the environment and that most people and animals will be exposed to cysts without developing clinical signs, subclinically infected people and animals should not be treated for *Giardia* spp. infection. In animals with diarrhea, treatment should be initiated. Fenbendazole (50 mg/kg PO q24h for 5 days) is effective in dogs. Metronidazole (10–15 mg/kg PO q12h for 5–7 days) can be used instead, but metronidazole-resistant strains of *Giardia* spp. exist and efficacy is lower than that of fenbendazole. In addition, high dosages of metronidazole can cause neurologic side effects.

In addition to the definitive treatment, fluid therapy is indicated for this particular dog, and a bland, highly digestible diet should be used until the diarrhea resolves.

2 Is environmental management indicated, and what recommendations should be made to the owner? *Giardia* spp. cysts can persist in the environment for several months if conditions are wet and cold. Environmental decontamination is essential for successful treatment of *Giardia* spp. infection. Animals ingesting cysts from the environment or their own hair coats can reinfect themselves and shed cysts within 5 days after their most recent drug treatment.

Environmental management should consist of the following:

- Treat all animals with drug therapy as described above and move them out of the environment to a holding area.
- Clean organic debris from all surfaces and potential fomites in the environment.
- Disinfect surfaces and potential fomites in the environment using a quaternary ammonium compound according to manufacturer's instructions.
- Bathe all animals with a general pet shampoo, taking care to remove all fecal material from the hair coat and perineum.
- After shampooing, bathe animals again with a quaternary ammonium compound (particularly the perineum). Do not leave quaternary ammonium compounds on animals for longer than 3–5 minutes. Rinse thoroughly.
- Return animals to the disinfected environment after bathing.

CASE 37

1 How common is canine herpesvirus infection, and how is it transmitted? Canine herpesvirus occurs worldwide. Only canids (dogs, wolves, coyotes) are susceptible. Antibody prevalence in the dog population varies from 20% to nearly 100% depending on the population studied. Transmission usually occurs because of contact with oral, nasal, or vaginal secretions from infected dogs. Most dogs that shed the virus do not show clinical signs. Pregnant bitches without specific immunity are at risk of infection, which can be transmitted to the fetuses or to neonatal puppies. Previously infected bitches are unlikely to transmit infection. The most significant systemic disease occurs in fetuses or neonatal puppies as a result of *in-utero* infection or infection within the first 3 weeks of life. After this time, age-related resistance to infection develops as puppies mature and are able to maintain a higher body temperature.

2 What clinical signs occur after infection? Canine herpesvirus can cause severe disease in puppies, often with a mortality of 100% in affected litters. If bitches are acutely infected during pregnancy, they can abort a litter or deliver a partially stillborn litter, but they usually do not show other clinical signs. If older dogs are infected, they can develop a mild rhinitis, conjunctivitis, and/or ocular dendritic ulcers, which can be part of the canine infectious respiratory disease complex. Sometimes adult dogs can develop a vesicular vaginitis or posthitis. Once a dog is infected, it will develop a lifelong latent infection.

CASE 38

1 What are your primary differential diagnoses for PU/PD in this dog? Before the results of laboratory testing were available, the differential diagnoses for

PU/PD in this dog that should have been considered are chronic kidney disease, hyperadrenocorticism, hypercalcemia (including hypercalcemia of malignancy), diabetes mellitus, and diabetes insipidus. Bacterial pyelonephritis can be associated with PU/PD even in the absence of renal failure, because bacterial endotoxins can lead to a secondary nephrogenic diabetes insipidus. Endotoxin competes with antidiuretic hormone for binding sites on the tubules, leading to decreased resorption of water.

2 **How would you interpret the laboratory results?** The detection of increased serum creatinine concentration together with a urine specific gravity of 1.018 indicates renal azotemia. However, bacterial pyelonephritis could also be contributing to the low specific gravity, and there could also be a prerenal component to the azotemia given the high albumin concentration, making dehydration likely.

3 **How common are bacterial urinary tract infections in dogs?** It has been estimated that about 14% of dogs have a urinary tract infection during their lifetime. Older female dogs are predisposed. The presence of pathogenic bacteria together with a breach of the normal host defense mechanisms are required for infection of the lower urinary tract to become established. Host defense mechanisms include normal micturation, normal anatomic structures, an intact mucosal defense barrier, and antimicrobial properties of the urine (e.g. high or low pH).

4 **What are the most common bacteria causing urinary tract disease in dogs?** By far the most common bacterial species found in urinary tract infections is *Escherichia coli*. Other bacterial pathogens that are frequently detected include *Enterococcus* spp., *Staphylococcus* spp., *Proteus* spp., *Klebsiella* spp., *Pseudomonas* spp., and *Enterobacter* spp.

5 **How would you treat this dog?** Treatment is indicated in this dog given the likelihood of pyelonephritis. The choice of antimicrobial agent should be based on the results of susceptibility testing. While awaiting culture results, use of a fluoroquinolone would be an appropriate choice for treatment of pyelonephritis. Data regarding the correct duration of antimicrobial treatment are lacking. In the past, treatment for 4 weeks has been recommended for pyelonephritis, but shorter treatments (10–14 days) are likely to be effective.

CASE 39

1 **How would you interpret the CBC?** The CBC shows leukocytosis characterized by mature neutrophilia and monocytosis.

2 **What imaging abnormalities are present in the radiograph?** Moderate hilar lymphadenopathy is present along with interstitial infiltrates located primarily in the hilar region. Mild caudodorsal interstitial infiltrates are also present.

3 **What differential diagnoses should be considered?** Interstitial lung disease with hilar lymphadenopathy in a young dog in an endemic area is most consistent

with fungal pneumonia or pulmonary lymphoma. Actinomycosis or nocardiosis should also be considered. Given the travel history to Arizona, coccidioidomycosis would be highest on the list for this dog, followed by histoplasmosis.

4 What other diagnostic tests should be performed? A biochemistry panel and urinalysis are indicated to assess the overall health of the animal. A positive coccidioidomycosis antibody titer in conjunction with typical clinical signs is suggestive of this infection. Histoplasmosis urine antigen testing could also be considered. If these tests did not provide a diagnosis, bronchoscopy with bronchoalveolar lavage would be indicated. In this case, the histoplasmosis urine antigen test was positive, making histoplasmosis very likely in the dog. Although this test cross-reacts with *Blastomyces* antigen, blastomycosis was considered very unlikely on the basis of the dog's travel history.

CASE 40

1 How would you interpret the CBC results and radiographs? The thoracic radiographs reveal an alveolar pattern affecting the dependent portions of the cranial and middle lung lobes, suggestive of bronchopneumonia. The CBC, with a neutrophilic leukocytosis with a mild left shift and monocytosis, supports the possibility of bacterial infection.

2 Which differential diagnoses are highest on your list? The radiographic infiltrates in this dog could be related to pneumonia (infectious, aspiration, or foreign body inhalation), hemorrhage, or neoplasia. Fungal infection would be less likely given the distribution of the alveolar pattern and lack of hilar lymphadenopathy.

CASE 41

1 What tests would you recommend on this fluid? Given the likely presence of pus in the fluid, aerobic bacterial, anaerobic bacterial, and *Mycoplasma* spp. cultures should ideally be performed. Although the dog was recently treated with amoxicillin, any resistant bacteria should still be identifiable on culture. Cytologic examination of the bronchoalveolar lavage specimem should also be performed to identify the inflammatory infiltrate and look for intracellular bacteria. Cytology revealed a purulent exudate, and pure culture of *Mycoplasma* spp. was recovered. DNA sequencing of the isolate revealed *Mycoplasma cynos*. Given the fastidious nature of mycoplasmas, they might not remain viable when specimens are sent to laboratories by mail. Therefore, an alternative for veterinarians in private practice would be to request PCR for mycoplasmas (and other respiratory viruses and bacteria) on the bronchoalveolar lavage specimen. Because *M. cynos* appears to be more pathogenic than other airway mycoplasmas, use of a laboratory that offers a specific PCR assay for *M. cynos* (and differentiates it from other mycoplasmas) is recommended. The possibility of concurrent viral infection in this dog cannot be excluded based on the results of the bronchoalveolar lavage.

2 What underlying diseases should be considered? In adult animals with pneumonia, a search should be performed for predisposing systemic or respiratory conditions. In an adult, large-breed dog, the most common underlying diseases are foreign body inhalation and aspiration pneumonia, often associated with laryngeal dysfunction. Underlying immunosuppression due to diabetes mellitus or Cushing's disease should also be considered. In younger animals, exposure to viruses (canine distemper virus, adenovirus, parainfluenza virus, or respiratory coronavirus) can predispose to secondary bacterial pneumonia. In adult dogs, infection with canine influenza virus or canine herpesvirus can also facilitate development of bacterial pneumonia. Given the history of multiple animals affected and exposure to multiple new animals in the household, whole blood was submitted for canine distemper virus PCR and was positive. While false-negative tests are common, a positive test is supportive of infection. It was suspected that the vaccines purchased from the local supply store might have been improperly stored or administered, resulting in lack of protection from distemper.

CASE 42

1 What is your ECG diagnosis? At the beginning of the strip, the ECG shows wide and bizarre looking complexes. At the end of the ECG strip, there is a sinus rhythm. The wide complexes are of ventricular origin, so one could think that this would resemble a ventricular tachycardia. However, because the rate of the ventricular complexes is relatively slow (about 130/min), the correct term for this rhythm is an accelerated idioventricular rhythm. Accelerated idioventricular rhythm is a ventricular rhythm with a rate between 60 and 160/min, which places it between idioventricular (i.e. ventricular escape) rhythms (<60 bpm) and true ventricular tachycardia in terms of rate. Accelerated rhythms can be seen with almost any severe systemic diseases, such as gastric dilatation–volvulus, sepsis, pancreatitis, or pain.

2 How would you treat the ECG abnormality? This dog does not need antiarrhythmic therapy. Treatment of the underlying disease will abolish the arrhythmia. In this case, ultimately blood cultures revealed growth of a *Staphylococcus* sp., and bacteremia explained the ECG changes and the fever. The dog was treated with antimicrobial drugs, selected on the basis of susceptibility test results. The fever resolved 24 hours after initiating antimicrobial drug therapy, and a recheck ECG performed 3 days later revealed no more abnormalities.

CASE 43

1 What is the most likely diagnosis? Given that there was no history of trauma and the puppy otherwise appeared well, the most probable reason for the clinical signs was an infection with human mumps virus (a paramyxovirus). This virus causes a common disease in children, and is widespread in many regions of the world. Even in countries where vaccination is performed, mumps outbreaks still occur. Although humans are primary natural hosts of the mumps virus, other animal species can be experimentally infected. On rare occasions, puppies (and kittens) can develop a similar disease following close contact with infected humans. There are a few reports of parotid gland enlargement in dogs from households in which children had suffered concurrently or recently from mumps.

2 What diagnostic tests could be considered? Recent exposure of the puppy to a child with mumps makes this diagnosis likely. However, in humans, an estimated 20–25% of infections are asymptomatic and, in sick individuals, only 30–40% have the typical acute parotiditis while the others show respiratory or non-specific symptoms. Thus, a healthy human can also be a source of infection. In human medicine, several laboratory techniques are used to confirm mumps, although in many cases the diagnosis is based on typical clinical signs only. In veterinary medicine, this disease is very rare, and the diagnosis is made on the basis of history and typical clinical signs (salivary gland enlargement, normal mentation or mild lethargy, and a self-limiting course of the disease).

3 What is the prognosis? The prognosis is good, because mumps is usually a self-limiting disease that resolves within 1–2 weeks.

CASE 44

1 What are the possible differential diagnoses? Enlargement of the salivary gland can occur after trauma or foreign body penetration. However, in this case, there were no signs of injury or fistula suggesting such a condition and the problem was bilateral. Infection with canine distemper virus would also be a possibility. However, there were no other signs of distemper in this patient, and PCR for canine distemper virus and was negative. Idiopathic sialoadenitis and phenobarbital-responsive sialoadenosis have also been reported and can be bilateral, but these conditions occur in adult dogs and therefore would be unlikely in a 3-week-old puppy without any other clinical signs.

2 What treatment is needed? Mumps in children is usually a mild, self-limiting disease and only supportive care is indicated (warm or cold packs to the swollen salivary gland region, and in some patients analgesics). As the puppy was otherwise well, observation only was indicated. The parotid enlargement persisted for 7 days. During that time the dog's appetite, growth rate, and behavior were normal and similar to those of its littermates. No other puppy in the litter became sick.

3 What complications can develop in the course of mumps in dogs? In humans, mumps is usually a mild disease that involves the parotid gland. However, the virus also replicates in other organs, which on rare occasions can result in orchitis, meningitis, or encephalitis, and less frequently in a systemic inflammatory disease. Meningoencephalitis caused by mumps virus has been described in dogs, in some cases without parotid gland enlargement. Experimental infection in cats resulted in parotiditis and orchitis.

4 Can a dog suffering from mumps transfer this infection to humans or other animals? In humans, mumps is usually transmitted by the airborne route, because the virus is shed in saliva. Sporadic disease in dogs is thought to result from transmission from humans, usually as a result of close contact with affected children. There are no reports of transmission from one animal to another or from animals to humans, although the saliva of sick dogs does contain mumps virus.

CASE 45

1 What is your ocular diagnosis? The ocular diagnosis is a descemetocele with mild anterior uveitis in the right eye. Descemet's membrane is a hydrophobic structure and does not take up fluorescein stain (which is hydrophilic).

2 What diagnosis of the eyelid lesions might you suspect based on the clinical presentation? The age of the dog and clinical presentation are suggestive of papillomatosis. Papillomas are benign lesions caused by papillomaviruses and are most frequently seen in younger dogs. Cutaneous papillomatosis is most commonly observed, but ocular papillomas occur occasionally. The lesions usually regress spontaneously over time; however, if they cause other problems (as seen in this dog), removal is advised. Surgical excision, cryotherapy, or laser surgery are suitable options.

3 What treatment do you suggest for this dog? In this patient, the papillomas were removed with cryotherapy (liquid nitrogen) and the corneal ulcer was treated with a grafting procedure (pedicle conjunctival graft). The postoperative ocular treatment consisted of antibiotic drops and atropine.

CASE 46

1 What are the differential diagnoses for acute hemorrhagic diarrhea, and what diagnostic tests would you perform? First, gastrointestinal bleeding due to coagulation disorders has to be considered (e.g. by evaluating clotting times, platelet count). Extraintestinal disorders causing acute diarrhea (e.g. hypoadrenocorticism, renal and liver failure) may be less likely based on history (e.g. intoxication) and the results of physical examination, hematology, biochemistry panel, and urinalysis. Hemorrhagic diarrhea caused by infectious agents, including parasites, has to be considered in young and immunocompromised dogs, in diarrhea outbreaks occurring in multiple animals, and in patients with concurrent evidence of sepsis. In these cases, fecal examinations (e.g. flotation, *Giardia* spp. antigen ELISA) and blood cultures should be performed. Parvovirus infection is suspected in patients (especially in young and unvaccinated animals) with sudden onset of vomiting and hemorrhagic diarrhea, especially dogs with concurrent neutropenia. Fecal ELISA for parvovirus antigen is regarded as a very specific, but only moderately sensitive, diagnostic test. Therefore, PCR for diagnosis of parvovirus infection could also be considered.

2 What is the definition of hemorrhagic gastroenteritis syndrome? A presumptive diagnosis of a "hemorrhagic gastroenteritis syndrome" can be made based on typical clinical findings associated with an increased hematocrit (usually >0.5–0.55 l/l) and a rapid clinical improvement with adequate fluid therapy. However, diagnosis of hemorrhagic gastroenteritis syndrome is mainly based on exclusion of other diseases known to cause acute hemorrhagic diarrhea.

3 Which dogs are predisposed to hemorrhagic gastroenteritis syndrome? In several studies, it has been shown that young to middle-aged dogs of small breeds (e.g. Yorkshire Terrier, Miniature Pinscher, and Miniature Schnauzer) are more commonly affected with "hemorrhagic gastroenteritis syndrome".

CASE 47

1 What information from the history is important for interpretation of the fecal culture? The owner reported that the dog was on a raw meat diet. The prevalence of *Salmonella* spp. in feces of healthy dogs has been reported to be between 0 and 3.6%. However, the prevalence was shown to be much higher in dogs that are fed raw food diets, and *Salmonella* spp. were isolated from 30% of fecal samples in Greyhounds fed raw chicken diets and from 69% of fecal samples in healthy Alaskan sled dogs. This indicates that the mere isolation of *Salmonella* spp. from feces is insufficient to make a diagnosis of *Salmonella* spp.-induced enteritis.

2 What bacterial species are currently considered primary enteropathogenic bacteria? *Clostridium difficile*, *Clostridium perfringens*, *Campylobacter* spp., *Salmonella* spp., and *Escherichia coli* (associated with granulomatous colitis in Boxer dogs) are included in the list of potential primary enteropathogenic bacteria.

3 Which bacterial species is believed to play a primary role in dogs with hemorrhagic gastroenteritis syndrome? To date, the etiology of this syndrome is not fully understood, but there is evidence that *Clostridium* spp. and their toxins might be involved in the disease process. In necropsy reports of dogs with hemorrhagic gastroenteritis syndrome, the adherence of large gram-positive bacilli, identified as *Clostridium perfringens*, to the necrotic mucosal surfaces of the intestinal tract was described. Since these histologic evaluations had been performed post mortem, interpretation of these abnormal findings is difficult. However, a recent study reported similar findings in intestinal biopsy samples prospectively collected antemortem. *Clostridium* spp., identified by culture as *C. perfringens* in most cases, were detected on the small intestinal mucosa in all dogs with hemorrhagic gastroenteritis syndrome, but not in any control dogs.

CASE 48

1 Why is fluid therapy considered life saving in this case? Given the rapid and intense loss of fluid into the gut lumen, dogs with hemorrhagic gastroenteritis syndrome are frequently severely dehydrated. This dog showed signs of severe dehydration, with tachycardia, pale mucous membranes, and prolonged capillary refill time. Therefore, a volume of fluid sufficient to stabilize these cardiovascular parameters is considered the most important life-saving treatment.

Hypothermia, tachycardia, and tachypnea are criteria for sepsis as well as for hypovolemic shock. Therefore, it is important to identify those few patients with hemorrhagic gastroenteritis syndrome that would benefit from early antibiotic therapy. In dehydrated patients, parameters that are not typically associated with hypovolemia, such as hyperthermia, leukocytosis, and left shift, should be evaluated to identify septic patients.

2 How much fluid would you give over the first 24 hours? In this dog, 6 liters of crystalloid solutions should be administered over the first 24 hours. This is calculated as follows:

- **Hydration deficit (replacement requirement):**
  body weight (kg) × % dehydration as a decimal = deficit in liters: **3,000 ml**
- **Maintenance requirement (40–60 ml/kg/day)** **1,500 ml**
- **Ongoing losses (e.g. vomiting, diarrhea, polyuria)** **1,500 ml**

This amount of fluid should be divided into three aliquots and be given very rapidly, with reassessment of the clinical status of the patient after administration of each aliquot.

3 Would you treat this dog with antibiotics? A recently published study showed that in dogs with aseptic hemorrhagic gastroenteritis syndrome, antibiotics do not change the outcome or shorten the time to recovery, and septic events seem to be rare in dogs with hemorrhagic gastroenteritis syndrome. Inappropriate use of antibiotics can also promote risk of antimicrobial resistance and unnecessary adverse drug reactions. Therefore, antimicrobial administration is not recommended as routine treatment in dogs with hemorrhagic gastroenteritis syndrome. However, ruling out an enteropathogenic bacterial infection can be challenging and bacterial translocation is a potentially life-threatening complication; therefore, dogs with acute hemorrhagic diarrhea of unknown cause that are not treated with antibiotics should be monitored very closely.

CASE 49

1 What ophthalmic findings are present? There is epiphora and blepharospasm in both eyes, and the dog has diffuse corneal edema. Glaucoma and buphthalmia are present in the left eye, with congested scleral and episcleral vessels. The cornea has 360-degree deep neovascularization close to the limbus, which is a typical finding in anterior uveitis. The pupil in the left eye is dilated and non-responsive. The iris is swollen and hyperemic. The posterior segment cannot be evaluated in either eye.

2 What further diagnostic tests would you suggest? Ocular ultrasound would be helpful in evaluating the intraocular structures, which cannot be examined otherwise because of the profound corneal edema.

CASE 50

1 What is the diagnosis? The ocular ultrasound revealed complete retinal detachment (which was present bilaterally) with subretinal hyperechoic mass-like infiltrates, suggestive of fungal granulomatous lesions. Cytologic examination of the lymph node aspirate revealed yeast organisms that were recognized by their thick wall, lack of capsule, and broad-based budding. Other diagnostic tests that could be performed are histopathology of lymph node biopsies and fungal culture. PCR and antibody/antigen tests for infectious diseases can be helpful if yeast organisms cannot be found on aspirates.

The clinical signs are highly suggestive of blastomycosis, which is a systemic mycotic infection caused by a dimorphic fungus (*Blastomyces dermatitidis*). The organism is a thick-walled yeast that reproduces by budding in infected tissues (yeast phase). In nature, it is most likely a soil saprophyte, which produces infective spores (conidia). Infection occurs through inhalation from the environment, and sporting dogs and dogs living near water are at increased risk of blastomycosis. A primary infection is established in the lungs and eventually disseminates throughout the body, with the preferred sites being the skin, eyes, bones, lymph nodes, subcutaneous tissue, external nares, brain, and testes. Ocular involvement is common and has been reported to occur in up to 50% of cases. Anterior uveitis, panophthalmitis, secondary glaucoma, subretinal granulomas, and retinal detachment are most commonly reported.

2 What treatment would you suggest? Oral itraconazole (5 mg/kg q12h for at least 60 days) is currently considered the treatment of choice for blastomycosis. In one study, up to 80% of dogs were successfully treated.
3 What is the prognosis for vision in this dog? The prognosis for vision is guarded in dogs with anterior uveitis and glaucoma, and enucleation of painful blind eyes is recommended. However, the eyes of dogs with posterior segment involvement can recover with appropriate treatment.

CASE 51

1 What are the differential diagnoses for the problems identified? Cough can be of respiratory or cardiac origin. The nature of the cough and lack of signs of heart failure on physical examination (such as tachycardia, delayed capillary refill times, and poor pulse quality) made cardiac disease less likely in this case. Respiratory abnormalities can be localized to the upper or the lower respiratory tract. In this dog, there were no signs of upper respiratory disease (such as stridor), but increased lung sounds over the lung field suggested the possibility of lower respiratory tract disease. The cutaneous ecchymoses could be traumatic or secondary to a coagulation disorder. The latter was suspected because there was no history of trauma. Coagulation disorders can result from defects of primary hemostasis (vasculopathy, thrombocytopenia, thrombocytopathy) or secondary hemostasis (lack of coagulation factors).
2 What diagnostic tests would you perform? Thoracic radiographs are indicated for further work-up of the cough. In addition, a CBC should be performed to evaluate for anemia and thrombocytopenia, as well as signs of infection or inflammation in the leukogram. Serum biochemistry and urinalysis should be performed to evaluate liver function (production of coagulation factors) and to assess for evidence of other systemic disorders that might contribute to coagulopathy. In addition, a coagulation profile should be performed. In heartworm endemic regions or dogs with a travel history to those regions, a heartworm antigen test would also be indicated.

CASE 52

1 What is your assessment of the diagnostic test results? The thoracic radiographs reveal a severe bronchointerstitial lung pattern with micronodular infiltrates. This could be seen with neoplasia, infectious diseases (especially fungal or parasitic diseases), or inflammatory disorders such as eosinophilic bronchopneumopathy. The peripheral eosinophilia could be seen with parasitic infection as well as in hypersensitivity disorders and is commonly found in dogs with eosinophilic bronchopneumopathy. The combination of increased PT and aPTT and increased D-dimers suggests consumption of coagulation factors due to DIC. The two pulmonary diseases that are most likely to be associated with coagulation abnormalities in dogs from this region are infection with the parasite *Angiostrongylus vasorum* and a neoplastic process.

2 What additional diagnostic work-up would you suggest? Diagnosis of *A. vasorum* infection requires collection of a fecal specimen on three consecutive days for analysis using the Baermann technique. Alternatively, larvae sometimes can be detected microscopically in bronchoalveolar lavage fluid. Measurement of antigen using ELISA on serum and detection of the organism in whole blood using real-time PCR can also be used for diagnosis. If there is no evidence of infection with either of these diagnostic methods, diagnosis should focus on neoplastic disease (usually through bronchoalveolar lavage or fine needle aspiration of the lung). Given the presence of a micronodular lung pattern, which suggests metastatic neoplasia, a search for a primary tumor in another location would also be indicated.

CASE 53

1 What treatment would you suggest for this dog? In this dog, treatment should first stabilize the patient and then address the infection. For stabilization, the dog received intravenous fluids and two units of fresh frozen plasma for replenishment of coagulation factors. Three drugs can be used for treatment of canine angiostrongylosis: milbemycin oxime, moxidectin, or fenbendazole. The advantage of milbemycin oxime and moxidectin is that they can be administered less frequently than fenbendazole. However, in a study on naturally infected dogs, fenbendazole was as effective as moxidectin combined with imidacloprid. In the case described here, the dog was treated with fenbendazole (50 mg/kg PO for 14 days) (recommended dose: 25–50 mg/kg PO q24h for 7–21 days).

2 What should you recommend to the owner to prevent reinfection? To prevent recurrent infection in dogs living in endemic areas, owners should prevent their dogs from eating snails and slugs, which act as intermediate hosts for *A. vasorum*. Treatment in the prepatent period with milbemycin oxime or moxidectin can decrease the establishment of adult parasites and therefore can be recommended as prophylaxis for dogs that reside in endemic areas.

CASE 54

1 What is the most likely diagnosis? Given the signs of mild nasal depigmentation on the right side, aspergillosis should be highest on the differential diagnoses list.

The depigmentation is thought to result from production of a dermonecrotic toxin that destroys pigment along the drainage path of the fungus. It occurs in approximately 40% of dogs with nasal aspergillosis.
2 What physical examination features would be expected in this dog? Nasal aspergillosis is associated with turbinate destruction in dogs and it should be anticipated that nasal airflow will be preserved bilaterally or there could be increased nasal airflow on the affected side. Ocular retropulsion and soft palate palpation should be normal because there is no mass effect in the nasal cavity. The dog could exhibit pain on palpation of the muzzle or the frontal sinus region. Ipsilateral lymphadenopathy might be present, although aspiration cytology of the draining node would typically reveal a reactive population of lymphocytes and plasma cells with absence of organisms.

CASE 55

1 What is the most likely diagnosis? These exophytic warts are typical of canine oral papillomatosis. Papillomaviruses (family Papillomaviridae) infect keratinizing epithelia and mucous membranes. They cause no lysis of the cells but can induce proliferative disorders. At least nine types of canine papillomavirus have been identified, in association with exophytic warts (such as in canine oral papillomatosis), endophytic (inverted) warts, pigmented plaques (common in Pugs), and, in some cases, squamous cell carcinomas. Canine papillomavirus-1 often induces a subclinical infection, but sometimes it can cause oral papillomatosis. Single or multiple verrucous lesions develop, typically located on the oral mucosa and on the mucocutaneous junctions. Less frequently, the eyelids can be affected. In some cases, the warts spread to the esophageal mucosa, perioral haired skin, and even other cutaneous sites. Such severe and/or recurrent lesions are usually associated with defects in host immunity.
2 Are there other differential diagnoses? The clinical presentation of canine oral papillomatosis is so typical that hardly any disease looks similar. When cauliflower-like lesions are identified on the oral mucosa of a young dog (<2 years old) with no other abnormalities, canine oral papillomatosis is extremely likely.
3 How can the diagnosis be confirmed? Usually no other tests are necessary. If the identity of the lesions is unclear, excisional biopsies, which include some adjacent normal tissue, can be submitted for histopathology. This typically reveals hyperplasia of the epidermis with extensive orthokeratotic hyperkeratosis. Typical features are clumped keratohyalin granules in the stratum spinosum, koilocytes (keratinocytes with swollen, clear cytoplasm and a pyknotic nucleus), clear cells (keratinocytes with swollen, blue–gray cytoplasm and enlarged nuclei), and in some cases intranuclear inclusion bodies. Immunohistochemistry has also been used to confirm the diagnosis. PCR has been established for the detection of viral DNA

in biopsy or cytobrush samples. However, papillomavirus DNA can be found in the skin of many healthy dogs; therefore, interpretation of the PCR results can be difficult.

CASE 56

1 What is the prognosis? In young dogs, the prognosis is usually good, because canine oral papillomatosis is typically a self-limiting disease.

2 What treatment is indicated? In immunocompetent animals, spontaneous wart regression usually occurs within 4–8 weeks, so no treatment is needed. After recovery, the dogs are immune to subsequent infections. Immunosuppressed animals of any age can suffer from recurrent or persistent disease. If the warts do not disappear or cause reluctance to eat, airway obstruction, or hemorrhage due to their size or location, surgical removal by excision, cryosurgery, or electrosurgery can be performed. However, surgery has the potential to lead to a higher rate of recurrence. Treatment with autogenous vaccines (a homogenate of fresh warts inactivated with formalin) has been performed in the past, but data confirming efficacy of this procedure are lacking. Similarly, treatment with interferon or immunomodulators, and recently with azithromycin or taurolidine, has been suggested, but the outcome of these treatments remains unclear. Any reports of effective treatment without a placebo control group should be reviewed with caution, because self-regression is difficult to distinguish from therapeutic effect.

3 Can dogs be vaccinated against oral papillomatosis? Many decades ago, a vaccine containing inactivated virus in crude wart extract was demonstrated to be effective for prevention of canine oral papillomatosis, and was used to protect against the disease or to facilitate recovery. More recently, an experimental subunit vaccine containing immunogenic proteins of canine papillomavirus-1 and a DNA vaccine have been shown to induce both humoral and cellular immunity. A recombinant adenoviral vaccine expressing canine papillomavirus antigens was also shown to prevent or reduce disease burden in dogs after challenge. However, no canine papillomavirus vaccine is currently available commercially.

CASE 57

1 Can this dog spread the disease to other dogs? Infective virions occur in the upper stratum granulosum and stratum corneum and are probably released during normal death of cells in these layers. This is the suggested mechanism of transmission. Occasionally, mass outbreaks have been observed in dog colonies. However, on most occasions, the disease is sporadic. Papillomaviruses establish persistent infection of the squamous epithelium, but only in dividing cells. This means they must be introduced into the basal cell layer, which is normally protected by many layers of keratinocytes. Thus, it is believed that trauma is required to the skin before papillomaviruses can infect a new host. Even if this happens, many dogs remain subclinically infected, because about 50% of apparently healthy dogs harbor the DNA of papillomaviruses within clinically normal skin. The risk of disease after papillomavirus infection is higher in immunocompromised dogs (severe combined immunodeficiency, chronic canine monocytic ehrlichiosis, or dogs on glucocorticoids or cyclosporine).

2 Are other animals and humans at risk of becoming infected? To date almost 200 distinct types of papillomavirus have been recognized. They are extremely host species-specific viruses, therefore crossing of the species barrier is a very rare event. Canine papillomaviruses do not appear to infect humans.

CASE 58

1 What further diagnostic tests should be performed? Common causes of lymphohistiocytic pleocytosis in the CSF are viral or protozoal encephalitis and meningoencephalitis of unknown origin. The most frequent viral encephalitis in dogs is canine distemper. There are few reports of other viral encephalitides (rabies, Aujeszky's disease, arbovirus infections restricted to certain geographic regions), and the clinical course in these is usually acute and rapidly progressive. The most frequent protozoal encephalitides in dogs are neosporosis and toxoplasmosis. Other CNS infections that can result in a lymphohistiocytic pleocytosis are ehrlichiosis, hepatozoonosis (caused by *Hepatozoon canis*), fungal infections in certain geographic regions (e.g. cryptococcosis, blastomycosis, coccidioidomycosis), and protothecosis. Neoplastic diseases, such as lymphoma, should also be considered. Diagnostic testing should include assays for canine distemper virus infection, neosporosis, and toxoplasmosis. These pathogens can sometimes be detected in CSF using PCR assays. For distemper, conjunctival scrapings, blood, and urine can alternatively be used for PCR. PCR should be performed on non-centrifuged CSF to increase sensitivity. Concurrent use of antibody testing can be useful to support results of other assays, but positive antibody test results do not prove active infection.

2 What treatment should be started while results of diagnostic tests are pending? Treatment for suspected neosporosis should be initiated while diagnostic results are pending. Chronic cerebellitis with cerebellar atrophy and lymphohistiocytic pleocytosis in the CSF has been reported as a manifestation of neosporosis in adult dogs. Other manifestations of neosporosis are polyradiculoneuritis in young dogs, and myositis, encephalitis, and myelitis in adult dogs with clinical signs of ascending paralysis and cerebellar disease. Polyradiculoneuritis in young dogs results in characteristic rigid extension of the pelvic limbs and arthrogryposis due to development of muscle contracture during skeletal growth. Commonly used drugs for treatment of neosporosis are clindamycin (15 mg/kg PO q12h) or a trimethoprim/sulfonamide combination (15–20 mg/kg PO q12h) for a minimum duration of 6 weeks (up to 3–4 months). Trimethoprim/sulfonamides might be more effective for treatment of CNS infections than clindamycin because they cross the blood–brain barrier more effectively. Folinic acid should be added if long-term treatment with trimethoprim is prescribed.

3 Why might glucocorticoids be contraindicated for treatment of this disease? *Neospora caninum* cysts persist lifelong in the tissues, mostly in muscle and the CNS. Defects in cell-mediated immunity and immunosuppression appear to be associated with the development of clinical disease. Thus, use of glucocorticoids in immunosuppressive dosages is contraindicated in any dog with suspected neosporosis because it can negatively influence the chance of resolution of the clinical signs.

CASE 59

1 How would you initially manage this case? The first priority for this dog is to provide supplemental oxygen using an oxygen cage or mask, and then evaluate the cardiac arrhythmia to determine whether it is life-threatening and needs to be treated. Acute respiratory distress and cough in dogs result from disease of the upper or lower airway, or can be of cardiac origin. Radiographs are therefore recommended in this case as soon as the dog is more stable, to help localize the cause.

2 The client is concerned about costs; therefore, what diagnostic tests would you perform? At a minimum, three-view thoracic radiographs and an ECG should be recommended as initial diagnostics. Echocardiography might be required depending on these findings. A CBC, biochemical profile, and urinalysis should also be recommended to evaluate the dog's general health status.

3 What are the primary differential diagnoses for the problems? Based on the signalment, history, and physical examination findings, the most likely cause of respiratory distress is pulmonary parenchymal disease (e.g. pulmonary edema, pneumonia) or vascular disease (thromboembolism, lung lobe torsion). A right-sided apical heart murmur would not be expected to be caused by a disease that would result in cardiogenic pulmonary edema, but further diagnostics are required to determine the relationship between the abnormal cardiovascular findings and the respiratory signs. Pale mucous membranes could be a sign of poor perfusion, but must be differentiated from anemia.

CASE 60

1 Describe the thoracic radiographic findings. The thoracic radiographs show right-sided cardiomegaly with a mixed interstitial–alveolar lung pattern in the caudodorsal lung lobes. The pulmonary arteries are enlarged and tortuous.

2 How do these findings affect the differential diagnoses list in this case? The radiographic findings suggest the presence of pulmonary hypertension with secondary right-sided cardiomegaly. Despite the presence of a right-sided cardiac murmur and cardiomegaly, signs of right-sided congestive heart failure (such as jugular distension, hepatomegaly, ascites, or pleural effusion) were not present in this dog. Likely causes of pulmonary hypertension in this case are chronic pulmonary parenchymal disease, heartworm disease, and pulmonary thromboembolism.

3 What is your diagnostic plan? Echocardiography is needed for definitive diagnosis of pulmonary hypertension and to assess the risk of pulmonary thromboembolism, which is a life-threatening condition that is difficult to diagnose ante mortem. Normal D-dimer concentrations would suggest the absence of pulmonary thromboembolism (negative predictive value of 60–100%), but dogs with pulmonary thromboembolism can have normal coagulation profiles. Heartworm antigen testing is recommended. Urinalysis should be performed to assess for proteinuria, because chronic dirofilariasis can lead to glomerulonephritis caused by antigen–antibody complex deposition. Once the dog has been stabilized, bronchoalveolar lavage could be performed for further work-up of pulmonary parenchymal disease if other diagnostic tests do not identify the cause.

CASE 61

1 What are other important consequences of the infection with this parasite? When multiple adult heartworms partially obstruct the blood flow in the right atrium and block the tricuspid valve, caval syndrome may occur. This syndrome is characterized by intravascular hemolysis, hemoglobinemia, hemoglobinuria, regenerative anemia, and increases in AST, ALT, ALP, bilirubin, and BUN. A CBC, biochemistry panel, and urinalysis were performed in this dog, and evidence of all of the above abnormalities was detected.

2 How would you classify the stage of heartworm disease in this case? This dog is classified with heartworm disease stage 4 (caval syndrome).

3 How would you treat this dog? Dogs with caval syndrome require surgical extraction of adult heartworms, otherwise death can follow within a few days. Dogs with stage 1 to 3 heartworm disease should be treated with the adulticide melarsomine. This is the only US Food and Drugs Administration-approved therapy for adult worms. For 2 months before commencing adulticide therapy, it is recommended by the American Heartworm Society that dogs be treated with strict exercise restriction, prednisone (0.5 mg/kg PO q12h for 1 week followed by tapering over 4 weeks), doxycycline (10 mg/kg PO q12h for 4 weeks) to kill the filarial endosymbiont *Wolbachia pipientis*, and a heartworm preventive (ivermectin, selamectin, moxidectin) to reduce the microfilaria burden.

When adulticide therapy is commenced, a tapering dose of prednisone is again administered, together with strict exercise restriction, close observation, and other supportive therapy as required.

4 What is the prognosis? The prognosis for heartworm disease depends on the stage of the disease. Low parasite burdens are associated with a good prognosis, whereas caval syndrome causes death in approximately 40% of cases, despite appropriate therapy.

CASE 62

1 What is the most common composition of uroliths in dogs? The two most common stones in dogs are calcium oxalate and struvite, which account for around 88% of stones worldwide. A global shift was reported from predominantly calcium oxalate stones to struvite stones between the years 1999–2000 and 2009–2010; currently, the percentages of both stone types are approximately equal. Calcium oxalate stones occur more often in male dogs (around 74% of stones), while struvite stones are more common in females (around 86% of stones). Most dogs with calcium oxalate stones are between 5 and 11 years old, while dogs with struvite stones are between 2 and 8 years old. Most struvite uroliths in dogs are associated with urinary tract infection.

2 What further tests would you recommend in this dog? Urinalysis and aerobic bacterial urine culture (via cystocentesis) are important tests for work-up of urolithiasis. Dogs with struvite stones tend to have alkaline urine, whereas dogs with calcium oxalate stones tend to have acidic urine. The presence of specific types of crystalluria is not always predictive of the stone type present. In addition, storage of urine between collection and laboratory analysis can be associated with crystal formation. Abdominal radiographs and ultrasound of the urinary tract should be performed to ensure no new stones are present.

CASE 63

1 Considering the results of the urinalysis, how would you treat this dog? Struvite stones were most likely present in the past in this dog; these can be dissolved with dietary therapy. Dissolution diets should be fed for 1 month after stone dissolution has occurred. Antimicrobial drug therapy, selected based on culture and susceptibility results, should be given throughout the dissolution period, and it is currently recommended that it be continued for 1 month after dissolution of the stone, although this requires further evaluation because shorter periods of treatment might be sufficient. Efficacy of the therapy should be monitored by serial urinalysis with culture and susceptibility testing starting 1 week after initiation of therapy. The goal is to maintain acidic urine with a specific gravity below

1.015, and negative urine cultures. Monthly ultrasound of the urinary bladder to assess size and number of uroliths is recommended. Expected dissolution time is 2–3 months.

2 What methods of stone removal other than surgical cystotomy after laparotomy would be possible in this dog? Depending on urethra and stone size, voiding urohydropulsion, stone basket removal, lithotripsy, and laparoscopic-assisted cystotomy are potential alternatives to open laparotomy and cystotomy to remove stones from the urinary bladder.

3 The dog was stone free but bacteriuria was present. What is the difference between bacteriuria and urinary tract infection? List possible reasons for recurrent urinary tract infections in dogs. Bacteriuria is the presence of bacteria in the urine, with or without clinical signs. A urinary tract infection is defined as bacteriuria together with clinical signs of lower urinary tract disease, and typically antimicrobial treatment is indicated only for this situation. Recurrent urinary tract infection results from relapse of an existing infection or a reinfection. Relapse means that the same bacterial isolate as previously isolated causes the infection. When relapse occurs, it is often shortly after discontinuation of antimicrobial therapy and reflects failure to eliminate the infection. This can be due either to inappropriate antimicrobial therapy (type, dose, or duration of therapy) or failure of antimicrobial drugs to adequately penetrate the site of infection. Reinfections with a different organism usually occur later than a relapse. These indicate the existence of abnormal host defenses (e.g. diabetes mellitus, ectopic ureters, sphincter mechanism incompetence), which allow pathogenic bacteria to enter the urinary tract continuously.

CASE 64

1 What is the risk of infection to other animals and humans? Tetanus is always a consequence of contamination of a wound with spores from the environment. *Clostridium tetani* replicates in the gastrointestinal tracts of healthy animals and humans worldwide, and is excreted with feces. Thus, the spores are ubiquitous in soil, manure, feed, dust, mud, etc. If swallowed, they do not cause disease. In healthy tissues, clostridial spores are unable to germinate to vegetative forms that produce toxin. In wounds, spores germinate as a result of low oxygen concentration due to the presence of necrosis, impaired local perfusion, or infection with accompanying bacteria that consume oxygen. Thus, tetanus is a non-contagious disease.

2 Should dogs be vaccinated to prevent tetanus? Effective vaccines to prevent tetanus are available worldwide for humans and horses. Tetanus is uncommon in the dog, which is attributed to a natural resistance in this species. Although young animals are more susceptible, tetanus is rare even in puppies. Therefore, tetanus vaccines are not recommended generally for dogs, although some horse vaccines in selected countries are also licensed for dogs.

3 **How can tetanus be prevented in dogs?** The best way to prevent tetanus is early and appropriate management of any wounds. Hydrogen peroxide cleaning is recommended because it not only reduces the number of bacteria, but also increases oxygen concentration in the wound area.

CASE 65

1 **What is your interpretation of the thoracic radiographs?** The thoracic radiographs show a diffuse nodular soft tissue pattern that coalesces to alveolar infiltrates in the left caudal lung lobe and right cranial lung lobe. Mild tracheobronchial lymphadenopathy is evident and mild cardiomegaly is present.
2 **What differential diagnoses should be considered?** The primary differential diagnoses in this patient are fungal pneumonia and neoplasia, particularly lymphoma. Given the travel history within California, coccidioidomycosis is a possibility. Other fungal infections, such as blastomycosis and histoplamosis, would be more common with travel to the Ohio or Mississippi river valleys. *Pneumocystis* and *Toxoplasma gondii* infection could also be considered as potential causes for this pulmonary infiltrate, but they are extremely rare causes of pneumonia in dogs from this region.
3 **What diagnostic tests should be performed?** A CBC, biochemistry panel, and urinalysis would be indicated to assess the overall health of the animal. Given the degree of respiratory difficulty and cyanosis, pulse oximetry or an arterial blood gas analysis is indicated to determine the severity of gas exchange abnormalities. Positive fungal antibody tests for *Coccidioides* spp. could confirm a diagnosis; however, serum antibody tests for *Histoplama capsulatum* and *Blastomyces* spp. have low sensitivity and specificity for diagnosis of these infections. Urine antigen testing would be preferred for the diagnosis but does not differentiate between *H. capsulatum* antigen and *Blastomyces* spp. antigen owing to cross-reactivity. A transtracheal wash or bronchoscopy with bronchoalveolar lavage should be considered to look for cytologic evidence of infection or neoplasia. Documentation of *Pneumocystis* infection can be possible by detecting the organisms cytologically in bronchoalveolar lavage fluid or through PCR. *T. gondii* might be found in bronchoalveolar lavage fluid or antibody testing could be performed.

CASE 66

1 **Given the tissue tropism of this organism, what other examinations might be indicated?** Given the tissue tropism of this organism, a dilated fundic examination is indicated. This was performed, but was normal. Thorough palpation of the skin for skin lesions would also be recommended.
2 **What treatment options should be considered?** Given the severity of the clinical and radiographic findings, hospitalization is recommended and oxygen

supplementation is advised to alleviate the respiratory distress. Antifungal drugs to consider include deoxycholate amphotericin B, or lipid-complexed amphotericin B, and azole drugs (itraconazole, fluconazole, posaconazole, voriconazole). Concerns for using a highly active agent, such as amphotericin B, would be the risk of rapid and extensive kill of fungal organisms with associated inflammation, leading to acute respiratory distress syndrome. Also, deoxycholate amphotericin B can be nephrotoxic and saline diuresis with close monitoring of renal parameters is indicated. Lipid-complexed products are less toxic but more expensive. The azole drugs could be safer to use in this case but if used alone might not result in rapid and efficient control of disease and restoration of pulmonary function.

CASE 67

1 What is your most likely diagnosis? The most likely diagnosis for a unilateral alopecic lesion that has negative skin scrapings and no clear indication of a bacterial infection in a young dog is dermatophytosis. Bacterial infection was unlikely because there were only a few bacteria, they were extracellular, and low numbers of extracellular bacteria are to be expected on a distal limb.

2 What further tests are indicated in this dog? The first test to identify fungal spores and hyphae could be a trichogram. If this is negative, fungal culture and/or PCR for dermatophytes would be the next steps.

3 How would you treat this dog based on your most likely diagnosis? The level of antimycotic therapy instituted depends on the number of animals in the household, the degree of contact with the animal(s), and the immune status of the owner(s). Topical treatment with enilconazole, lime sulfur rinses, or a shampoo that contains miconazole and chlorhexidine twice weekly is always indicated. If there are more in-contact animals in the household, those animals also should be rinsed or shampooed at least weekly. Systemic antifungal therapy with an azole antifungal drug (itraconazole is the registered treatment of choice in many countries), griseofulvin, or terbinafine should be recommended to accelerate recovery and reduce the chance of transmission, especially if immunocompromised humans or young children live in the household or if there is a high level of owner–dog contact. After 4 weeks, a second fungal culture should be submitted and treatment continued until these culture results are available. If a negative culture result is obtained, therapy could be discontinued, particularly if an infection caused by a geophilic fungus, such as *Microsporum gypseum*, is present. However, if owners are immunocompromised, treatment should be continued until after a second negative monthly culture, as recommended in some guidelines. If the culture is positive, treatment is continued and another culture should be submitted 4 weeks later.

CASE 68

1 What are your primary differential diagnoses for the new clinical presentation? Cutaneous hemorrhages can occur as a result of thrombocytopenia, which in turn may result from decreased platelet production, increased destruction (primary or secondary immune-mediated disease), splenic sequestration or increased consumption. They can also result from impaired platelet function (which might result from non-steroidal anti-inflammatory drugs or von Willebrand's disease), or endothelial damage (vasculitis). The possibility of disorders of secondary hemostasis (decreased coagulation factors) should also be considered. A variety of infections can also be associated with cutaneous hemorrhage, including ehrlichiosis and other rickettsioses. In this puppy, a consumptive coagulopathy might have resulted from septic complications of parvovirosis or co-infections with other pathogens that might cause cutaneous hemorrhage, such as infectious canine adenovirus-1.

2 What diagnostic tests should be done first? Tests of coagulation function should be performed first, such as a CBC (to evaluate the platelet count) and a coagulation profile. A biochemistry panel should also be considered to evaluate serum proteins and serum markers of liver function.

CASE 69

1 What is the most likely diagnosis in this puppy? The history, clinical signs, and laboratory findings in this young unvaccinated dog are suggestive of infectious canine hepatitis (ICH) caused by canine adenovirus-1 (CAV-1). Adequate and safe protection against ICH is obtained by vaccination with attenuated live CAV-2 vaccines. CAV-2 belongs to the canine infectious respiratory disease (CIRD) complex, but vaccines containing CAV-2 cross-protect against CAV-1. Attenuated live CAV-2 is a component of vaccines that contain other core antigens (such as canine distemper virus and parvovirus).

2 What tests could be performed to confirm the diagnosis? A diagnosis of ICH can be confirmed by performing PCR on tissues or secretions from animals with clinical signs. Urine is an ideal specimen for PCR in dogs early in the course of infection. In the later stages of the disease, antibody testing can be used to support the diagnosis in unvaccinated animals, but subclinical exposure can occur, therefore a positive antibody test result does not prove a diagnosis of ICH.

3 Why are confirmatory tests necessary? An attempt to make a diagnosis of ICH is important for prognosis and to establish adequate control strategies. CAV-1 remains viable for months in the environment at low temperature and for many days at room temperature on contaminated fomites. It is shed in all secretions (vomit, feces, and urine) in the acute phase of disease, and urinary excretion lasts for months. Transmission to other dogs through oronasal exposure to virus in the environment should be prevented by use of effective chemical disinfectants

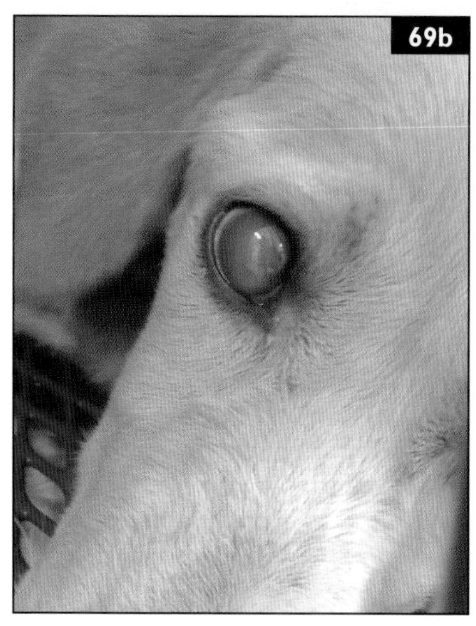
69b

(accelerated hydrogen peroxide, bleach-based disinfectants).

4 What is the prognosis for this dog? The dog experienced severe ICH because he was young and unvaccinated and also suffered from parvovirosis. The hepatic necrosis was complicated by DIC, making the short-term prognosis poor. Dogs with ICH can have a hyperacute fatal course with death before the onset of clinical signs. Some other lethal cases have been associated with viral encephalitis, manifested by lethargy, disorientation, seizures, cranial nerve deficits, ataxia, and other neurologic signs. Conversely, in some other cases, a mild febrile disease can be the only clinical manifestation. In all dogs surviving the acute phase, a clinical consequence can be the so-called "blue eye", observed about 2 weeks after the onset of disease, when the corneal endothelium is damaged by immune-complex deposition (**69b**). Long-term prognosis is linked to the possible development of chronic active hepatitis and immune-complex glomerulonephritis with secondary renal failure.

CASE 70

1 What differential diagnoses should be considered for nasal discharge in this patient? In this young otherwise healthy dog, sinonasal aspergillosis (SNA) would be the most likely cause of the nasal discharge; however, a chronic foreign body or dental problems (e.g. oronasal fistula, tooth root abscess) should also be considered. Neoplasia would be another differential diagnosis, but seems less likely because of the young age of the dog. Given the unilateral character of the nasal discharge, inflammatory diseases, such as lymphoplasmacytic rhinitis, seem less likely as well. Therefore, more diagnostic steps are necessary in this case to obtain a definitive diagnosis.

2 Why did the patient not respond to antimicrobial treatment? In most cases of nasal discharge in dogs, bacterial cultures of nasal swabs are not helpful in establishing a diagnosis. Multiple bacterial organisms can be cultured from the noses of healthy dogs, therefore bacteria causing secondary infections when host defense mechanisms are impaired are thought to derive from the physiological microflora and are not primary pathogens. However, this secondary bacterial infection explains improvement of nasal discharge with antibiotic treatment in some cases, even if the underlying disease is not bacterial in origin. To treat the patient successfully, diagnosis and treatment of the underlying primary disease process should be attempted.

3 How would you proceed to work-up the case? For further investigation of the problem, the oral cavity should be thoroughly examined for signs of dental disease or masses protruding from the hard or soft palate. In most cases, routine bloodwork is not helpful in establishing a diagnosis, but it is necessary prior to anesthesia. In addition, the platelet count and coagulation status should be evaluated before obtaining biopsies, to assess the risk of hemorrhage. Diagnostic imaging is indicated to localize a disease process within the nasal cavity and characterize possible bony or soft tissue abnormalities. Both CT and MRI are more sensitive than radiographs in detecting lesions typical of SNA. If dental disease is suspected, dental radiographs can also be helpful. Imaging should be followed by rhinoscopy to visualize the disease process, to identify and remove foreign material, and to obtain biopsy samples for histopathology and fungal culture. To confirm a diagnosis of suspected SNA, a combination of findings is usually required, including one or more findings such as presence of destructive rhinitis on CT or MRI, visualization of fungal plaques on rhinoscopy, identification of fungal structures on cytologic or histologic examination, positive fungal culture for *Aspergillus* spp., and/or detection of *Aspergillus* spp. antibodies in serum. False-negative results can occur with any of these tests and can complicate the diagnosis.

CASE 71

1 What is your diagnosis? Even with the results of histopathology and fungal culture still pending, a diagnosis of sinonasal aspergillosis (SNA) is very likely in this dog. Typical CT findings of SNA include destruction of the turbinates and increased soft tissue opacity in the nasal cavity, and thickened reactive frontal, maxillary, or vomer bones. Frontal sinus abnormalities can be detected in more than 70% of CT studies. This dog also had typical findings on rhinoscopy, including destruction of the turbinates and visualization of fungal plaques. The sensitivity of histopathology for diagnosis of SNA depends on the sampling site. If biopsy specimens are taken directly from fungal plaques, fungal organisms can be detected in most cases; if specimens are taken from unaffected mucosal areas, the likelihood of detection of the fungus is lower. Cytology has a good sensitivity for diagnosis of SNA if impression smears or brush cytology of biopsy samples from plaque material are performed; sampling of nasal discharge and blindly collected samples of the nasal cavity yield a low diagnostic value. To increase the sensitivity of fungal culture, biopsy samples of fungal plaques should be submitted (sensitivity of 44–77%).

2 What do you recommend for treatment in this case? The currently accepted treatment is topical administration of the antifungals clotrimazole or enilconazole in 1% or 2% solution. Enilconazole is less irritating to mucosal surfaces, but treatment with enilconazole is more likely to be followed by aspiration pneumonia, due to its lower viscosity. Either drug is instilled into the nasal cavity and frontal sinuses via catheters for a 1-hour infusion treatment, which includes a 90-degree rotation of the patient every 15 minutes to guarantee optimal contact of the antifungal drug with all affected mucosal surfaces. Debridement of all accessible mucosal plaques should be performed endoscopically before infusion treatment and is critical in order to ensure effective drug penetration. If the frontal sinus cannot be accessed endoscopically, trephination or surgical access to the frontal sinus should be recommended for debridement of plaques and instillation of antifungals. Tubes can be placed blindly or endoscopically into the nasal cavity or frontal sinus. Nasal discharge, epistaxis, and sneezing are short-term and self-limiting adverse effects seen in most dogs after the procedure. Endoscopic re-evaluation and a second treatment are recommended 3–4 weeks after the procedure. As a less time-consuming alternative treatment, clotrimazole cream can be instilled directly into the frontal sinuses after trephination and a 5-minute flush with clotrimazole solution (**71b**). This protocol was associated with an 86% success rate in a recent study, although success rates varied from one study to another depending on the length of follow-up. Many dogs have persistent nasal discharge due to recurrent bacterial infections secondary to extensive loss of nasal turbinates.

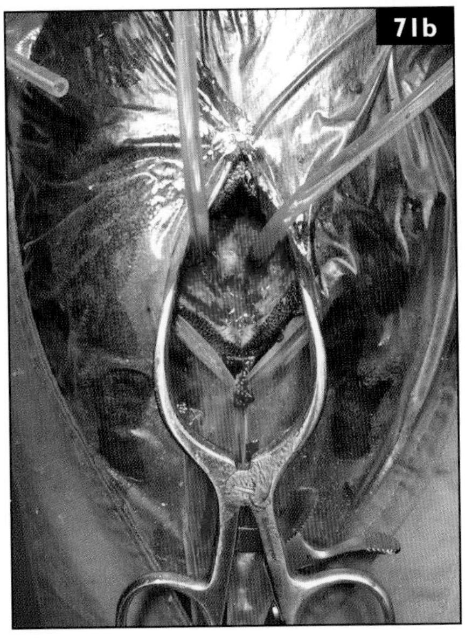
71b

CASE 72

1 What are the most likely differential diagnoses in this dog? In this case, exfoliative cutaneous lesions, alopecia, and systemic signs were observed. There was also a mild anemia, hyperproteinemia, hyperglobulinemia, and hypoalbuminemia, suggesting chronic immune stimulation. Renal failure was evidenced by the azotemia combined with isosthenuria. The increased UPCR together with a benign urine sediment raised concern for the possibility of glomerular disease. Differential diagnoses include chronic inflammatory diseases with dermatologic involvement, such as leishmaniosis, immune-mediated diseases (especially systemic lupus erythematosus), and neoplasia (e.g. cutaneous lymphoma).

2 What diagnostic tests should be done next? Further diagnostic tests to confirm a diagnosis of leishmaniosis include cytologic examination of impression smears of the skin lesions; biopsy of the skin lesions; fine needle aspiration and cytology of the lymph nodes; antibody tests for *Leishmania* spp.; or PCR of skin, blood, conjunctival swabs, or bone marrow. To diagnose immune-mediated diseases, antinuclear antibody tests or skin biopsies might be indicated. Skin biopsies would also be required for diagnosis of cutaneous lymphoma.

CASE 73

1 Describe the cytologic findings in the lymph node aspirate. Cytology showed many protozoal amastigotes inside the cytoplasm of a macrophage as well as extracellularly, together with some small lymphocytes. The amastigotes are consistent with those of *Leishmania* spp. The sensitivity of cytology is about 80% in dogs with clinical signs and is lower in subclinically infected dogs. Organisms can sometimes also be found in aspirates of the spleen, liver, skin nodes, bone marrow, or other tissues and body fluids.

2 What factors can influence with the results of *Leishmania* spp. antibody tests? Most antibody tests used to diagnose leishmaniosis have good specificity, but antibodies cannot be detected in about 30% of infected dogs. Sensitivity and specificity depend on the antigens used in the test. Tests that use whole-parasite extracts are more sensitive, but have a lower specificity, because cross-reactions with other species, such as *Trypanosoma cruzi*, can occur. However, this is generally only a problem in areas where both *Leishmania* spp. and *Trypanosoma* spp. infections are endemic. Tests that use recombinant antigen are very specific but lack sensitivity, especially in subclinically infected dogs.

CASE 74

1 What are the treatment options, and what is the prognosis for this dog? Stage III of canine leishmaniosis has a guarded to poor prognosis. This is because *Leishmania* spp. can be resistant to antileishmanial drugs, there can be frequent relapses, and secondary renal tubular injury can occur. This dog already had glomerular disease and secondary renal tubular failure (chronic kidney disease; IRIS stage II). Treatment should address fluid and acid–base balance. Nutrition is important and feeding a diet with reduced protein content is recommended. The first-line antileishmanial drugs include a combination of allopurinol (10 mg/kg PO q12h, usually lifelong) and meglumine antimoniate (100 mg/kg SC q24h for 4 weeks) or miltefosine (2 mg/kg PO q24h for 4 weeks).

2 The owner has two other dogs and three young children. What actions are indicated to prevent human infection in this situation? Leishmaniosis is a zoonotic disease. In humans, the disease can be fatal, especially in young children and immunocompromised people, including those that are malnourished. The primary means of transmission of *Leishmania* organisms to humans from dogs is through sandfly bites; although the possibility of transmission through direct contact with ulcerative lesions has been suggested, there are no proven cases in the literature. The other two dogs in the household should be tested for *Leishmania* spp. infection. Sandfly bites can be prevented by regular use of collars, spot-on solutions, or sprays containing insecticides (e.g. permethrin). In some countries, a vaccine is now available. Leishmaniosis is not endemic in UK and there are no sandflies, therefore the risk of transmission from the dog to the children is low.

CASE 75

1 What is your first assessment of this dog's problems? Respiratory distress can result from disorders of the upper respiratory tract, lower respiratory tract, or pleural space. In this dog, there was no stridor, but tachypnea and increased lung sounds on expiration suggested lower respiratory tract disease. Cough can be respiratory, cardiac, or rarely extrapulmonary but intrathoracic in origin. The suspected right ventricular concentric hypertrophy reported by the referring veterinarian could be seen with pressure overload, for example due to pulmonic stenosis or tetralogy of Fallot. However, cardiac disease was considered less likely as a cause of the dog's clinical signs on the basis of the physical examination findings (lack of a murmur, normal pulse quality and capillary refill time).

2 What diagnostic steps should you perform next? The next diagnostic steps would be thoracic radiography, as well as reassessment of the echocardiography findings.

CASE 76

1 What is your assessment of the radiographic findings, and what is the differential diagnosis? The thoracic radiographs reveal a severe interstitial lung pattern. In the caudal lung lobe, the pattern appears almost alveolar. This could be seen with pulmonary edema, hemorrhage, or infectious (fungal, parasitic, *Pneumocystis* spp. infection) or inflammatory (eosinophilic bronchopneumopathy) lung disease.

2 What is your assessment of the echocardiographic study? Echocardiography shows a slightly dilated right ventricle with mild hypertrophy of the right ventricular wall. The pulmonary artery appears dilated in comparison with the aorta. Pulmonary hypertension was suspected but could not be confirmed based on these findings.

CASE 77

1 How can pulmonary hypertension be confirmed by echocardiography? Usually, pulmonary hypertension is associated with a dilated right ventricle with or without right ventricular wall hypertrophy. In addition, the pulmonary artery is frequently dilated. Diagnosis is confirmed by identifying a tricuspid insufficiency jet velocity of >3.0 m/s and by exclusion of pulmonic stenosis (pulmonic velocity <2.5 m/s). An alternative method to identify pulmonary hypertension is to identify a pulmonic insufficiency jet with a velocity >2.5 m/s. However, this dog had neither a tricuspid nor a pulmonic insufficiency jet. The acceleration time/ejection time ratio of the pulmonary artery flow velocity was 0.23, which is also suspicious of pulmonary hypertension, but pulmonary hypertension could not be confirmed in this dog.

2 What other tests are available to identify pulmonary hypertension? If echocardiography cannot prove the presence of pulmonary hypertension, the pulmonary artery pressure can be measured invasively by introducing a catheter into the pulmonary artery and measuring the pressure directly. In this patient, the pulmonary artery pressure was severely increased, with a pressure of 85 mmHg.

3 What are the main differential diagnoses for pulmonary hypertension? Pulmonary hypertension can result from several congenital diseases (e.g. patent ductus arteriosus or a ventricular septal defect), and can be secondary to left-sided heart failure. Pulmonary hypertension can also be caused by primary pulmonary hypertension, which is rare in dogs. Secondary pulmonary hypertension can be seen with severe pulmonary disease, lung torsion, thromboembolic diseases (secondary to IMHA, sepsis, DIC, Cushing's disease, protein-losing nephropathy/enteropathy), or parasites, such as heartworm or lungworm.

4 What further tests do you recommend? At this point, the next step would be to test for *Dirofilaria immitis* and *Angiostrongylus vasorum* infection. As the dog had never been outside Germany, heartworm disease was considered unlikely. Therefore, the dog was first tested for *A. vasorum*, by Baermann fecal examination, and this test was positive. The dog was treated with fenbendazole (50 mg/kg PO q24h for 14 days), and with sildenafil (1 mg/kg PO q8h) for the pulmonary hypertension.

CASE 78

1 What are the three most likely differential diagnoses for this dog, based on your review of the image provided? Based on the presence of comedones, the disease seems to be follicular, and the three most likely differential diagnoses are bacterial folliculitis, demodicosis, and dermatophytosis.

2 What diagnostic tests should be done immediately? An impression smear and deep skin scrapings should be the first tests to be conducted, to assess for bacterial pyoderma and demodicosis.

CASE 79

1 What questions need to be asked to guide your further diagnostic testing? The cytology shows many segmented neutrophils. Cocci are seen intracellularly and extracellularly. In addition, there are a few macrophages. This is diagnostic for bacterial pyoderma. In the skin scraping, one *Demodex* mite is visible. The cause of bacterial pyoderma and adult-onset demodicosis usually is an underlying immunosuppressive disease. In a 10-year-old dog, endocrine diseases, such as hypothyroidism and hyperadrenocorticism, should be considered as well as neoplastic disease elsewhere in the body. Questions should try to identify clues that might suggest hypothyroidism (is the dog heat seeking, exercise intolerant, gaining weight?), hyperadrenocorticism (is the dog showing increased thirst and urination, polyphagia, panting?) or other signs of systemic illness.

2 If there are no additional clues in the history, what other diagnostic tests should be considered for this patient? A CBC and biochemistry panel can provide clues to underlying diseases. A disproportionate increase in ALP activity and an increase in serum glucose and cholesterol concentrations can suggest hyperadrenocorticism. An increase in serum triglycerides and cholesterol can suggest hypothyroidism. A thyroid panel could also be considered, although a low T4 concentration in this dog could be due to euthyroid sick syndrome and would only be relevant in association with either a high TSH concentration, high anti-thyroglobulin antibodies, or other clinical or biochemical clues for the disease. An abdominal ultrasound examination and a radiograph of the thorax should be suggested to evaluate for possible underlying neoplastic disease.

CASE 80

1 How would you treat the dog's demodicosis? The demodicosis needs to be treated with either amitraz rinses or with macrocyclic lactones (ivermectin or moxidectin, 300 mg/kg PO q24h). For amitraz rinses, the dog needs to be clipped completely and thoroughly rinsed once weekly in a well-ventilated area. Ideally, this should occur a few hours after using an antibacterial shampoo containing chlorhexidine or benzoyl peroxide to remove crusts and debris and treat the bacterial skin infection. The dog must not get wet between rinses. Macrocyclic lactones are not registered for systemic treatment of canine demodicosis owing to the potential for neurologic adverse effects with potentially fatal outcome. Collies are particularly sensitive to these toxic effects owing to a deletion mutation of the *MDR-1* gene. However, adverse effects can also be seen in dogs without that defect. Thus, the ivermectin or moxidectin doses should be gradually increased from 50 mg/kg to 300 mg/kg over 3–4 days to identify sensitive dogs; such dogs initially will show mild effects, such as tremors, ataxia, and lethargy, which should resolve once the drug is discontinued. Dogs are re-evaluated clinically and skin scrapings evaluated every 4 weeks, and miticidal treatments ideally are continued until 8 weeks past the first negative skin scraping. In this particular dog, systemic antibacterial therapy could also be considered. In a dog with severe skin disease, a culture and susceptibility test should be performed before antibiotic therapy to confirm the suitability of the empirically chosen antibiotic.

2 How would you monitor and adjust the thyroid hormone supplementation? Ideally a post-pill T4 concentration should be determined 1 month after initiating treatment, 6 hours after the administration of the morning dose. This should be in the upper end of the normal range. Clinical improvement will be difficult to judge in this dog, because a positive response is expected due to the miticidal therapy alone.

CASE 81

1 What are your differential diagnoses in this dog? The top differential diagnoses for an acute onset of generalized lower motor neuron (LMN) tetraparesis in a dog are immune-mediated acute polyradiculoneuritis (idiopathic or Coonhound radiculitis), botulism, and myasthenic crisis. Tick paralysis should also be considered in the USA and Australia. Acute rhabdomyolysis, protozoal polyradiculoneuritis, poliomyelitis (paralytic form of rabies, tick-borne encephalitis virus), and coral snake poisoning have also been reported in rare circumstances. Severe metabolic disease (hypothyroidism, Addison's disease, hypoglycemia, hypo- or hyperkalemia) can also cause acute LMN weakness and should be excluded with laboratory analyses.

2 What are the next diagnostic steps? A thorough history should be taken for any dog with acute onset of severe LMN paresis to assess the possibility of intake of dead animal carcasses or spoiled food, which could give rise to a suspicion of botulism. Botulism should also be considered if several animals in a group are affected. In addition, history and physical examination of dogs with acute LMN paralysis should investigate potential exposure to ticks (in the USA and Australia), raccoon bites (Coonhound radiculitis), or coral snake poisoning.

In this dog, botulism was strongly suspected based on the history. Rapid onset of paralysis with subtle cranial nerve involvement with mydriatic pupils reflects the typical course with onset of clinical signs within 12–72 hours. Polyradiculoneuritis and myasthenic crisis have a more protracted onset. Botulism is commonly reported in the literature as outbreaks in groups of several affected dogs (e.g. in sled hounds, hunting foxhounds), or around lakes due to the ingestion of dead waterfowl. Botulism is caused by ingestion of the preformed toxin of *Clostridium botulinum* in spoiled food. Seven types of *C. botulinum* toxin are known (A–G), but up to now only toxin type C and, rarely, type D have been associated with botulism in dogs. Confirmation of botulism requires demonstration of the toxin in serum, feces, vomitus, or carrion, or a rising antibody response to botulinum toxins in acute and convalescent sera. This usually requires submission of specimens to specialized laboratories. Specimens should be handled with care and packages labeled as dangerous. Currently, the most sensitive test is a mouse inoculation assay. Mice are inoculated with the test material. Thereafter, the specific toxin type is assessed by repeating the test with antitoxin protection. Results are usually only available with a delay of at least a week and, therefore, do not assist with the initial management of the dog.

When the initial diagnosis of botulism remains unclear, other diagnostic tests that should be considered are a thyroid hormone panel, antibody tests for protozoal infection, and acetylcholine receptor antibodies. Furthermore, electrodiagnostic examination with inclusion of specific tests for neuromuscular transmission (repetitive nerve stimulation) and proximal nerve root function (F-waves) can assist in the diagnosis and specific localization of neuromuscular disease. Cerebrospinal fluid examination should be considered for diagnosis of rare cases of poliomyelitis. In this dog, the only abnormal findings were mild abnormalities on electrodiagnostic examination (low amplitude of the compound muscle action potential, borderline decrement on repetitive stimulation). Type C botulism, which was already suspected based on the history, was further confirmed by the presence of botulinum toxin type C in the serum.

3 What treatment is indicated? Treatment of botulism is mostly supportive and focuses on maintaining respiratory function. Death can occur as a result of paralysis of the diaphragm and intercostal muscles and, therefore, intubation and ventilation may be necessary. Botulinum toxin is internalized into peripheral nerve endings, but unlike tetanus toxin it does not undergo retrograde axonal transport. In the nerve endings it inactivates SNARE proteins and interferes with the release of acetylcholine in the synaptic cleft. The use of botulinum antitoxin is of questionable value because it antagonizes only the toxin in the systemic circulation and not the toxin that is already internalized in the peripheral nerve endings. Thus, antitoxin will not reverse any clinical signs that are already present, but it has the potential to prevent further progression of paralysis. Only toxin-specific antitoxin is useful. As most published clinical cases in dogs have been attributed to botulinum toxin type C, botulinum antitoxin type CD should be used in dogs.

CASE 82

1 What would be the next diagnostic steps to further work-up the dog's major problems? Nervous system involvement is present with ataxia and proprioceptive deficits. Neurologic and ophthalmologic examinations would be the next appropriate steps for localization. Further diagnostic testing, such as CBC, radiographs, CT or MRI, and CSF collection and analysis would be indicated depending on the site of localization.

2 What are the differential diagnoses for generalized lymphadenomegaly, and what is the first step in a diagnostic work-up? Neoplasia, hyperplasia, infiltrative protozoal or fungal infections, and suppuration are four processes that cause generalized enlargement of lymph nodes. Fine needle aspiration and cytology of the nodes is the most direct and easiest step to determine which problem is present. In addition, a CBC should be performed to assess the white blood cell count and differential.

3 What disease processes can be associated with miosis and aqueous flare? Disease processes that can be associated with miosis include neurologic dysfunction with increased parasympathetic or decreased sympathetic input as well as intraocular injury or inflammation. The presence of aqueous flare suggests that a primary ophthalmologic process is present. This further supports the need for a thorough ophthalmologic and fundic examination.

CASE 83

1 What is the site of neurologic localization, and what further tests would be indicated? A lesion in the spinal cord from T3 to L3, more localized to the left side, would be expected. Spinal radiographs should be taken, if possible under anesthesia. Should these results be uninformative, CSF analysis, contrast myelography, or imaging with CT or MRI might be needed while the dog is anesthetized.

2 What infectious diseases of dogs can be associated with inflammation in the anterior and posterior eye segments? Systemic bacterial, fungal, and protozoal infections that spread in the circulation can either lodge in the uveal or chorioretinal vasculature or cause immune complex deposition at these sites.

3 What further diagnostic tests would you suggest to confirm one of these infections? Blood culture or PCR, aqueous or vitreous cytologic examination, or antibody testing can be performed to identify a specific etiologic agent.

4 What does electrophoresis suggest about the cause of the globulin increase? Electrophoresis shows polyclonal hyperglobulinemia, which is most characteristic of chronic antigenic stimulation, usually from a chronic persistent intracellular infection (e.g. *Brucella canis*, *Ehrlichia canis*, *Leishmania* spp.) or chronic persistent extracellular infections that are not being controlled by humoral or cell-mediated immunity (e.g. heartworm disease, aspergillosis, deep mycotic infections). Monoclonal gammopathy would be more indicative of a plasma cell or B-cell myeloma. Myeloma often causes spinal lesions; however, these are usually osteoproliferative and osteolytic, involving the vertebral bodies and spinous processes.

CASE 84

1 What are the most common etiologic agents that cause discospondylitis in dogs? Discospondylitis, especially at multiple sites, is most likely to be caused by circulating infectious agents (bacteremia or fungemia). *Staphylococcus* spp., *Brucella canis*, and *Aspergillus* spp. are commonly incriminated.
2 How would you interpret the *Brucella canis* test results? The results are highly suggestive of brucellosis; however, false-positive test results can occur and, therefore positive blood culture results would have been more definitive.
3 What other signs would be expected in a neutered or intact dog with brucellosis? Neutered animals usually show few if any signs of brucellosis, but can develop problems associated with systemic infections such as discospondylitis. Intact female dogs can show signs of infertility, abortion, stillbirth, or can give birth to pups with a febrile disease. Intact male dogs can show signs of epididymal enlargement, scrotal dermatitis, and infertility. Given the insidious nature of the disease, dogs that are congregated in shelters can become infected and carry the organism despite being neutered prior to rehoming.

CASE 85

1 What are the typical clinical signs of large and small intestinal diarrhea, and how would you categorize the diarrhea in this dog? The typical clinical signs in small bowel diarrhea are weight loss, moderate frequency in defecation, and a moderate to large amount of feces. In addition, melena can be present. The typical clinical signs in large bowel diarrhea are tenesmus, mucus or fresh blood in the feces, and frequent defecation of small amounts of feces. This dog had tenesmus, hematochezia, and mucus in the feces, which are typical signs for large bowel diarrhea. Concurrent small bowel involvement is possible but less likely, because the dog had not lost weight.
2 Do you think coccidiosis is a likely explanation for the chronic diarrhea in this dog? *Isospora* spp. can be a primary pathogen, but infections are generally only associated with clinical signs in puppies or in adult dogs in association with concurrent gastrointestinal or immunosuppressive diseases. This coccidian parasite replicates in the small intestine and generally causes self-limited acute diarrhea. Therefore, it is unlikely that clinical signs in this dog can be explained by coccidiosis.
3 What part of the physical examination is missing, but absolutely indicated in this case? A rectal examination was not mentioned in the description of the physical examination. However, this is the first step in the diagnostic work-up of a dog with large intestinal signs. Rectal polyps, infiltrative disorders, and strictures can be identified or suspected with a thorough digital examination.

CASE 86

1 What causes of large bowel diarrhea are still on your differential diagnosis list? Given that the fecal examination was negative and the dog had been treated with antiparasitic drugs several times, a parasitic infection (e.g. *Trichuris vulpis*) was considered unlikely as cause of the chronic large intestinal signs. Fungal diseases (e.g. histoplasmosis) were unlikely, because this dog lived in an area where these fungi were not endemic. A chronic bacterial infection remained a possibility. The dog had been fed with two different hypoallergenic diets without significant improvement. Therefore, a food allergy was also considered unlikely. However, some dogs with chronic large bowel diarrhea respond to fiber-supplemented diets and, therefore, treatment for fiber-responsive colonic dysfunction could be attempted. Extraintestinal diseases (e.g. uremia, pancreatitis, or hypoadrenocorticism) were unlikely, because the dog did not show any signs of systemic illness. Lymphoma can occasionally occur in young dogs, but is not likely at this age. Anatomic disorders (e.g. strictures, ileocolic or cecocolic intussusception) should also be considered in young dogs with chronic large bowel diarrhea unresponsive to anthelmintics and food trials and should be worked-up by further imaging studies.

2 How would you manage an idiopathic inflammatory bowel disease involving the large intestine? Some dogs with idiopathic inflammatory bowel disease respond to antibiotics that also have an immunomodulatory component, such as metronidazole or tylosin. Anti-inflammatory drugs, such as sulfasalazine or mesalamine, could be tried because this group of drugs is thought to cause fewer adverse effects than immunosuppressive drugs. Tear production should be monitored, because sulfa-based drugs can cause keratoconjunctivitis sicca. In dogs not responding to fiber supplementation, immunomodulatory antibiotics, and anti-inflammatory drugs, the next line of treatment would be immunosuppression. Frequently used immunosuppressive drugs include prednisolone, azathioprine, and cyclosporine. However, a diagnostic work-up to investigate the possibility of anatomic abnormalities, neoplastic infiltrations, and infectious agents should ideally be performed before starting the immunosuppressive therapy.

3 Why might colonic biopsies be indicated before starting immunosuppressive therapy, especially in this case? French Bulldogs are one of several breeds predisposed to granulomatous colitis. It is mandatory to rule out this disease first, because immunosuppressive therapy would be contraindicated in dogs with granulomatous or neutrophilic infiltrates until infectious agents have been excluded.

CASE 87

1 What test would you perform to differentiate idiopathic neutrophilic inflammatory bowel disease from histiocytic colitis? The pathognomonic lesion of histiocytic ulcerative colitis in dogs is mucosal infiltration with large numbers of macrophages staining positively with periodic acid–Schiff (PAS). Large numbers of PAS-positive macrophages could be detected on histopathology in this dog, confirming a diagnosis of histiocytic colitis.

2 What is the cause of histiocytic ulcerative colitis? Histiocytic ulcerative colitis is primarily seen in Boxers. However, this form of colitis has also been reported in English and French Bulldogs. By fluorescent in situ hybridization, invasive *Escherichia coli* within the colonic mucosa and macrophages can be detected in affected Boxers. Correlation between clinical remission and eradication of mucosally invasive *E. coli* during treatment with enrofloxacin has supported the causal involvement of *E. coli* in the development of histiocytic ulcerative colitis.

3 How would you treat a dog with histiocytic ulcerative colitis, in contrast to idiopathic inflammatory bowel disease? In contrast to idiopathic inflammatory bowel disease, poor clinical response is observed in all dogs with histiocytic ulcerative colitis treated with various combinations of immunosuppressive and anti-inflammatory drugs (e.g. prednisolone, sulfasalazine). Clinical improvement and eradication of mucosally invasive *E. coli* is most likely achieved with prolonged (≥8 weeks) enrofloxacin treatment. Short-term treatment with amoxicillin–clavulanic acid, based on the results of antimicrobial susceptibility testing, can result in a reduction in intramucosal *E. coli* and partial histopathologic improvement. However, this does not translate to clinical improvement. Some invasive *E. coli* strains can be resistant to enrofloxacin (especially in dogs that have previously received short courses of fluoroquinolones), therefore colonic mucosal cultures with susceptibility testing can help optimize treatment.

CASE 88

1 What is the most likely cause of the cardiac murmur? A new murmur in a sick adult dog should be promptly investigated, because it is suggestive of infective endocarditis (IE). The absence of fever should not rule out this diagnosis. The most common pathogens of IE are *Streptococcus* spp., *Staphylococcus* spp., gram-negative rods, *Enterococcus* spp., and *Bartonella* spp. Other causes of diastolic murmur at the left heart base include congenital dysplasia of the aortic or pulmonic valves, which is very unlikely in this case given the patient's age.

2 Are the other abnormalities in this case associated with the cardiac disease? Arterial thromboembolism frequently occurs with IE, so clinical signs and laboratory abnormalities are extremely variable depending on the site affected by thromboemboli. All the laboratory abnormalities found in this case could be explained by IE.

3 What are the next diagnostic steps? Thoracic radiographs, echocardiography, and blood pressure measurement are indicated in this case. Three aerobic bacterial blood cultures should be collected from separate sites within a 24-hour period.

Bartonella spp. cannot be isolated using routine blood culture, and successful isolation requires special *Bartonella* isolation techniques such as a combination of pre-enrichment culture and PCR testing. In dogs with IE due to *Bartonella* spp., specific antibody to different *Bartonella* species can often be detected.

CASE 89

1 How are the valvular vegetations formed, and how do they cause cardiac murmurs? Vegetations are formed by a matrix of fibrin, fibronectin, and platelets, where bacteria adhere and grow protected from the phagocytic activity of leukocytes. Vegetations cause improper valve coaptation with consequent regurgitation, and can create stenosis in severe cases. The diastolic murmur in this case is caused by the regurgitation of blood from the aorta. Infective endocarditis (IE) most commonly involves the mitral valve and/or the aortic valve.

2 What factors predispose to endocarditis? There is no consistent evidence that dental or oral surgical procedures cause IE. Chronic mitral valve disease does not predispose to IE, while congenital valvular malformation and underlying immune system dysfunction can be predisposing factors, but are not often identified. Contaminated indwelling catheters or other sources of chronic bacteremia (e.g. discospondylitis, abscesses) are sometimes associated with development of IE.

3 What are other systemic signs of endocarditis? Other systemic signs include fever and sequelae of thromboembolism, including polyarthritis, neurologic abnormalities, peripheral edema, organ infarction, lameness, lack of a peripheral pulse, and cold limbs.

4 Should any therapy be considered pending microbiologic tests? Empiric antimicrobial therapy is recommended while blood culture and susceptibility testing are pending. Parenteral ampicillin (20 mg/kg IV q6–8h) combined with enrofloxacin (5 mg/kg IV q24h) or ampicillin combined with an aminoglycoside for 1–2 weeks should be used, with careful monitoring of renal function should an aminoglycoside be selected. When results of culture and susceptibility testing are available, antimicrobial treatment should be modified if needed and continued for several months, based on echocardiographic monitoring.

CASE 90

1 How did this dog become infected with *B. vinsonii* subspecies *berkhoffii*? The cat flea (*Ctenocephalides felis*) is the main vector of *Bartonella* spp., but many blood-sucking arthropods including other fleas, ticks, lice, and biting flies also have the potential to transmit these pathogens. There is some epidemiologic evidence that *B. vinsonii* subspecies *berkhoffii* can be transmitted by ticks, such as *Rhipicephalus sanguineus*.

2 What are the most common *Bartonella* species that infect dogs, and what are their reservoir hosts? At least fourteen species of *Bartonella* can infect dogs. The most common in dogs are *Bartonella henselae* (for which cats are the reservoir) and *B. vinsonii* subspecies *berkhoffii* (for which dogs are the reservoir). Wild canids, raccoons, voles, wild mice, squirrels, and cattle are reservoirs of other *Bartonella* spp. capable of infecting dogs.
3 What are other signs of *Bartonella* spp. infection in dogs? A wide range of disorders have been associated with *Bartonella* spp. infection in dogs, including myocarditis/endocarditis, peliosis hepatis, bacillary angiomatosis, and pyogranulomatous disease. *Bartonella* spp. infection has also been suspected as an underlying cause of meningoradiculoneuritis, polyarthritis, uveitis, skin lesions, epistaxis, and cavitary effusion, although evidence linking *Bartonella* spp. infection to these conditions in dogs is weaker.
4 What is the recommended therapy for endocarditis caused by *Bartonella* spp.? The optimal treatment protocol for *Bartonella* spp. endocarditis is unknown. In human patients, a combination of penicillin and an aminoglycoside has been used, usually followed by valve replacement. Other possible treatments include a combination of a parenteral fluoroquinolone (e.g. enrofloxacin) or an aminoglycoside and doxycycline in hospital for 1–2 weeks, followed by treatment after discharge with doxycycline combined with enrofloxacin or rifampin for 4–6 weeks. Longer therapy might be required in some cases.
5 What are the public health implications of this diagnosis? *Bartonella* spp. are zoonotic pathogens but direct transmission from dogs to humans has not been proven. Human infection occurs via blood-sucking arthropods; therefore, ectoparasite control in dogs is crucial. Dogs can be subclinically infected by several species of *Bartonella*.

CASE 91

1 What is your assessment of the dermal lesion? Non-pruritic papules mainly originate from infiltration of the skin by inflammatory or neoplastic cells. As the dog is still young, inflammatory processes (potentially secondary to infection) are higher on the list of differential diagnoses. Solitary papules with this appearance can occur with leishmaniosis, which is transmitted by sandfly bites. These lesions are typically found in young dogs in endemic areas that are exposed to *Leishmania infantum* for the first time and develop a protective cell-mediated immune response.
2 What further diagnostic tests are indicated? Fine needle aspiration of the papule should be performed to differentiate between neoplastic and infectious causes. A fine needle aspirate could also be submitted for *L. infantum* PCR.

CASE 92

1 What treatment do you recommend for this dog? Although *Leishmania infantum*-associated papular dermatitis can be self-limiting, treatment is recommended with allopurinol monotherapy (10 mg/kg PO q24h). Domperidone (2 mg/kg PO q24h), a drug recently licensed for veterinary use in Europe, can be used as adjuvant treatment. Domperidone is a dopamine D2 receptor antagonist that has antiemetic properties (for which it is available in human medicine). As prolactin release is inhibited by dopamine, domperidone increases the prolactin concentration. This stimulates a Th1 cellular immune response, which can help to clear *L. infantum* infection.

2 How should the dog be monitored in the future? In an otherwise healthy dog with *L. infantum* infection, a CBC, biochemistry panel, and urinalysis should be performed every 6 months; if clinical signs or laboratory changes are present, every 3 months. Urinalysis allows early detection of proteinuria as a marker of glomerular disease. In addition, urinalysis should be used to monitor for xanthine crystalluria, which can occur as a result of allopurinol therapy. Antibody titer to *Leishmania* should be measured every 6 months to determine whether continued allopurinol treatment is needed and for prognostication. Treatment can be discontinued if the titer becomes negative. A 3-fold increase in titer is associated with progression of disease and recurrence of clinical signs in dogs that have previously responded to treatment.

CASE 93

1 What is the dog's most life-threatening problem? The dog is in decompensated hypovolemic shock.

2 What initial treatment would you perform to address this problem? Initial therapy should include oxygen supplementation and intravenous or intraosseous fluid therapy with boluses of crystalloid (10–30 ml/kg) and/or colloid (5–15 ml/kg) fluids. After an initial fluid bolus, the dog should be re-evaluated and, if needed, additional boluses should be given.

3 What laboratory parameters should be assessed in order to optimize treatment? Initial laboratory work should include: (1) hematocrit to assess for anemia; (2) a white blood cell and differential count to assess for neutropenia; (3) serum glucose concentration to assess for hypoglycemia; (4) potassium to guide potassium supplementation; (5) serum creatinine concentration to assess for prerenal azotemia; and (6) total protein and albumin to assess for hypoproteinemia/hypoalbuminemia, which are mainly caused by enteral loss.

CASE 94

1 What should be the fluid therapy plan for the next 10 hours? The dog was about 10% dehydrated, which equates to a fluid deficit of 50 ml. The maintenance fluid requirement for a puppy is about 4 ml/kg/h. The dog has ongoing losses, estimated to be about 10 ml/h (which ideally should be measured). Thus, fluid therapy should include: (1) rehydration over 10 hours = 5 ml/h; (2) replacement of ongoing losses = 10 ml/h; (3) maintenance = 2 ml/h. Therefore, the dog should initially receive 17 ml/h of crystalloid fluids intravenously (or intraosseously). The dog's reduced mental status could be explained by hypoglycemia. Therefore, the dog should receive a glucose bolus of 0.5 g/kg 50% glucose diluted 1:2 with crystalloids to a concentration of <20% to reduce osmolality (0.5 ml of 50% glucose diluted with 1 ml lactated Ringer's solution intravenously or intraosseously). Usually, one would also add glucose at a concentration of 5% to the intravenous fluids. As the dog is rehydrated and losses are replaced, the glucose concentration should be reduced to 1.2–2.5% and monitored on a regular basis (e.g. every 2–4 hours). The dog's serum potassium concentration is very low and so potassium should also be added to the fluids. The rate of potassium administration should not exceed 0.5 mmol/kg/h, which is 12 ml/h of a 20 mmol/l solution or 6 ml/h of a 40 mmol/l solution for this dog. Alternatively, the dog could receive potassium at 0.5 ml/kg/h (0.25 ml/h/dog). With these high potassium administration rates, serum potassium concentration should be monitored closely.

2 What should be the nutritional plan when the vomiting is under control? When vomiting is under control, the the dog should ideally be fed enterally. Therefore, the resting energy requirement (RER) should be calculated using the formula RER = 70 × $kg^{0.75}$. Puppies have a higher energy requirement; therefore, a correction factor of 2–3 × RER should be used. Thus, the energy requirement for this puppy is 42 kcal/day. The dog should be fed in small portions every 2–4 hours. If appetite is poor, a nasoesophageal or esophagostomy tube could be placed. When persistent vomiting is present, parenteral nutrition might be necessary.

CASE 95

1 What is the ocular diagnosis based on the clinical findings? The ocular findings in the right eye are consistent with anterior uveitis. Key findings of an inflammatory process of the anterior uvea include flare in the anterior chamber, iris hyperemia (rubeosis iridis), and a low intraocular pressure. Inflammation of parts or the entire uveal tract (iris, ciliary body, choroid) is caused by tissue damage and disruption of the blood–aqueous barriers. Hyphema and fibrin accumulation can sometimes be detected in more severe cases. Anterior uveitis in the dog can have multiple underlying etiologies and, among these, infectious diseases are the most common.

2 What further tests would you recommend? Further tests should include a fundic examination as well as a CBC, biochemistry panel, and urinalysis.

CASE 96

1 What is your interpretation of the findings in the left retina? There are multifocal intraretinal hemorrhages in the tapetal area of the retina.

2 What is your interpretation of the laboratory findings? The CBC shows severe thrombocytopenia. The biochemistry panel reveals hyperproteinemia with hyperglobulinemia and hypoalbuminemia, suggestive of a chronic persistent infection or inflammatory process.

3 What underlying disease would you suspect, based on the physical examination, the ophthalmic findings, and the laboratory results? What additional diagnostic tests would you recommend? Based on the physical examination, the ophthalmic findings, and the laboratory results, ehrlichiosis should be suspected as an underlying disease. Diagnosis of ehrlichiosis includes direct visualization of morulae in peripheral blood smears, detection of *Ehrlichia canis* antibodies, or detection of *Ehrlichia* spp. DNA by PCR testing.

CASE 97

1 What *Ehrlichia* species infect dogs, and how are they transmitted? Ehrlichiosis is a tick-borne disease, caused most often by *Ehrlichia canis* (the cause of canine monocytic ehrlichiosis) or *Ehrlichia ewingii* (the latter primarily occurring in the United States). Other species that infect dogs are *Ehrlichia chaffeensis* and an *Ehrlichia muris*-like agent. The distribution of canine ehrlichiosis is mainly related to the geographical distribution of the ticks that act as vectors for these bacteria. *E. canis* is transmitted by the brown dog tick (*Rhipicephalus sanguineus*).

2 Describe the different phases of canine monocytic ehrlichiosis, including the typical clinical signs. Canine monocytic ehrlichiosis presents in three phases: (1) an acute phase that lasts 2–4 weeks; (2) a subclinical phase that lasts months to years; and (3) a chronic phase that can last years. The clinical signs (which can be transient) in the acute phase are usually general malaise, anorexia, fever, or petechial bleeding. Laboratory findings in this phase include thrombocytopenia and, less commonly, neutropenia and non-regenerative anemia. During the chronic phase, clinical signs can include petechial bleeding, pale mucous membranes, lymphadenopathy, splenomegaly, uveitis, and weight loss. Laboratory findings in the chronic phase include pancytopenia due to bone marrow hypoplasia, hyperproteinemia, hyperglobulinemia, hypalbuminemia, and proteinuria due to glomerulonephritis.

3 What is the most common ocular finding in dogs with canine monocytic ehrlichiosis, and what is the pathogenesis? Ocular lesions are reported to occur in 10–37% of dogs with canine monocytic ehrlichiosis. The lesions can include ocular, retinal, or orbital hemorrhages that result from thrombocytopenia or vasculitis. Uveitis is one of the most common ocular findings.

4 What systemic and ophthalmic treatment would you recommend? The treatment of choice for ehrlichiosis is oral doxycycline. Treatment for anterior uveitis in dogs with ehrlichiosis should additionally include topical glucocorticoids and atropine.

CASE 98

1 How likely is rabies in this dog, considering that a bite wound was not seen? Rabies virus is shed almost exclusively in saliva up to 10 days before death from rabies, and a bite is the only relevant route of infection for dogs. However, due to the long incubation time (1–3 months or more) owners might not remember a bite wound or even realize that a bite occurred. Thus, rabies should always be considered in a unvaccinated dog that lives in, or has traveled to, an endemic area when there is a sudden change in behavior and/or onset of unexplained acute, progressive CNS signs.

2 How can a diagnosis of rabies be made? In humans, rabies virus can be detected using molecular methods in saliva or dermal tissues antemortem. However, attempts to make an antemortem diagnosis of rabies are not allowed in non-humans because of the low sensitivity of the test and the public health risk. The preferred method is post-mortem detection of viral antigen in the brain using direct immunofluorescence. For confirmation of inconclusive results, mouse inoculation testing and virus isolation have been used, which are now increasingly replaced by the use of molecular methods (reverse-transcriptase PCR).

3 How would you treat a dog suspected to have rabies? In most countries rabies is a notifiable disease, so local regulations must be followed. Considering the public health risk, in many countries the law requires euthanasia of a dog with suggestive signs of rabies. If an unvaccinated dog bites a human, public health authorities generally recommend isolation and observation of the dog in approved facilities. If the dog is shedding rabies virus in saliva, progressive neurologic signs and death will develop within 10 days of the bite. After death or euthanasia, diagnostic testing for rabies on brain specimens should follow. No supportive or antiviral treatment has proved to be effective in rabid animals, so treatment is not recommended and, because of the public health risk, in many countries it is prohibited.

CASE 99

1 What is the most likely diagnosis? Dermatophytosis is the most likely diagnosis. The most probable dermatophyte involved is *Microsporum gypseum*, a geophilic fungus, given the dog's signalment and the localization of the lesions.

2 Name three other differential diagnoses. One other differential diagnosis is vasculopathy. Mildly ischemic lesions can be characterized by alopecia and scaling on the distal extremities, and Jack Russell Terriers are predisposed to vasculopathies. Often the tips of the ears and tail are also affected in these cases and these areas should be inspected closely in this dog. Demodicosis and bacterial pyoderma are two other important differential diagnoses for alopecia and scaling in dogs.

3 What diagnostic tests are indicated in this dog? Wood's lamp examination and trichograms are indicated to assess for dermatophytosis. Positive fluorescence along the hair shafts is diagnostic for dermatophytosis caused by *Microsporum canis*. Hair shafts with adhering spores and hyphae do not provide information on the fungal species involved. If these tests are negative, a deep skin scraping for demodicosis and an impression smear or tape preparation to assess for bacterial infection are the next steps. If skin scrapings are negative and there are no intracellular bacteria on cytology, a fungal culture is indicated, particularly when numerous macrophages are present. In addition, should the owner's finances permit, collection of multiple punch biopsies of the skin can be performed at the same visit. Alternatively, skin biopsies can be recommended at a later stage, if fungal culture is negative.

CASE 100

1 How should this dog be treated? The extent of antifungal therapy instituted depends on the number of animals in the household, the degree of contact of the owner(s) with the animal(s), and the immune status of the owner(s). Topical treatment with enilconazole, lime sulfur rinses, or a shampoo that contains miconazole and chlorhexidine twice weekly is always indicated. If there are more in-contact animals in the household, these animals also should be rinsed or shampooed at least weekly. Systemic antifungal therapy with an azole antifungal drug (itraconazole is the registered treatment of choice in many countries), griseofulvin, or terbinafine should be recommended to hasten recovery and reduce the chance of transmission, especially if immunocompromised humans or young children live in the household, or there is a high level of owner–dog contact. After 4 weeks, a second fungal culture should be submitted and treatment continued until these culture results are available. If a negative culture result is obtained, therapy could be discontinued, particularly if an infection caused by a geophilic fungus such as *Microsporum gypseum* is present. However, if owners are immunocompromised, treatment should be continued until after a second negative monthly culture, as recommended in some guidelines. If the culture is positive, treatment is continued and another culture submitted 4 weeks later.

2 How would you treat the environment around this dog? Environmental decontamination also depends on the type of dermatophyte, the number of animals in the household, the immune status of the owner(s), the severity, duration, and extent of the disease, and the dedication of the owner(s). Therefore, if a zoophilic fungus such as *Microsporum canis* is identified, there are a large number of animals in the household, disease is severe and of long duration, or immunocompromised people are present, more aggressive environmental therapy is indicated. Vacuuming regularly and thoroughly and discarding the vacuum bags carefully is indicated in all situations, as is frequent washing of the dog's bedding and blankets in hot water. Disinfecting surfaces with bleach is effective and realistic in kennels, but not possible for materials in many private households. In some countries, enilconazole foggers are available to treat environmental contamination and are effective within the bounds of the fogger treatment (i.e. areas covered by furniture will not be treated). Steam-cleaning with steam at 85°C or greater will also reduce the presence of viable spores and hyphae.

3 What recommendations should be provided to the owner to minimize the chance of zoonotic transmission? In addition to the abovementioned measures, owners should avoid direct contact with the dog as much as possible and wash or sanitize their hands thoroughly after each contact during the therapy. In some situations (particularly with immunocompromised owners or young children) direct contact should be prevented and the environment should not be shared.

CASE 101

1 What is your assessment of the ocular lesions? There are conjunctival and scleral ecchymoses in both eyes.

2 What is the MRI diagnosis? On MRI, there are multifocal parenchymal and ventricular hemorrhages with secondary vasogenic edema.

3 What would be the primary infectious agent to test for, and what is the test of choice? The primary infectious agent to test for would be *Angiostrongylus vasorum*. Baermann faecal flotation of three fecal samples is considered the test of choice.

CASE 102

1 What is the epidemiology and pathophysiology of angiostrongylosis? *Angiostrongylus vasorum* is a metastrongylid nematode parasite that inhabits the pulmonary arteries and right heart of dogs and wild carnivores in Europe, Africa, and Asia. Dogs become infected by ingesting intermediate hosts (e.g. snails, slugs). Third-stage larvae pass from the gut to the liver, transform to fourth-stage larvae and then migrate to the heart and pulmonary arteries. The larvae are coughed up, swallowed, and passed in the feces. Infected dogs can appear healthy or can have different clinical signs, including cough, right-heart failure, and spontaneous hemorrhages due to bleeding diathesis. The cause of the bleeding is poorly understood, but is believed to be a consumptive coagulopathy initiated by the parasite. Ocular signs can result from aberrant migration of larvae inside the eye, with severe granulomatous uveitis and secondary glaucoma.

2 What treatment would you suggest? The drug of choice is fenbendazole (25–50 mg/kg PO q24h for 10–20 days). Other drugs (e.g. ivermectin, milbemycin oxime, imidacolprid 10%, moxidectin 2.5%, levamisole) have also been suggested. In this dog, treatment with fenbendazole was started immediately. The ocular ecchymoses slowly improved and completely disappeared within 2 weeks of treatment, and the dog fully recovered.

CASE 103

1 How would you interpret the radiographic findings? The thoracic radiographs reveal a severe, diffuse bronchial pattern with marked widening of multiple bronchi. The most visible bronchi fail to taper along their course. There are dependent alveolar infiltrates in the left and right cranial lung lobes as well as within the ventral aspect of the right middle lung lobe. These findings are suggestive of bronchiectasis with concurrent pneumonia.

2 What underlying disease process could be present? Bronchiectasis is an irreversible pathologic dilatation of the airways that can result from any chronic infectious or inflammatory disease that is not adequately controlled with medical therapy. Potential causes include bronchopneumonia that is treated with an inappropriate antibiotic or for an inappropriate length of time, resistant bacterial infection, overuse of cough suppressants in the face of uncontrolled infection or inflammation, foreign body obstruction of an airway with secondary infection, or long-standing airway inflammation. It can also be seen in association with primary ciliary dyskinesia.

3 What complications are possible? Hypoxemia is possible, so pulse oximetry or arterial blood gas analysis would be useful to determine the severity of gas exchange abnormalities. Secondary bacterial infections are also possible. Initially, a CBC, biochemistry panel, and urinalysis are indicated to assess the overall health of the animal.

CASE 104

1 How would you interpret the pulse oximetry reading? Pulse oximetry represents a crude estimation of the partial pressure of arterial oxygen. The principle of pulse oximetry is based on the red and infrared light absorption characteristics of oxygenated and deoxygenated hemoglobin. The instrument uses two light emitting diodes opposite a detector to determine the relative absorptions of red light (absorbed by oxygenated blood) and infrared light (absorbed by deoxygenated blood) during pulsatile flow. Measurements of relative light absorption are made multiple times every second and are processed by the instrument to provide an average of the readings over the previous 3 seconds. False readings are common because of pigmented skin or mucous membranes, poor peripheral pulse, vasoconstriction, or anemia. If the pulse oximeter emits a strong regular pulsation that matches the heart or pulse rate found, the readings are likely to be more accurate. A pulse oximeter reading of 87% correlates with a PaO_2 of less than 60 mmHg (**104**), indicating hypoxemia.

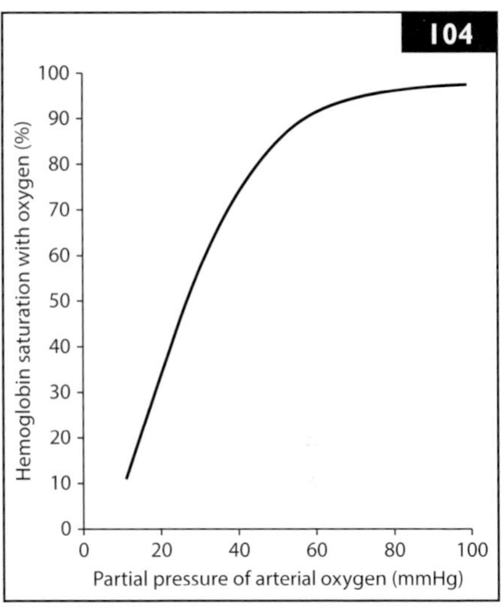

2 How would you interpret the CBC? The leukogram was characterized by moderate eosinophilia and marked basophilia. Heartworm disease as well as other internal parasites (gastrointestinal or respiratory) and external parasites should be considered. Other considerations for eosinophilia and basophilia include mast cell neoplasia or inflammatory conditions of large epithelial surfaces (e.g. respiratory tract, gastrointestinal tract, and skin). A heartworm antigen test was positive in this case and therefore heartworm infection was diagnosed.

CASE 105

1 How would you interpret the rhinoscopy findings? The mucosa appears hyperemic and edematous. Multiple white plaque lesions, most likely consistent with fungal infection, can be seen.

2 How would you interpret the cytologic findings in this dog? Long, septate hyphae 5–7 μm wide with parallel walls are evident along with an admixture of neutrophils. These are consistent with the hyphae of *Aspergillus* spp., which can also be identified based on their branching at 45-degree angles; however, branching was not observed in this case.

3 What treatment should be considered? Topical therapy with clotrimazole or enilconazole is reportedly most efficacious against nasal aspergillosis. A CT scan should be performed to assess the integrity of the cribriform plate because such drugs can cause toxicity if they leak into the CNS. Meticulous debridement of all fungal plaques followed by a 1-hour topical treatment with antifungal medication is indicated. For dogs that have a breach in the cribriform plate or frontal bone, or for those that cannot tolerate prolonged anesthesia for topical treatment, consideration can be given to use of an oral azole antifungal agent; however, efficacy for cure is questionable. Newer agents such as voriconazole and posaconazole are favored over itraconazole. Fluconazole is not active against *Aspergillus* spp.

CASE 106

1 What is your differential diagnosis for the non-healing wounds? The differential diagnosis for the chronic non-healing wounds in this dog include sterile nodular panniculitis, cutaneous mycobacteriosis, nocardiosis, sporotrichosis, infection with a cell-wall deficient bacterium (rare), or bacterial infection secondary to a persisting foreign body (e.g. suture or drain material, or plant awn foreign body). In the latter case, infection with *Actinomyces* spp. can be involved. Other systemic fungal infections, such as coccidioidomycosis, blastomycosis, or histoplasmosis, could also be considered, although they are less likely given the appearance of the lesions.

2 What diagnostic tests would you recommend for this dog? Recommended diagnostic tests should include biopsy of the lesions for histopathology and culture of a macerated tissue specimen for aerobic and anaerobic bacteria, mycobacteria, and fungi. Special stains should be requested for the histopathologic examination, including Gram, Gomori's methenamine silver, periodic acid–Schiff, and acid-fast stains. An ultrasound examination of the region is indicated to evaluate for the presence of foreign material. A work-up for other systemic disease should also be considered (CBC, biochemistry panel, and urinalysis).

CASE 107

1 Which other rapidly growing mycobacterial species can infect dogs and cats? Other rapidly growing mycobacterial species that can infect dogs and cats include *Mycobacterium fortuitum*, *Mycobacterium smegmatis*, *Mycobacterium thermoresistible*, *Mycobacterium goodii*, and *Mycobacterium chelonae*.

2 How does the clinical presentation of disease caused by rapidly growing mycobacteria differ from that caused by *Mycobacterium avium*? Rapidly growing mycobacteria are thought to have a tropism for adipose tissue, and when inoculated by means of penetrating wounds, mycobacterial panniculitis develops. Underlying immunosuppressive disease is usually not present and most dogs are in good body condition or obese. Although disseminated infections with rapidly growing mycobacteria can occur, they are extremely rare. In contrast, *Mycobacterium avium* tends to cause disseminated infections in dogs, involving lymph nodes, liver, and spleen. The intestinal tract can also be involved. In general, *M. avium* tends to cause disease in immunocompromised animals (including humans). Although most infected dogs do not have obvious evidence of immunocompromise, some breeds seem to be predisposed as a result of underlying genetic immunodeficiency (e.g. Basset Hounds).

3 What is the zoonotic potential of this organism? Rapidly growing mycobacteria are not transmitted from one companion animal to another (or to humans) through routine contact, so zoonotic potential is insignificant.

4 How should this infection be treated? Most rapidly growing mycobacterial infections respond to treatment with fluoroquinolones or doxycycline, although high doses of doxycycline (10 mg/kg PO q12h) are recommended. Some rapidly growing mycobacteria can be resistant to multiple antimicrobial drugs and require combination therapy. This dog should be treated based on the results of culture and susceptibility testing of the isolate, which is generally performed at specialized laboratories. Susceptibility testing in this case revealed susceptibility to amikacin, kanamycin, cefoxitin, imipenem, clarithromycin, azithromycin, and clofazamine; intermediate susceptibility to tobramycin, gentamicin, and cefotaxime; and resistance to ceftriaxone, cefepime, ciprofloxacin, doxycycline, moxifloxacin, and amoxicillin–clavulanic acid. The dog was treated with clarithromycin and the wounds subsequently healed slowly over the following 12 months.

CASE 108

1 How would you interpret the laboratory results? There is a mild normocytic normochromic anemia and evidence of renal disease based on the presence of azotemia and isosthenuria. Moderate to severe proteinuria is present, the magnitude of which is suggestive of glomerular protein loss, and also can explain the hypoalbuminemia (i.e. a protein-losing nephropathy is present). Casts in the urine are common in dogs with glomerular disease, and are usually hyaline casts. All together, these laboratory results are suggestive of a glomerulopathy that is accompanied by decreased renal tubular function. According to the suggestions of the International Renal Interest Society Glomerular Disease Study Group, this dog's disease can be classified as tier III C, which is the most severe form.

2 What further work-up would you suggest? Further work-up should include a search for underlying chronic persistent infections or other systemic diseases, such as neoplasia, that can cause glomerular disease. Other underlying infectious causes include infections caused by *Ehrlichia canis*, *Dirofilaria immitis*, *Leishmania* spp., *Borrelia burgdorferi*, *Babesia canis*, and chronic bacterial infections of specific sites, including discospondylitis and endocarditis. The diagnostic work-up should include imaging (thoracic radiographs and abdominal ultrasound) and specific tests for these pathogens depending on the region. Given that high blood pressure occurs in up to 80% of dogs with glomerular disease, blood pressure measurement should be performed. If tests for infectious diseases are negative, renal biopsies could be recommended to differentiate between immune-complex glomerulonephritis and other forms of glomerular disease, such as amyloidosis.

CASE 109

1 Does leishmaniosis explain the clinical abnormalities in this dog? In this dog the glomerular disease could be explained by leishmaniosis. Dogs with leishmaniosis-associated renal disease usually have advanced disease.

2 How would you treat this dog? Treatment consists of specific therapy for leishmaniosis with appropriate medications, such as allopurinol in combination with antimonial compounds or miltefosine. For the glomerular disease, treatment involves inhibition of the renin–angiotensin–aldosterone system to reduce proteinuria, antithrombotic therapy in dogs with low antithrombin III concentrations, and use of diets with a reduced protein and sodium content and high amounts of omega-3 polyunsaturated fatty acids. Antihypertensive drugs can also be required.

3 What is the prognosis? Considering the severity of the glomerular disease, the prognosis for this dog is poor. According to one study, dogs with glomerular disease with azotemia had a median survival time of 13 days, but with appropriate medical therapy longer survival times are possible.

CASE 110

1 Is this lesion consistent with dermatophytosis? Dermatophytosis can mimic many different skin diseases and therefore should always be considered. Lesions typical of dermatophytosis are patchy and usually non-pruritic skin lesions with alopecia, erythema, papules, scaling, and crusting. Lesions often appear on the face or limbs. Usually the lesions are single or few in number and are 1–4 cm in diameter, but they can sometimes be multiple, or coalesce. Occasionally, they are well demarcated, with active inflammation at the periphery, and central crusting or healing ("ringworm"). In most cases, dermatophytosis causes focal lesions. However, in immunosuppressed animals, generalized dermatophytosis can develop with large alopecic areas, often complicated by secondary bacterial infections.

2 What is a "dermatophyte"? In contrast to single-celled yeasts, dermatophytes (literally: "skin plants") are complex fungi that form a mycelium. Owing to their keratinolytic properties they cause superficial skin infections in dogs and many other species, including humans. The most prevalent dermatophyte species in dogs is *Microsporum canis*. Other species include *Trichophyton* spp. and *Microsporum gypseum*.

3 What tests should be done if dermatophytosis is suspected? A simple and rapid screening test for *M. canis* infection is Wood's lamp examination of lesions in a dark room. However, only about 50% of *M. canis* strains fluoresce under UV illumination and other dermatophyte species do not fluoresce at all. Furthermore, lint and topical medications (e.g. tetracycline), debris, or scale, can produce false-positive results. Thus, a Wood's lamp examination should be followed by other testing methods. Direct microscopic examination of affected hairs plucked under Wood's lamp illumination or from the edge of a lesion can be very helpful and is simple and rapid. Hair specimens can be treated with a clearing agent such as 10–20% potassium hydroxide before examination. Potassium hydroxide solutions must be gently heated for 10 minutes for clearing to occur. Hairs or hair fragments with hyphae and arthrospores are thicker than normal hair shafts, with a rough and irregular surface. Direct microscopic examination is insensitive. A more sensitive diagnostic method is fungal culture of hairs or scales from the margin of new lesions on Sabouraud agar, which also allows identification of the infecting species. Wherever possible, submission of specimens to a veterinary diagnostic laboratory that uses standardized methodology is recommended to ensure proper quality assurance for culture and identification of dermatophytes.

CASE 111

1 What was the likely source of *Microsporum canis* infection in this dog? Infections with *M. canis* result from direct contact with infected animals, a contaminated environment, or fomites, including dust particles, brushes, clothes, etc. Cats and dogs serve as reservoirs of dermatophytes, mostly *M. canis*. Many canine and feline infections are subclinical. In dogs and cats younger than 1 year of age, the prevalence of dermatophyte colonization is higher than that in older animals. Cats seem to be the principal reservoir for *M. canis*, because more cats than dogs are infected, and commonly without clinical signs. In the case described here, close contact with the recently introduced kitten is the most likely source of infection. Intact skin is resistant to dermatophyte infection, but any injury (such as a cat scratch) can facilitate the germination of arthrospores and infection of the skin.

2 What is the prognosis? Given that the lesion in this dog is small and localized, the prognosis is good, because in immunocompetent dogs dermatophytosis is a self-limiting disease that resolves spontaneously. However, this can take several weeks.

3 Can the dog transmit this disease to other animals or humans? Infected animals shed arthrospores of *M. canis* (or other dermatophytes) on scales and broken hairs. The arthrospores can survive in the environment for a year or longer. Other animals or humans can be infected and develop a similar skin disease. Children are more prone to developing dermatophytosis than adults, because young individuals of all species are less resistant to this infection, and children commonly have closer contact with pets.

CASE 112

1 What differential diagnoses should be considered for mucosal pallor, and what is your assessment for this dog? Pale mucous membranes can be caused by shock or by anemia. Shock is unlikely in this dog, as capillary refill time was normal and pulse quality was bounding, therefore anemia is likely.

2 What are the next diagnostic steps? The next diagnostic step is evaluation of the hematocrit. If the hematocrit is low, a reticulocyte count should be obtained to differentiate between regenerative and non-regenerative anemia. A blood smear to evaluate red blood cell morphology and a slide agglutination test to evaluate for hemagglutination are also indicated.

CASE 113

1 What is your diagnosis? The diagnosis is hemolytic anemia due to infection with a large *Babesia* species (most likely *Babesia canis*).

2 What factors have to be addressed and kept in mind before and during a blood transfusion? The donor dog should be healthy, test negative for blood parasites, be properly vaccinated, and should receive parasite prevention (especially for fleas and ticks) regularly. The hematocrit of the donor should be determined. The donor should ideally have the same blood group as the recipient. If the blood group is different or no blood typing is available, a cross-match of donor and recipient blood should be performed. The donor can donate up to 15 ml/kg blood (750 ml for this donor). The recipient's hematocrit will increase by 0.01 l/l for each 2 ml/kg of whole blood transfused. Therefore, about 300 ml of whole blood are needed to increase the recipient's hematocrit to 0.3 l/l. Blood should be collected into a sterile bag that contains anticoagulant (e.g. 1 ml sodium citrate to 9 ml blood). Blood should be administered using a transfusion set that includes blood filters, over a period of 4–6 hours. As transfusion reactions can occur, regular monitoring of the transfusion is mandatory. Following transfusion, the hematocrit should be re-evaluated.

CASE 114

1 What are two underlying pathophysiologic processes associated with hyperesthesia? Inflammation and compression are the two pathologic processes that are associated with increased sensitivity to physical stimulation or palpation.

2 What are the four anatomic structures associated with diffuse hyperesthesia? Diffuse or generalized hyperesthesia that is caused by inflammatory or compressive diseases is most likely to involve the nerve endings in bone (periosteum), joint (synovium), nerve (meninges), or muscle (perimysium).

3 What are the two underlying pathophysiologic processes associated with elevated rectal temperature? Rectal temperature can be increased as a result of fever from the body's resetting of its thermostat, or hyperthermia from sources of endogenous or exogenous heat.

CASE 115

1 Which organ systems are likely to be responsible for the hyperesthesia in this dog, and how can this be associated with fever? This dog has inflammation of the bones and muscles, which is the probable cause of fever via a resetting of the hypothalamic thermostat as a result of inflammatory cytokines, although increased muscle activity and rigidity can themselves lead to increased body temperature caused by diffuse prolonged muscle contractions. Inflammation, however, is the more likely cause when the high white blood cell count is considered.

2 Which type of organism is seen in the muscle biopsy (e.g. virus, bacterium)? The muscle biopsy shows a protozoal cyst.

3 Which infectious diseases caused by these types of organisms are associated with polymyositis? Protozoal diseases that can present with polymyositis include toxoplasmosis, neosporosis, sarcocystosis, and hepatozoonosis.

4 Which of these organisms can additionally cause polyperiostitis? *Hepatozoon* spp. can cause both polymyositis and polyperiostitis.

CASE 116

1 What drugs are used in the treatment of hepatozoonosis, and how long must treatment be continued? Treatment involves concurrent use of trimethoprim/sulfonamide, clindamycin, pyrimethamine, and decoquinate. The decoquinate treatment is initiated after the other drugs are started and it is continued thereafter. Adjunctive anti-inflammatory and/or analgesic therapy might be needed to suppress some of the inflammatory response and help alleviate the discomfort.

2 How do the clinical manifestations and diagnostic findings differ between *Hepatozoon canis* and *Hepatozoon americanum* infection? Dogs with *H. canis* infection more commonly have increased rectal temperature and lethargy; however, they more rarely have signs of hyperesthesia or gait dysfunction. Dogs with *H. americanum* infection more commonly have hyperesthesia and marked radiographic bone changes. Dogs with both infections can have marked neutrophilia with left shift. Circulating parasites within neutrophils are more commonly identified in dogs with *H. canis* infection.

CASE 117

1 What are the most likely differential diagnoses for this case? The history and clinical signs suggest inflammatory joint disease as the most likely cause, but metabolic or endocrine disorders should also be considered. Polyarthropathies can result from non-erosive immune-mediated disease or (less commonly) from processes that cause erosion of the joint surfaces. They can also develop as a result of bacteremia. Immune-mediated polyarthritis may result from primary autoimmune disease (systemic lupus erythematosus or idiopathic immune-mediated polyarthritis) or be secondary to infections, treatment with some drugs (especially sulfonamides), or potentially neoplasia. The history of access to wooded areas and the geographic location raise suspicion for infection with pathogens such as *Anaplasma phagocytophilum* or *Borrelia burgdorferi*. Fungal pathogens such as *Blastomyces dermatitidis* have also been associated with polyarthritis. Other pathogens that are less common in this region that could cause polyarthritis include *Ehrlichia canis*, *Rickettsia rickettsii*, and possibly *Bartonella* spp. (although the association of *Bartonella* spp. with polyarthritis is not clear). Pathogens such as *Ehrlichia chaffeensis* and *Ehrlichia ewingii* should be considered in southern and central areas of the USA. *Leishmania* spp. infection should be considered in other geographic areas of the world.

2 What diagnostic testing should initially be performed? A CBC to detect abnormalities associated with infectious or immune-mediated disorders (thrombocytopenia, anemia, leucopenia, or leukocytosis) is indicated, as well as a biochemistry profile and urinalysis to assess for metabolic or endocrine causes. Radiography of affected limbs can be performed to assess for erosive polyarthritis. Arthrocentesis of multiple joints with cytologic examination and culture of synovial fluid should be performed to characterize the disease process and rule out septic arthritis. Tests for antibodies against *Anaplasma* spp., *B. burgdorferi*, *E. canis*, and *E. ewingii* can be performed, and antigen testing for *Blastomyces* antigen should also be considered. However, given the acute history, antibody tests can still be negative, and so PCR for *A. phagocytophilum* and *Ehrlichia* spp. could also be performed.

CASE 118

1 What is the structure seen in the neutrophil? The blood smear shows an intracytoplasmic morula. This can be either *Anaplasma phagocytophilum* or *Ehrlichia ewingii*, because they have the same morphology and infect the same cells. Given the region, *A. phagocytophilum* is more likely. Morulae appear from 4–8 days post *A. phagocytophilum* infection. However, morulae are not always seen in dogs with granulocytic anaplasmosis or ehrlichiosis, and can be confused with cytoplasmic granules or artifacts. Therefore, antibody tests or PCR should be performed in addition, to confirm infection.

2 What conclusions can be made from the results of the synovial fluid analysis? The results of the analysis are consistent with neutrophilic polyarthritis. Idiopathic non-erosive polyarthritis is the most common form, representing 60–80% of all cases. Infections involving *A. phagocytophilum*, *Borrelia burgdorferi*, *E. ewingii*, and *Blastomyces* are potential causes of polyarthritis.

CASE 119

1 Does this result alone confirm a diagnosis of granulocytic anaplasmosis? A positive result on the in-clinic ELISA indicates the presence of antibodies against *Anaplasma phagocytophilum* or *Anaplasma platys*. The test does not differentiate between antibodies to different *Anaplasma* spp. Based on the geographic location and the presence of morulae, *A. phagocytophilum* infection is suspected in this dog. The antibody test does not distinguish between recent infection and past exposure, because antibodies can persist for many months. In fact, most dogs with acute anaplasmosis have negative antibody test results. Thus, diagnosis of anaplasmosis has to be based on direct detection of the organism, such as detection of morulae or positive PCR, or acute and convalescent phase antibody testing using immunofluorescent antibody tests (so that a 4-fold change in titer can be detected), together with compatible clinical signs and a positive response to treatment. In endemic areas, up to one-third of dogs have antibodies without ever showing clinical signs of infection.
2 What other tests could be performed? PCR could be performed because it is is highly specific and sensitive during the acute phase of infection, and can identify the *Anaplasma* spp. present if specific assays for *A. phagocytophilum* are used. *A. phagocytophilum* infection was confirmed by PCR in this case.
3 What is the treatment for this disease in dogs? Doxycycline (5 mg/kg PO q12h) should be given for 2 weeks. Clinical improvement as well as an increase in the platelet count is usually seen within 24–48 hours; otherwise, other causes should be considered. Pain could be managed with non-steroidal anti-inflammatories or opioids, but usually antimicrobial therapy alone is rapidly effective. Ectoparasite preventives should be used year-round.
4 What is the prognosis in this case? Anaplasmosis has an excellent prognosis when treated appropriately.

CASE 120

1 What is the likelihood that the dog was infected with *Mycobacterium tuberculosis*? *Mycobacterium tuberculosis* infection is extremely rare in dogs. *M. tuberculosis* is the major cause of tuberculosis in humans, who are the only reservoir hosts. Tuberculosis has become increasingly important in immunosuppressed people, especially with the spread of human immunodeficiency virus infection. If dogs are infected, it is through direct contact with infected humans (a reverse zoonosis). Infection with *M. tuberculosis* in dogs is often subclinical or insidious. It is unclear what factors contribute to the host's resistance. Cell-mediated immunity is typically associated with protection against facultative intracellular pathogens and seems to be associated with the enhanced capacity of activated macrophages to kill mycobacterial organisms or to inhibit their intracellular multiplication. In contrast to other *Mycobacterium* spp., *M. tuberculosis* has an affinity for tissues with high oxygen content, and this explains its common localization in the lungs. Pulmonary manifestations in dogs include bronchopneumonia, pulmonary nodule formation, and hilar lymphadenopathy, with associated clinical signs of fever, weight loss, anorexia, and a harsh, non-productive cough. Animals with tuberculous pneumonitis discharge organisms in the sputum, as do infected people and aerosolized droplets are the primary means of transmission of this disease. Although pets acquire *M. tuberculosis* infection from people, and spread from dogs to people has not been reported, infected animals represent a potential risk to their owners.

2 Are there diagnostic tests that can rule out the possibility of infection in this dog? There are no diagnostic tests in dogs that reliably rule out infection with *M. tuberculosis*. Antibody tests or intradermal tests do not work reliably in dogs and are commonly falsely negative. Detection of the organism by PCR or culture (e.g. in tracheobronchial lavage specimens) is only successful in dogs with clinical signs. Thus, in conclusion, although the risk is low, this dog might have become infected, and there is no definitive test to rule out infection. This risk has to be discussed with the family, especially as there is a baby in the household.

CASE 121

1 What is your interpretation of the thoracic radiographs? The thoracic radiographs show marked narrowing of the tracheal lumen on the left lateral view. A patchy interstitial to alveolar pattern is present in the cranioventral thorax and is worse in the right cranial lung lobe. There is a diffuse alveolar pattern with lobar sign and volume loss in the region of the left cranial lung lobe, causing a leftward shift in the mediastinum. A moderate, diffuse bronchial pattern is present caudodorsally. The esophagus is moderately dilated with gas.

2 What differential diagnoses should be considered? The primary differential diagnosis in this patient is aspiration pneumonia, likely as a complication of brachycephalic syndrome. Tracheal hypoplasia is most likely a component of brachycephalic syndrome in this breed of dog, although tracheal edema or inflammation should also be considered as a cause for narrowing of the lumen. Esophageal dilation could reflect aerophagia; however, esophageal dysfunction (megaesophagus or a hiatal hernia) cannot be ruled out. Although less likely, given the recent visit to a veterinary clinic, the possibility of canine infectious respiratory disease complex should also be considered.

3 What diagnostic tests should be performed? A CBC and biochemistry panel (and potentially urinalysis) are indicated to assess the overall health of the animal. If possible, pulse oximetry (or, alternatively, blood gas analysis) would be useful to determine the severity of pulmonary dysfunction. PCR for canine distemper virus infection could be considered. Further diagnostic testing should be delayed pending stabilization of the patient.

CASE 122

1 How would you interpret the CBC? The CBC showed a mild regenerative anemia, which may be consistent with the age of the dog. The white blood cell count demonstrated marked leukocytosis, characterized by neutrophilia with a left shift and monocytosis. The platelet count was increased, consistent with a reactive thromobocytosis.

2 What stabilizing treatment should be provided? Given the severity of the clinical findings and radiographic changes consistent with aspiration pneumonia, hospitalization would be recommended. Intravenous fluids should be employed along with intravenous antibiotics. Antimicrobial drug choices should be based on the organisms considered most likely in aspiration pneumonia, including enteric bacterial species, *Mycoplasma* spp., and anaerobic bacteria. A short course of terbutaline could be considered to counteract acid-induced bronchoconstriction. Oxygen supplementation would be advised to alleviate respiratory distress. Antiemetic medications and gastrointestinal protectants could be helpful during the initial observation period. Nebulization could be used to hydrate airway secretions; however, coupage should not be performed on a vomiting patient because increased intrathoracic pressure could exacerbate emesis.

3 What follow-up tests should be considered? A follow-up CBC would be advised in 2–5 days to assess response to therapy. Pulse oximetry should be monitored for improvement or deterioration in gas exchange. Recheck thoracic radiographs would be recommended in 2 weeks to assess tracheal size, pulmonary infiltrates, and the esophageal changes. Videofluoroscopy could be considered in the future to investigate the possibility of a hiatal hernia given the breed predisposition to this condition.

CASE 123

1 What is a likely explanation for the edema, based on the history? Given the previous diagnosis of leishmaniosis, low oncotic pressure due to hypoalbuminemia secondary to a protein-losing glomerulonephritis should be suspected. This is a common complication of the disease. A CBC, serum biochemistry panel, and a urinalysis with UPCR revealed proteinuria (UPCR 6, RI <0.5) with a serum albumin concentration of 12 g/l (RI 29–37 g/l).

2 How could the problem and its clinical consequences be addressed? Protein loss in this dog can be managed through administration of an angiotensin converting enzyme inhibitor (e.g. benazepril). Plasma colloid osmotic pressure can be improved by administering a constant rate infusion of colloids (e.g. hydroxyethylstarch 130KD/0.4 at 2 ml/kg/h). Albumin production may be improved by enteral nutrition. If the appetite is reduced, esophagostomy tube feeding should be discussed with the owner. It is difficult in a dog this size to increase serum albumin concentration by plasma transfusion (a dose of 45 ml/kg is needed to increase albumin by 10 g/l). Transfusion of human albumin or canine albumin is more effective at raising the albumin concentration, but administration of human albumin is associated with a high risk of anaphylactic reactions. Plasma antithrombin concentration should be determined, and if low, antithrombotic treatment (e.g. clopidogrel) should be recommended.

CASE 124

1 What is your interpretation of the physical examination, and what are the differential diagnoses for the described heart murmurs? The main problem identified on physical examination was the new continuous heart murmur with point of maximal intensity over the left heart base. The previously documented left basal systolic murmur could result from pulmonic stenosis (PS) (infundibular, sub, supra, or valvular), aortic or subaortic stenosis (AS/SAS), tetralogy of Fallot, obstructive outflow disorders, or an atrial septal defect (ASD) leading to a relative pulmonic stenosis. Given the loud murmur intensity and the fact that it had been present for several years, an ASD was considered unlikely. The continuous left basal heart murmur could be due to a congenital persistent ductus arteriosus (PDA) or a coexisting systolic and diastolic murmur (e.g. AS/PS along with severe aortic or pulmonic insufficiency, respectively). As the continuous murmur was newly reported, an acquired cause was more likely than PDA.

2 What further diagnostic procedure should be recommended? Echocardiography should be performed to identify the cause of the heart murmur.

CASE 125

1 What is your interpretation of the echocardiographic images? Figure **125a** shows a hyperechogenic vegetative oscillating lesion on the septal aortic valve cusps. The left ventricle appears slightly volume overloaded. Figure **125b** shows a severe aortic regurgitation jet in diastole, approaching the center of the left ventricle, due to a vegetative lesion on the septal cusps. This explains the diastolic murmur. Figure **125c** shows the continuous wave Doppler of the aortic velocity. The systolic velocity is about 4 m/s, which resembles a pressure gradient of 64 mmHg according to the modified Bernoulli equation ($4 \times v^2$). Normal velocity is <2.0 m/s, so there is evidence of moderate aortic stenosis. This explains the systolic component of the murmur.

2 What is your main differential diagnosis? Taking the echocardiographic findings together, there is a high suspicion of aortic valve endocarditis causing a systolic and diastolic murmur due to aortic stenosis and aortic valve insufficiency. Both murmurs together auscultate as a continuous murmur. The main underlying reason could be congenital aortic stenosis. In this dog, the aortic valve is severely thickened and there is a vegetative lesion, which makes congenital aortic stenosis less likely. However, aortic valve stenosis can be a predisposing factor for the development of endocarditis. Although many dogs with endocarditis are presented with a history of fever (60%), this dog did not have fever at the time of evaluation.

3 What further tests would you recommend? Other diagnostic tests that could be performed in this dog to assess the severity of disease and determine whether there are complications of endocarditis (such as thromboembolic disorders) include evaluation of laboratory parameters (CBC, biochemistry panel, and urinalysis), thoracic radiographs, abdominal ultrasound, urinalysis, and bacterial urine culture, bacterial blood cultures (three specimens from different sites), and diagnostic tests for *Bartonella* spp.

CASE 126

1 What are the suggested criteria for diagnosis of infective endocarditis? Diagnosis of infective endocarditis (IE) is often established by identification of major and/or minor critera for IE. A scoring system, adapted from the modified Duke's criteria for IE in people, has been proposed to determine the diagnosis of IE in dogs.

Major criteria	Minor criteria	Diagnosis
Positive echocardiogram: vegetative or erosive lesion or abscess	Fever Medium to large dog (>15 kg) Subaortic stenosis	**Definitive** Histopathology of valve 2 major criteria 1 major and 2 minor criteria
New valvular insufficiency: > mild aortic insufficiency without subaortic stenosis or annuloaortic ectasia	Immune-mediated disease: • polyarthritis • glomerulonephritis Thromboembolic disease	**Possible** 1 major and 1 minor criterion 3 minor criteria
Positive blood culture: ≥2 positive blood cultures ≥3 if common skin contaminant	Positive blood culture not meeting major criteria listed in this table Detection of *Bartonella* spp. infection	**Rejected** Other disease diagnosed Resolution of regurgitation or valvular abnormality within 4 days of treatment No pathologic evidence of endocarditis on post-mortem examination

In this dog, a diagnosis of endocarditis could be established from three major (vegetative lesion, new severe aortic insufficiency, positive blood culture) and one minor (large dog >15 kg) criterion.

2 What are known predisposing factors for endocarditis? Predisposing factors that should raise suspicion for IE are discospondylitis, prostatitis, pneumonia, urinary tract infection, pyoderma, periodontal disease, infected wounds, abscesses, or long-term indwelling central venous catheters, as well as immunosuppressive drug therapy such as with glucocorticoids, aortic stenosis, or recent surgery, especially in conjunction with trauma to mucosal surfaces in the oral or genital tract. Most dogs with IE do not have underlying congenital cardiac defects. No link has been made between dental prophylaxis and IE in dogs.

3 What is the general prognosis for dogs with endocarditis? The prognosis for IE depends on several factors. Factors indicating a poor prognosis include aortic valve involvement, thromboembolic complications, thrombocytopenia, elevation of serum ALP, and hypoalbuminemia. A slightly better prognosis is reported for isolated mitral valve involvement, gram-positive infections, and when underlying wounds or skin infections are present.

CASE 127

1 What are the body systems in which problems were identified in this dog? Problems were identified in the gastrointestinal tract, in the nervous system, and in the eye.

2 Where would you suspect the neurologic localization? The abnormal mental status with asymmetric neurologic signs suggests an intracranial location. The right-sided cranial nerve deficits indicate a problem in the right brainstem. Visual responses were abnormal, suggesting a neurologic and/or an intraocular disease process.

3 What would be your diagnostic plans for the various problems? Given the history of diarrhea, tenesmus, and hematochezia, large bowel disease is present. Defecation should be observed and feces collected. Tests should include a fecal microscopic examination for helminths and protozoal pathogens. A stained rectal scraping cytology should be performed. A complete ophthalmologic examination as well as a full neurologic examination is needed. A CBC, biochemical profile, and urinalysis should be performed as a screen for systemic disease and to ensure organ function is normal before anaesthesia. Under anaesthesia, a CSF tap should be obtained. Imaging of the brain with CT or MRI should precede the CSF collection, because there is a risk of brain herniation if intracranial pressure is increased.

CASE 128

1 What organisms can be seen on the rectal scraping cytology? On the rectal scraping cytology, large numbers of oval organisms demarcated by an unstained halo are surrounded by inflammatory cells. The organisms are *Prototheca* spp. These unicellular achlorophyllous algal organisms are found in the environment in organically enriched soil, water, and vegetation, and in cow's milk. Based on the location of lesions, spread of infection is thought to be by ingestion or contact with injured skin or mucosal surfaces. Typically, involvement of the colon results in large bowel diarrhea. This is followed by dissemination in immunocompromised hosts with typical localization in the eyes and CNS. Clinical manifestations of uveitis, retinitis, and panophthalmitis are accompanied by meningoencephalitis with a variety of neurologic signs.

2 What diagnostic tests could be performed for definitive diagnosis of this disease? A diagnosis can be made by microscopic identification of the organism in cerebrospinal fluid, rectal scrapings, or aspirates or biopsies of the eyes, colon, lymph nodes, or skin. Culture or PCR can be performed to definitively identify the *Prototheca* species involved.

The dog had a progressive deterioration in neurologic function. The owner decided not to pursue further treatment and the dog was euthanized. At necropsy, grossly the colon had a dark hemorrhagic color to the mucosal surface and enlarged ileocolic lymph nodes were identified. Multiple focal dark brown to gray pinpoint foci were visible on the cut surface of the midbrain, hindbrain, and cortical regions. The histopathologic examination showed multifocal lymphoplasmacytic to histiocytic meningoencephalitis with intralesional organisms consistent with *Prototheca* spp. The organisms were oval, refractile, 10–15 µm in diameter with a 2–3 µm-thick cell wall, and stained with Gomori's methanamine silver stain. Similar lesions and organisms were observed histologically in the mucosal and submucosal regions of the large bowel and in the ileocolic lymph node.

3 Are there any treatment options for this disease? In a few cases, a positive response to therapy has been seen with a combination of amphotericin B and itraconazole. Relapses were common in the few dogs that responded; therefore, continuous treatment with itraconazole is usually needed.

CASE 129

1 Can such titers result from previous vaccination with *Leptospira* vaccines? Older leptospirosis vaccines contain Canicola and Icterohaemorrhagiae serogroup antigens, and many of the newer vaccines contain these as well as Grippotyphosa and Bratislava or Pomona serogroup antigens. Thus, antibodies to these serogroups can result from vaccination. However, cross-reactivity with strains of other serogroups also occurs. Titers resulting from vaccination can be very high (exceeding 1,600 several months after vaccination) and be detectable for more than a year after vaccination; therefore, the presence of a titer to any serogroup alone is not diagnostic. Thus, diagnosis of leptospirosis requires demonstration of a 4-fold (2 titer steps) titer increase over a 1–2-week period.

2 What is the diagnostic significance of MAT results in a non-vaccinated dog? Unvaccinated dogs can have antibodies to *Leptospira* spp. due to subclinical exposure. Therefore, acute and convalescent titers are still required to document recent infection, in association with typical clinical signs. Although MAT is widely used, it has many limitations. Owing to the subjective endpoint determination, titers can be highly discordant among laboratories. Even in the same laboratory, the reproducibility can be poor, so the same laboratory should perform the acute and convalescent titers. Nevertheless, early antibiotic treatment is strongly indicated in suspected cases.

3 What other tests could help to confirm or rule out leptospirosis? Dark field examination of urine for viable (moving) leptospires has been performed in the past, but has very low sensitivity, and the same is true for culture of leptospires from urine. PCR of blood or urine is increasingly used for detection of leptospiral DNA. As these bacteria are usually shed intermittently and sometimes in low numbers, a negative result never excludes infection. In this dog, a second MAT titer was obtained 2 weeks later, and at that time the Grippotyphosa titer was 1:6,400. Thus, a diagnosis of leptospirosis was confirmed.

CASE 130

1 What is your differential diagnosis for the leucopenia? The leukopenia in this dog is caused by a neutropenia. The neutropenia is severe and is due to insufficient production or destruction of neutrophilic precursors in the bone marrow because no band neutrophils (thus no signs of regeneration) are present. Neutropenia without regeneration also can be caused by a shift from the central neutrophil pool to the marginal pool within the blood vessels.

2 Can a vaccinated dog develop parvovirosis? This dog received his last vaccination against parvovirus at 10 weeks of age. Maternal antibodies that interfered with effective immunization were likely still to be present at that time. It is advised to administer vaccines to puppies every 3–4 weeks from 6–8 weeks of age until at least 16–18 weeks of age, because interference by maternal antibodies can last up to 18 weeks of age. Therefore, vaccination was likely ineffective in this dog.

3 Could a dog become infected with parvovirus from a cat? Dogs cannot be infected with feline panleukopenia virus. However, because a cat with panleukopenia can be either infected with a feline or with a canine parvovirus, cats with panleukopenia should be considered a potential risk to dogs that do not have antibodies against parvoviruses. It has also been shown that healthy cats can shed canine parvovirus and, thus, can pose a risk to unprotected dogs.

CASE 131

1 What supportive treatment is appropriate in a dog with parvovirosis? A dog with parvovirosis should be kept in isolation and receive intensive care. Appropriate supportive therapy and good nursing care significantly decrease mortality. Restoration of fluid, electrolyte, and acid–base balance by IV continuous-rate infusion is the most important aspect of supportive treatment. Fluid therapy should be continued as long as vomiting and/or diarrhea persist. Metabolic acidosis and hypokalemia are common and should be corrected through IV fluid supplementation. Hypoglycemia should also be addressed if present. Although withholding food and water were general recommendations in earlier days for treating gastrointestinal diseases, including parvovirosis, recent information suggests this is contraindicated. Thus, oral intake of water and food should only be restricted if severe vomiting persists and should be restarted as early as possible. A highly digestible diet is preferred but if the patient does not eat it, any restricted-fat diet is better than no food intake at all. If nausea is present or persistent vomiting occurs, antiemetics should be administered. Antiemetic drugs are helpful to reduce fluid loss, decrease patient distress, and make enteral nutrition possible. Dogs that develop hypoproteinemia may benefit from plasma or whole blood transfusions to restore oncotic pressure. A whole blood transfusion will help to resolve the problem, but if erythrocytes are not needed, plasma transfusion is a more appropriate therapy. Plasma transfusion, in combination with heparin, is also helpful to treat DIC, as it replaces depleted antithrombin and provides other important factors to counteract the systemic inflammatory response syndrome. Ideally, serum albumin concentration should be maintained at 20 g/l or higher. If edema caused by decreased albumin is present and is not corrected by a plasma transfusion, synthetic colloids, such as hetastarch, should be considered. Colloids should not be given until dehydration is corrected and should always be used with additional fluids. Central parenteral nutrition also can correct hypoproteinemia if it contains a sufficient amount of amino acids, and it is indicated in dogs that are persistently anorectic or show severe vomiting.

Co-infection with intestinal parasites can exacerbate parvovirosis by enhancing intestinal cell turnover and subsequent viral replication. Appropriate anthelmintic therapy should be initiated as soon as vomiting ceases.

2 Which antibiotics should be used? As the gut barrier is often destroyed in dogs with parvovirosis, intestinal bacteria can translocate into the bloodstream. Bacteremia can ensue, facilitated by the existing neutropenia, leading to sepsis in these immunocompromised patients. Thus, prevention of sepsis is essential. As the bacteria usually derive from the gut, antibiotics with good activity against gram-negative and anaerobic bacteria are recommended. Antibiotics should be administered parenterally, ideally IV. The patient should be fully rehydrated before a nephrotoxic drug, such as an aminoglycoside, is administered.

CASE 132

1 Is treatment with recombinant feline interferon-ω useful? Feline interferon-ω is licensed in Europe, Asia, and Australia for treatment of viral infections in cats and dogs. In experimental as well as in field studies, feline interferon-ω has been effective in dogs with parvovirosis. Given that feline interferon-ω may reduce mortality, treatment with 2.5×10^6 IU/kg IV q24h for 3 consecutive days has been recommended in severely sick dogs with parvovirosis.

2 Is administration of specific antibodies useful? Specific antibodies can be used not only for prevention but also for treatment of parvovirus infection. Commercial products containing highly concentrated immunoglobulins (multivalent hyperimmune immunoglobulin preparations) are available in some European countries for dogs and cats (heterologous preparation produced in horses). However, a placebo-controlled double-blinded field study was not able to show efficacy of this type of commercial product in the treatment of dogs with parvovirosis.

3 Are drugs that increase the neutrophil count available and useful? Filgastrim (recombinant human granulocyte colony-stimulating factor [G-CSF]) has been used for treatment of severe neutropenia in dogs. The human product increases blood neutrophil counts in healthy dogs and in dogs with several specific neutropenic conditions. Filgrastim has been used in both dogs and cats with parvovirus-associated neutropenia, but was not shown to be effective. The lack of efficacy of exogenous G-CSF is probably the result of an already existing high level of endogenous G-CSF and massive necrosis of bone marrow progenitor cells. Filgastrim could also lead to an increase in parvovirus replication and therefore is not recommended.

CASE 133

1 How is the anemia in this dog classified, and what are the main differential diagnoses? The high reticulocyte count, the high MCV, and the presence of polychromasia, normoblastemia, anisocytosis, and Howell–Jolly bodies indicate regenerative anemia. Increased red cell destruction and hemorrhage should be considered as possible causes. The icterus suggests the possibility of extravascular hemolysis, but icterus could be hepatic or posthepatic as well. Spherocytosis and agglutination of erythrocytes suggest the presence of primary or secondary immune-mediated hemolytic anemia (IMHA). IMHA can be secondary to a variety of underlying disorders, such as infections (e.g. *Mycoplasma haemocanis*, *Babesia* spp., *Ehrlichia* spp., *Rangelia vitalii*, chronic bacteremia), neoplastic diseases (e.g. lymphoma), and exposure to drugs, toxins (e.g. trimethoprim/sulphonamide, beta-lactam antibiotics, bee stings).

2 What diagnostic tests should be performed next? Further diagnostics should include cytologic examination of fine needle aspirates of the enlarged lymph nodes to evaluate the presence of infectious agents or lymphoma. In addition, tests for underlying infectious diseases should be performed. Tests of coagulation function should be considered given the subcutaneous hemorrhage. Should lymph node aspirates be non-diagnostic, ultrasound of the abdomen should be performed to evaluate the liver and spleen and obtain additional specimens (after ruling out coagulation disorders).

CASE 134

1 What are the cytologic findings in the lymph node aspirate? The cytology shows a predominance of small lymphocytes together with a high number of plasma cells. Within the cytoplasm of one cell, several parasitic organisms can be seen. There are also a few macrophages and lymphoblasts.

2 Can a definitive diagnosis be made? The geographic location, the physical examination findings, the laboratory results, and the presence of typical appearing organisms within the cytoplasm of a cell in the lymph node suggest a diagnosis of rangeliosis. Rangeliosis is a disease that only occurs in south and southeast regions of Brazil. It is also known as "nambiuvú" (which means "bloody ear margins") or bleeding plague. Rangeliosis can be associated with a secondary IMHA. PCR was performed to confirm the diagnosis in this case, and was positive for *Rangelia vitalii*.

CASE 135

1 What is the recommended treatment for this patient? Supportive treatment is indicated in order to correct the dehydration and address continuing losses. This includes intravenous administration of crystalloid fluids, use of antiemetics and antacids, and nutritional support. Some dogs require blood transfusions. Doxycycline (5 mg/kg PO q12h) together with either a single dose of imidocarb diproprionate (6 mg/kg SC) or diminazene aceturate (3.5 mg/kg SC) are the antiprotozoal drugs that are currently recommended for treatment of rangeliosis. Dogs treated with imidocarb dipropionate can be premedicated with atropine (0.5 mg/kg SC) 30 minutes before injection to avoid parasympathetic adverse effects, such as salivation, vomiting, and occasionally diarrhea. Doxycycline treatment should be continued until clinical abnormalities have resolved and PCR results on blood and lymph node aspirates are negative.

2 The owner has two other dogs. What preventive measures should be recommended? *Rangelia vitalli* is transmitted by *Amblyomma aureolatum* ticks and possibly also by *Rhipicephalus sanguineus*. Preventive measures for other dogs include regular application of long-acting acaricides as well as treatment of the environment for ticks.

CASE 136

1 What is your main differential diagnosis for the lesion on the aortic valve, including infectious agents potentially involved, and which pathogen seems most likely based on the clinical findings? The lesion seen on echocardiography is consistent with valvular infective endocarditis, which is causing congestive heart failure in this dog. Infectious agents that can cause infective endocarditis include streptococci (such as *Streptococcus canis*), staphylococci (such as *Staphylococcus pseudintermedius* and *Staphylococcus aureus*), other gram-positive bacteria (such as *Erysipelothrix* spp. and *Actinomyces* spp.), gram-negative rods (most commonly *Escherichia coli*, but also *Pseudomonas aeruginosa*, *Salmonella* spp., *Citrobacter* spp., *Klebsiella* spp., *Proteus* spp., *Pasteurella* spp., and *Brucella canis*), *Bartonella* spp., *Enterococcus* spp., and, rarely, filamentous fungi, such as *Aspergillus* spp. The location of the lesion on the aortic valve in this dog, together with the presence of congestive heart failure, raises suspicion for *Bartonella* spp. infection, because *Bartonella* has a predilection for the aortic valve and is more likely than other pathogens to be associated with congestive heart failure.

2 What additional diagnostic tests would you recommend? Other diagnostic tests that are indicated are routine bloodwork (CBC, biochemistry, and urinalysis), aerobic bacterial blood cultures, and *Bartonella* spp. antibody tests or culture and PCR. For blood cultures, ideally 10 ml of blood should be collected into blood culture bottles three times over a 24-hour period. A different vein should be used for collection each time, using aseptic technique (i.e. clip and prepare the site, wash hands, and wear sterile gloves when collecting the specimen). In unstable animals with signs of sepsis, two specimens should initially be collected

10 minutes apart, after which intravenous antimicrobial drugs can be given. The third specimen is collected just before the next dose of antibiotics (i.e. a trough specimen). Negative blood cultures further increase suspicion for bartonellosis. *Bartonella* spp. antibody tests are species-specific. Ideally, antibody tests for *Bartonella vinsonii* subsp. *berkhoffii*, *Bartonella clarridgeiae*, and *Bartonella henselae* should be performed at a minimum. *Bartonella* spp. culture is difficult in dogs. Specimens for culture should be sent to a laboratory with special expertise in *Bartonella* spp. culture. Use of *Bartonella* alpha-Proteobacteria growth medium (BAPGM) enrichment culture, with subsequent PCR from culture medium, is the most sensitive method for detection of *Bartonella* in the blood of dogs.

3 How should this dog be treated pending the results of those diagnostic tests? Pending blood culture results, this dog should be treated with intravenous antimicrobials, optimally a combination of a penicillin derivative and an aminoglycoside. Aggressive diuretic therapy as well as amlodipine to decrease systemic vascular resistance should also be recommended. The prognosis for dogs with *Bartonella* spp. endocarditis is poor and most humans with this condition require valve replacement.

CASE 137

1 Do the antibody test results prove that *Bartonella* spp. infection is the cause of endocarditis in this dog, and would it rule out *Bartonella* spp. infection as a cause of disease if the test results had been negative? The positive antibody test results alone do not prove active infection with *Bartonella* spp. However, this finding in combination with aortic valvular infective endocarditis with congestive heart failure and negative blood cultures is strongly suggestive of *Bartonella* spp.-associated endocarditis. False-negative antibody test results for *Bartonella* spp. can occur, so negative antibody test results do not rule out *Bartonella*-associated endocarditis.

2 What is the prognosis for recovery? The prognosis is guarded to grave. In human patients, valve replacement would be indicated. This dog unfortunately died 10 days after treatment initiation.

3 What is the zoonotic potential of *Bartonella* spp.? *Bartonella* spp., if transmitted from cats to humans, cause cat scratch disease in humans as well as a variety of other conditions that can be life threatening in immunocompromised humans. These include valvular endocarditis, optic neuritis, and vasculoproliferative syndromes, such as bacillary angiomatosis, and hepatic and splenic peliosis. It can also be responsible for other chronic disorders in humans such as chronic fatigue syndromes, parasthesias, arthralgias/myalgias, and memory loss. Although most transmission involves fleas (cats are thought to inoculate flea feces into humans via a scratch wound), suspected needle-stick infections have been reported in veterinarians, and infections have also been reported in humans with a history of dog bites.

CASE 138

1 What is the main differential diagnosis? Canine distemper is the main differential diagnosis in this dog given the concurrent presence of respiratory and gastrointestinal signs, footpad hyperkeratosis, and the history of other puppies dying with neurologic signs. Distemper is caused by canine distemper virus (CDV). The virus replicates in lymphoid tissues and then spreads hematogenously to epithelial cells of the respiratory tract, gastrointestinal tract, urogenital tract, and CNS. This organ predilection could explain the clinical signs of this dog, because conjunctivitis, cough, and diarrhea are commonly observed. In addition, nasal as well as digital hyperkeratosis can occur. In animals that develop acute or chronic encephalitis, hyperesthesia, vestibular signs, seizures, ataxia, cerebellar signs, paraparesis, tetraparesis, and myoclonus can be present. Lymphopenia is frequently seen during the early phase of infection. This dog had not been protected by vaccination and additionally might have been immunosuppressed as a result of malnourishment, parasites, and stress. CDV infection is frequently complicated by secondary bacterial infections.

2 What diagnostic tests should be considered? The most commonly used test to diagnose distemper is PCR, which is highly sensitive and specific. PCR can be performed on whole blood, conjunctival scrapings, CSF, and urine. Recent vaccination can also lead to positive diagnostic test results. Some laboratories perform quantitative PCR assays that may aid discrimination between vaccination and natural infection. Use of direct immunofluorescent antibody staining on conjunctival swabs is not recommended owing to the possibility of false-positive test results due to nonspecific fluorescence. If neurologic signs occur, CSF analysis typically reveals elevated protein concentrations (>25 mg/dl) and elevated nucleated cell counts (>10 cells/µl) with a predominance of lymphocytes.

3 What treatment is recommended, and what is the prognosis? There is no specific antiviral therapy to treat distemper. Fluid therapy is indicated to correct dehydration and ongoing fluid losses; in addition, it can help to mobilize respiratory secretions. Antimicrobial drug therapy should be given to treat secondary bacterial infections in dogs with bronchopneumonia. In dogs with CNS involvement, anticonvulsant therapy can be indicated. The prognosis for dogs with severe neurologic signs is grave. Neurologic manifestations can occur several weeks after the onset of other clinical signs, so owners should be educated to monitor their dog for neurologic signs. Hyperkeratosis often develops in conjunction with neurologic signs and thus is a negative prognostic indicator.

CASE 139

1 What would be your differential diagnoses for the clinical presentation in this dog (before radiographs were obtained)? Differential diagnoses for cervical pain in dogs in the absence of other neurologic abnormalities include: inflammation/infection as a result of discospondylitis or meningitis; vertebral fractures, luxations, or disc herniations; or compression of the spinal cord secondary to neoplasia. The fever in this dog is suggestive of an inflammatory or infectious cause.

2 What is your interpretation of the radiograph? On the spinal radiograph, a lesion consistent with discospondylitis is evident (lysis of vertebral endplates). Early lesions are not detectable with spinal radiographs and can require serial imaging or CT or MRI to be detected. Advanced cases can show severe osteolysis, associated with vertebral shortening, luxation, or osteophyte formation. Although this dog had a cervical lesion, the most common site of lesions in dogs with discospondylitis is L7–S1.

3 What diagnostic tests should also be performed? Other diagnostic tests should include a CBC, biochemical profile, urinalysis, full spinal radiographs (to determine whether or not other disk spaces are involved), and thoracic radiographs and abdominal ultrasound to search for evidence of disease in other organs. Urinalysis is important to assess for bacteruria in dogs with discospondylitis. Blood cultures are indicated, as well as tests for *Brucella* spp. (antibody tests) and *Aspergillus* spp. antigen.

CASE 140

1 What other common sources of infection can be associated with discospondylitis? Besides genitourinary tract infections, infections of the skin or the oral cavity can be a source of organisms that subsequently spread hematogenously and cause discospondylitis. However, often the primary source of infection is not evident.

2 What are the most common infectious agents associated with discospondylitis? *Brucella canis*, *Staphylococcus* spp., *Streptococcus* spp., or *Escherichia coli* are often implicated as a cause of discospondylitis in dogs. Fungi, such as *Aspergillus* spp. *or Paecilomyces* spp., can also cause discospondylitis.

3 What treatment should be recommended? While culture is pending or in case of a negative culture, antimicrobial therapy with a first-generation cephalosporin or

amoxicillin–clavulanic acid in combination with a fluoroquinolone is recommended. The high end of the dose range should be used and treatment should last for at least 8 weeks. Subsequent treatment should be based on the results of culture and susceptibility testing. Clinical improvement should be expected within a week unless infection is caused by resistant bacteria, fungi, or *Brucella canis*. Should negative blood culture results be obtained, culture of a fluoroscopically-guided disc aspirate can be performed and may help to identify the infecting pathogen. Cage rest and pain management with non-steroidal anti-inflammatory drugs are also indicated. Brucellosis has a guarded prognosis and treatment usually requires combination therapy with high-dose doxycycline and aminoglycosides. Combination therapy with doxycycline and a fluoroquinolone could also be considered. *Aspergillus* discospondylitis is usually treated with amphotericin B and azole antifungal drugs.
4 What is the likely composition of the urolith? Given the presence of *Staphylococcus* spp. bacteriuria and the morphology of the crystals in the urine, the likely composition of the urolith is struvite. Medical therapy should be used in an attempt to dissolve the stone.

CASE 141

1 What are your primary differential diagnoses? The signs support an infectious or inflammatory/immune-mediated disorder, in light of the fever and generalized pain. The geographic location, clinical signs, and history of tick bites could be suspicious for a tick-borne disease, which remains possible despite the negative infectious disease test results. Rocky Mountain spotted fever (RMSF) is prevalent in Oklahoma, and none of the tests performed included methods to detect infection with *Rickettsia rickettsii*. Lyme disease is highly unlikely because the C6 ELISA is generally positive when dogs have clinical signs. *Bartonella* spp. would also be possible as they require special enrichment culture for diagnosis, because bacteremia levels are very low in dogs. Leptospirosis and sepsis are unlikely based on the lack of neutrophilia on the CBC.
2 What would be the next diagnostic step? Tests for RMSF should be performed. A low titer (1:64) for *R. rickettsii* was initially obtained, followed by a 4-fold increase (1:256) 2 weeks later, confirming a diagnosis of RMSF. *R. rickettsii* infects endothelial cells, causing vasculitis. Common signs include polyarthritis, ocular signs, neurologic signs, hemorrhages, and peripheral edema. PCR was not performed. It has limited sensitivity for RMSF because *R. rickettsii* bacteremia is transient.
3 How should this dog be treated? Doxycycline (5 mg/kg PO q12h) was prescribed for 2 weeks, and a clinical response occurred within 2 days. Prognosis is excellent with correct antibiotic therapy, but guarded if the disease is misdiagnosed.

CASE 142

1 What are the two clinical phases of shock, and what phase was present in this dog? The two clinical phases of shock are: (1) compensated shock, characterized by mild mental obtundation, increased heart and respiratory rates, shortened capillary refill time, good pulse quality; and (2) decompensated shock, characterized by severe mental obtundation, increased heart and respiratory rates, prolonged capillary refill time, poor pulse quality. In this case, the good pulse quality and the short capillary refill time reflect a compensated shock.

2 What are the five pathophysiologic types of shock? The five pathophysiologic types of shock are: (1) hypovolemic shock with decrease in circulatory blood volume; (2) cardiogenic shock with decrease in forward blood flow from the heart; (3) distributive shock with loss of systemic vascular resistance (septic shock being the most common cause); (4) metabolic shock with derangement of cellular metabolic function; and (5) hypoxemic shock with decrease in oxygen content in arterial blood.

3 How would you characterize the pathophysiologic type of shock in this dog? The dog had severe fluid loss due to diarrhea, making hypovolemic shock very likely. However, dogs in hypovolemic shock due to gastrointestinal fluid loss typically are hypothermic or have a rectal temperature in the low normal range. This dog had an elevated rectal temperature. He had not been in a warm environment before evaluation and did not have increased muscle activity. Therefore, the high temperature was suggestive of true fever. In this case, the shock signs might be partly due to hypovolemia; however, mental obtundation and fever are more likely to be associated with septic shock. At this stage, the clinical assessment was that the dog's fever and acute diarrhea were most likely caused by an infection involving the gastrointestinal tract.

CASE 143

1 Which bacterial species are considered to be enteropathogenic? *Clostridium difficile*, *Clostridium perfringens*, *Campylobacter* spp., *Salmonella* spp., and *Escherichia coli*, associated with granulomatous colitis in certain breeds, such as Boxers, are categorized as primary enteropathogenic bacteria in dogs and cats. The elevated rectal temperature and the increased numbers of band neutrophils make a bacterial infection likely as a cause of the acute diarrhea in this dog.

2 What are limitations of a fecal culture? Although fecal cultures are commonly performed in dogs with diarrhea, their utility is questionable. The diagnostic yield of such cultures is quite low, because similar isolation rates for putative bacterial enteropathogens are present in animals with and without diarrhea. For example, *C. perfringens* is part of the normal canine intestinal microbiota and is readily cultured from more than 80% of non-diarrheic dogs. Molecular techniques are needed to detect pathogenic strains of *E. coli*, because nonpathogenic strains belong to the normal bacterial microbiota of dogs. In toxin-producing species, a combination of toxin testing by ELISA and organism detection (culture, antigen ELISA, or PCR) is currently recommended for the diagnosis of an enteric bacterial infection. There are, however, many limitations to performing toxin assays as well.

3 How might you make a diagnosis of an enteropathogenic bacterial infection in this case? In patients with sepsis, the source of the bacterial infection, as well as the bacterial species involved and its antibiotic susceptibility, should be determined in order to define the best treatment. According to the clinical signs and the ultrasound changes, the intestinal tract was suspected as the primary site of infection. Because interpretation of fecal cultures is complicated, culture of blood and/or lymph node aspirates from the affected intestinal area should be performed.

CASE 144

1 Should antibiotics be administered to every patient with acute diarrhea and suspicion of an enteric bacterial infection? The decision for antimicrobial treatment of suspected enteropathogenic bacterial infection should depend on the patient's clinical signs. Acute enteritis without systemic signs of illness can be treated with intravenous fluids and supportive care alone. Inappropriate use of antibiotics can increase the risk of antimicrobial resistance and unnecessary adverse drug reactions.

2 Do you think antibiotics were indicated in this case? Given that the dog had signs of systemic infection (fever and a left shift), antibiotic treatment was indicated.

3 Is there a potential zoonotic risk? Salmonellosis is a disease of major zoonotic importance. Therefore, there is a risk of transmission to owners.

4 What would your recommendations be to the owner? Isolation and proper cleaning and disinfection practices are the main control measures to prevent zoonotic transmission. Feeding raw meat to dogs increases the potential risk of transmission of *Salmonella* spp. to people. Therefore, feeding of a commercial dry food diet was recommended in this case. In addition, the owner was advised to walk the dog in an area where no other dogs are present and where feces can be promptly removed. Gloves should be worn when handling feces, and hand washing after contacting the dog and before eating was recommended. Although the benefit of probiotics is not clear in acute infectious diarrhea, administration of probiotics containing different strains of live microorganisms was suggested after cessation of antibiotic treatment.

CASE 145

1 What is the most likely diagnosis? Although neither the history nor the physical examination supported the presence of a wound, a presumptive diagnosis of generalized tetanus could be made in this dog based on typical clinical signs. Tetanus is an intoxication caused by a toxin (tetanospasmin) produced by the bacterium *Clostridium tetani* after colonization of a wound. The bacteria remain in the wound area; however, tetanospasmin migrates along the motor nerves to the spinal cord, where it prevents neurons from releasing inhibitory neurotransmitters. Muscle spasticity and autonomic signs are the consequence. The incubation period ranges from 3 to 18 days.

2 What are potential differential diagnoses? The differential diagnoses in such a dog include strychnine poisoning and hypocalcemia.

3 How is the diagnosis confirmed? Confirmation of the diagnosis of tetanus is difficult, and so it is usually diagnosed on the basis of clinical signs. Circulating antibody against tetanospasmin can be detected in the serum of some animals, but such antibodies also can be found in healthy dogs. Culture of *C. tetani* from a wound (if a wound can be found) has a very low sensitivity.

4 What is the prognosis? The mortality rate for dogs treated with tetanus has been reported as 8–50%. The more quickly the clinical signs progress, and the later treatment is initiated, the poorer is the prognosis. Abnormalities in heart rate or blood pressure are negative prognostic factors. Survival rates are also low if there is respiratory muscle involvement.

5 What are the most common complications of this disease? The most common complications of tetanus in dogs include decubital ulcers due to lateral recumbency, seizures, hyperthermia resulting from muscular hyperreactivity, dysuria, and aspiration pneumonia. Less commonly, hiatal hernia, laryngeal spasm, ventricular tachycardia, third-degree atrioventricular block, and joint luxations have been reported. In humans, traumatic fractures have been described as a consequence of seizures. The common occurrence of complications means that prolonged hospitalization and intensive care are necessary in most cases.

CASE 146

1 How is *Clostridium tetani* transmitted? *Clostridium tetani* forms spores that can be found in the soil worldwide. When introduced into skin or other wounds, even small or superficial ones, the spores germinate to vegetative forms that produce tetanospasmin. Necrotic and contaminated wounds, and those associated with grass awns, have been suggested as a risk factor. Surgical wounds can also result in tetanus. In many cases a wound is not found, therefore absence of a wound does not preclude a diagnosis of tetanus.

2 What could be the source of infection in this dog? In this dog, no wound was detected or reported by the owner. However, the dog's permanent dentition was noted to be erupting. Mucosal injury connected with teething has been described as a possible entry point of *C. tetani* resulting in tetanus in dogs.

3 What treatment would be recommended? If a wound is identified, it should be debrided and flushed with hydrogen peroxide. Systemic antimicrobial therapy is recommended to reduce further toxin production. Metronidazole (15 mg/kg IV or PO q12h) is the drug of choice, and is preferred over penicillin. To neutralize the tetanospasmin, antitoxin (100–1,000 IU/kg IV or IM) is commonly used. However, antitoxin is ineffective against toxin already bound to axonal terminals, and its efficacy is controversial. Antitoxin is derived from equine serum; thus, a skin test should be performed before administration to assess the possibility of anaphylactic reactions. Muscle relaxants and sedatives can also be helpful, such as methocarbamol, benzodiazepines, phenothiazines, or barbiturates. Fluid therapy should be provided to prevent dehydration. Patients should be kept in a quiet, dark room. All handling must be with minimal stimulation. A well-padded bed should be provided for recumbent dogs, and they should be turned frequently. If swallowing is difficult or impossible, nutrition through a nasogastric or esophageal tube is necessary. Dogs with involvement of the diaphragm and intercostal muscles require mechanical ventilation. Given the high risk of life-threatening autonomic signs, heart and respiratory parameters should be frequently monitored in recumbent animals. Dogs must also be repeatedly evaluated for hyperthermia, and the use of fans and cool fluids can help to reduce rectal temperature.

CASE 147

1 What is the geographic distribution of *Blastomyces* spp.? The geographic distribution of *Blastomyces* spp. is primarily in North America, especially the southeastern, south-central, and upper Midwestern states of the USA, Canadian provinces that border the Great Lakes, and a small area of the northeastern USA and southeastern Canada near the St. Lawrence River. In this case, the signalment and clinical signs together with the dog's origin were highly suggestive of blastomycosis, and other diagnoses (such as disseminated neoplasia) were much less likely.

2 What are other anatomic sites of predilection of this organism? Other sites of predilection include the eye (uveitis, chorioretinitis, and panophthalmitis), bone, and CNS.

3 Had the cutaneous lesions not been identified, what other diagnostic tests could have been used to obtain the diagnosis, and what are the limitations of these tests?

Had the cutaneous lesions not been identified, other diagnostic tests could have included cytologic examination of a respiratory lavage specimen (obtained either by transtracheal wash or bronchoalveolar lavage), fine needle aspiration of the lung, or a urine test for *Blastomyces* spp. antigen. Obtaining specimens from the lung for cytologic examination is invasive and can cause respiratory distress or pneumothorax (in the case of lung aspirates). Urine testing for *Blastomyces* spp. antigen is sensitive for the diagnosis of blastomycosis (93.5% in one study), but cross-reactivity with *Histoplasma* spp. antigen can occur, so a positive test indicates either blastomycosis or histoplasmosis.

4 What treatment should be recommended? The recommended treatment for this dog, at a minimum, should be with itraconazole, but concurrent use of amphotericin B should be recommended in this case because of the severity of disease and evidence of dissemination. Fluconazole is an alternative to itraconazole, but is less active than itraconazole. In human patients, the use of fluconazole is only recommended if itraconazole is not tolerated.

CASE 148

1 What are your differential diagnoses? The main differential diagnoses for diseases causing hair loss are follicular diseases, and in a young dog, infectious folliculitides are the most likely. Thus, bacterial folliculitis, demodicosis, and dermatophytosis are all on the top of the list.

2 What tests would you propose? Deep skin scrapings or trichograms to rule out demodicosis and an impression smear to identify evidence of bacterial pyoderma are the most important initial tests. If the scrapings or trichograms are negative and no or very few extracellular bacteria are seen on cytology, a Wood's lamp examination should be performed. Positive fluorescence along the hair shafts is diagnostic for a dermatophytosis caused by *Microsporum canis*. A negative result should be followed by fungal culture and/or PCR for dermatophytes.

CASE 149

1 What is the prognosis for the disease in this dog? As only two small areas on the dogs' body are affected (localized demodicosis), the prognosis is very good, because 95% of affected dogs have spontaneous remission. Dogs that develop generalized infections require specific miticidal therapy. Neutering is also recommended for dogs with generalized infections to prevent the breeding of susceptible animals.

2 How would you treat this dog? Dogs with localized demodicosis usually are not treated at all or only treated with an antimicrobial shampoo (e.g. one that contains chlorhexidine).

CASE 150

1 What is the most likely diagnosis in this dog, based on the history and clinical signs? This young previously healthy dog most likely became infected with one or more pathogens belonging to the 'canine infectious respiratory disease complex' (CIRDC). CIRDC describes infections of the upper respiratory tract caused by single or multiple infectious agents. The pathogenesis of CIRD is multifactorial, because dogs infected experimentally with a single respiratory pathogen often show only mild clinical signs, while more severe clinical disease, as commonly found in natural outbreaks, cannot be reproduced under these conditions. CIRDC is characterized by an acute onset of mild to severe episodes of paroxysmal dry cough with or without nasal discharge and fever. Owing to the highly contagious nature of the disease, dogs in crowded indoor situations, such as in shelters and day-care centres, are most susceptible to infection. Multiple viral and bacterial agents have been detected in dogs with CIRDC. While traditionally canine distemper virus, canine adenovirus type 2, canine parainfluenza virus, canine herpesvirus-1, and *Bordetella bronchiseptica* were the most common pathogens identified, recent studies have shown involvement of new viral and bacterial agents in CIRD, including canine respiratory coronavirus, influenza viruses, *Mycoplasma cynos*, and *Streptococcus equi* subspecies *zooepidemicus*.

2 How would you interpret the radiographs? The thoracic radiographs show a generalized bronchoalveolar lung pattern with air bronchograms, consistent with a diagnosis of bronchopneumonia.

3 What do you recommend for treatment? Given that the dog is febrile, the CBC shows a left shift, and there is radiographic evidence of bronchopneumonia, it is likely that there is primary or secondary bacterial involvement. This could be due to a severe infection with a primary respiratory pathogen, such as *B. bronchiseptica*, or due to secondary bacterial infection following primary infection with a viral pathogen such as canine distemper virus. Antimicrobial therapy is therefore indicated in this case. Underlying canine distemper virus infection should not be excluded as a differential on the basis of the vaccination history, because vaccinated dogs occasionally develop distemper. Since multidrug resistance has been identified in some *B. bronchiseptica* isolates, as well as in other secondary bacterial invaders, performing a bronchoalveolar lavage or transtracheal wash to obtain a sample for bacterial culture and susceptibility testing is recommended to guide antimicrobial therapy. Furthermore, cytology of airway lavage specimens to identify whether rods or cocci are present can aid selection of an antibiotic for initial treatment while culture and susceptibility tests are pending. Antimicrobial therapy should be given for at least 10 days. In addition to antimicrobial treatment, dogs can benefit from airway humidification by nebulization of saline, fluid therapy, and high-quality nutrition. Glucocorticoids and cough suppressants are considered contraindicated in patients with infectious bronchopneumonia.

CASE 151

1 What drugs can result in increased serum liver enzyme activity without liver damage? Drugs that can induce excessive production of liver enzymes without liver damage include glucocorticoids and barbiturates.

2 Which extrahepatic diseases can result in increased serum liver enzyme activity? Extrahepatic diseases that can result in elevated serum liver enzyme activities include: (1) endocrine disorders (e.g. diabetes mellitus, hyperadrenocorticism); (2) hypoxia (e.g. cardiac disorders, respiratory disorders, anemia); (3) pancreatitis; (4) severe gastrointestinal diseases (e.g. bacterial translocation, increased toxin load due to damaged gut barrier); and (5) severe systemic disease (e.g. sepsis).

3 What is the half-life of serum ALT and ALP in dogs? The half-life of both enzymes is 2.5–3 days.

4 Can a single insult to hepatocytes result in elevated liver enzymes for a period of 6 weeks? Acute insult to hepatocytes can cause elevated serum liver enzyme activity. However, if the insult is short term and hepatocytes regenerate, liver enzyme activities should return to normal by 6 weeks.

5 Which non-invasive diagnostic tests should be performed to assess the significance of a chronic increase in liver enzyme activities? Non-invasive diagnostic tests that should be performed to assess the significance of chronic serum liver enzyme activity increases include: (1) assessment of parameters that reflect synthetic and excretory capacity of the liver (e.g. bilirubin, glucose, cholesterol, albumin, BUN); (2) results of specific liver function testing (e.g. serum bile acids); and (3) imaging studies to assess liver size, focal changes, echogenicity, vascularity/portal vasculature, and the biliary system.

CASE 152

1 What is the most likely differential diagnosis based on the ultrasound examination findings? Owing to the prominent mass effect, a neoplastic disorder should be ranked highest on the differential diagnosis list; an inflammatory disorder is less likely.

2 What would be your next diagnostic step? Fine needle aspiration should be performed. Fine needle aspiration has a low risk and is inexpensive, but there are limitations to the technique and the relative diagnostic value of cytologic examination *versus* histopathology should be known for any specific liver disease. A poor overall agreement between liver cytologic examination and histopathology of biopsy specimens has been reported. However, cytologic examination is more reliable when there is diffuse involvement of the liver parenchyma without architectural alterations. Frequently, round cell tumors (e.g. lymphoma, mast cell tumor), hepatic lipidosis, and some infectious diseases (e.g. aspiration of bile for diagnosis of bacterial cholangitis) can be diagnosed with fine needle aspiration. Histopathology of biopsy specimens is generally required for diagnosis of parenchymal liver diseases, such as hepatitis and inflammatory biliary tract disease (more common in cats). In addition, diagnosis and grading of malignancy for solid tumors can only be made by evaluation of adequately sized tissue specimens.

CASE 153

1 What is the diagnosis in this dog, and what forms of this disease are known? The diagnosis is echinococcosis. There are two forms of echinococcosis: (1) cystic echinococcosis, also termed “hydatid disease”, which is caused by *Echinococcus granulosus*; and (2) alveolar echinococcosis, caused by the larval stage of *Echinococcus multilocularis*.

2 Is cytologic identification sufficient to define the species involved, and what tests would be superior? Both parasitic forms can be identified by cytologic examination of fine needle aspirates, but the *Echinococcus* species involved cannot be determined. On histopathologic examination, *E. granulosus* has thicker membranes than *E. multilocularis*. PCR is required for definitive identification.

3 What is the life cycle of this agent and the required hosts? The adult worm lives in the gastrointestinal tract of a carnivore. Eggs in feces of carnivores are ingested by an intermediate host (e.g. sheep, goats, small rodents). Oncospheres are released in the intestinal tract of the intermediate host and penetrate the intestinal wall. They move through the circulatory system into different organs, particularly the liver and lungs, where they form slowly growing cysts. The definitive host then becomes infected by ingesting the cyst-containing organs of the intermediate host.

4 How did the dog in this case fit into the life cycle? Dogs and other carnivores are the definitive hosts in this parasitic infection. In this case, however, the dog was an incidental host.

5 What treatment is indicated? Treatment requires surgical removal of the cysts combined with medical treatment using albendazole and/or mebendazole before and after surgery.

CASE 154

1 What are the differential diagnoses for the petechiation and ecchymoses? Bleeding at different locations with petechiation and ecchymoses is a sign of a disorder of primary hemostasis involving platelets (number or function) or the vascular endothelium. In this case, the most likely causes are thrombocytopenia (caused by tick-borne diseases or immune-mediated thrombocytopenia), thrombocytopathy (due to drugs, infection, metabolic abnormalities, or von Willebrand's disease [vWD]), or vasculitis. Poodles can possess a genetic mutation related to type I vWD. Female poodles are also predisposed to immune-mediated thrombocytopenia. Severe coagulation factor problems usually do not cause petechial bleeding, but more likely bleeding into subcutaneous tissue, body cavities, muscles, or joints. Because of the history of tick infestation, infectious causes such as *Anaplasma platys* or *Ehrlichia canis* infection, or Rocky Mountain spotted fever were suspected in this case.

2 What diagnostic tests should be recommended? The first step should be to perform a CBC to assess platelet count and differentiate anemia from impaired perfusion as the cause of the pallor. If the platelet count is normal, plasma levels of von Willebrand factor (vWF), as well as coagulation times (e.g. PT and aPTT) should be measured. Blood smear evaluation might reveal infectious agents, but sensitivity and specificity are limited when compared with molecular techniques such as PCR. A biochemistry panel and urinalysis should be performed to evaluate for evidence of other disease, such as liver disease, that might be associated with a coagulopathy.

CASE 155

1 What conclusions can you make based on the laboratory test results? Laboratory testing showed pancytopenia, elevated liver enzyme activities, hypoalbuminemia, and hyperglobulinemia. Pancytopenia can result from infectious diseases, drugs, toxins, infiltrative neoplasia, and immune-mediated disease. The marked hyperglobulinemia suggests chronic antigenic stimulation from infectious, immune-mediated, or neoplastic disease. The blood smear showed morulae within monocytes, which could be *Ehrlichia canis* or *Ehrlichia chaffeensis*, because these species have the same morphology and target the same cells. Chronic *E. canis* infection can cause pancytopenia and hyperglobulinemia.

2 What initial treatment is required in this case? The history, physical examination, and laboratory findings support the diagnosis of canine monocytic ehrlichiosis. Doxycycline (5 mg/kg PO q12h) for at least 4 weeks is indicated, but the duration needed in chronic cases can be much longer, up to several months. Clinical improvement usually occurs within 24–48 hours, but cytopenias might only resolve after several months of therapy, or they might fail to respond at all. Severely anemic dogs require blood transfusion, but this does not significantly increase platelets counts.

CASE 156

1 What are the important findings from the ECG and urinalysis? The ECG shows sinus rhythm at 120 bpm and two ventricular premature contractions (VPCs) (black arrows). *Ehrlichia canis* infection can be associated with myocarditis in dogs, associated with the systemic inflammation and reduced tissue oxygenation secondary to anemia. This is uncommonly recognized clinically. Protein-losing nephropathy secondary to glomerulonephritis can also occur in dogs with canine monocytic ehrlichiosis. The UPCR confirmed significant proteinuria in this case, most likely of glomerular origin given its magnitude (>5). Ultimately, glomerulonephritis can lead to chronic renal tubular failure and hypertension, which were not present in this case. Chronic proteinuria can also predispose to thrombotic disease. Plasma antithrombin III concentration should be measured to determine whether specific antithrombotic therapy is needed.

2 Is specific therapy required for these findings? The VPCs might require specific therapy if they affect cardiac output or if they progress to life-threatening arrhythmias (ventricular tachycardia). Generally, if isolated VPCs are present, with similar morphology, no R-on-T phenomenon, and are less frequent than 1,000 per 24 hours, no therapy is required. Enalapril (0.25 mg/kg PO q24h initially) is recommended to reduce proteinuria. Clopidogrel (1–2 mg/kg PO q24h) is recommended if plasma antithrombin is <80%.

3 What is the prognosis in this dog? Chronic ehrlichiosis has a guarded prognosis. Prognosis is worse if severe leukopenia and severe anemia are present.

CASE 157

1 What are the main differential diagnoses, including specific infectious agents that might be involved? The main differential diagnoses for this dog are bone neoplasia (especially osteosarcoma) and bacterial or fungal osteomyelitis. Specific infectious agents that might be present in a dog with this history would include *Coccidioides* spp., *Histoplasma capsulatum*, *Aspergillus* spp., and other molds (such as *Paecilomyces*). Coccidioidomycosis is most likely based on the history of travel to Arizona. Bacterial osteomyelitis would be less likely, based on the history of no previous trauma or surgery, but should also be considered. Atypical bacteria, such as *Nocardia* spp. or *Mycobacterium avium*, should also be considered as rare causes of bacterial osteomyelitis.

2 What other diagnostic tests should be recommended for this dog? Other diagnostic tests that should be considered are fine needle aspirates of the lesion, and if this is not diagnostic, bone biopsy should be considered. In addition, thoracic radiographs should be performed to evaluate for metastatic disease (in the case of osteosarcoma) or pulmonary involvement by a fungal pathogen. A serum antibody test for *Coccidioides* spp. should be performed. In addition, routine bloodwork (CBC, biochemistry panel, and urinalysis) is indicated to determine whether there is evidence of other organs involved, to ensure there is no evidence of renal dysfunction because of the non-steroidal anti-inflammatory drugs, and before sedation or anesthesia is performed for bone biopsy.

CASE 158

1 What is the significance of the positive *Coccidioides* spp. antibody test? A positive *Coccidioides* spp. titer of this magnitude is consistent with a diagnosis of coccidioidomycosis, and it is extremely likely that a *Coccidioides* spp. is the cause of the osteomyelitis. Lower titers (1:4 or lower) might be consistent with previous exposure and not active infection, especially in a dog that resides in an endemic region. However, in general, presence of antibodies correlates with active infection because the immune system is unable to eliminate the pathogen.
2 Are any additional diagnostic tests indicated? No other diagnostic tests are indicated given the clinical signs and the magnitude of the titer.
3 What is the recommended treatment for this patient, and what are the possible adverse effects of therapy? The recommended initial treatment for this dog is single agent therapy with itraconazole, which has good bone penetration and is active against *Coccidioides* spp. The initial dose should be 5 mg/kg PO q12h, which could be reduced to 5 mg/kg PO q24h after the first week. Possible adverse effects of therapy are hepatotoxicity and cutaneous vasculitis (which tends to occur with higher doses of itraconazole). Liver enzymes should be monitored monthly, and treatment might need to be discontinued if increases in liver enzymes are accompanied by lethargy and/or inappetence. In that case, other antifungal drugs need to be considered as alternatives, such as fluconazole. Continued therapy with non-steroidal anti-inflammatory drugs for pain relief is also recommended, with periodic monitoring of renal values.

CASE 159

1 What are likely reasons that the *Giardia* spp. test remained positive? There are several possible explanations for the repeatedly positive *Giardia* test. Either the *Giardia* infection was never eliminated, or reinfection was occurring. A possibility for a lack of elimination is that the dog was infected with a *Giardia* strain that was resistant to metronidazole and/or fenbendazole. While metronidazole-resistant strains are relatively common, fenbendazole-resistant strains are unlikely, and fenbendazole is usually effective. It is possible that hygiene measures were not applied consistently; these include cleaning organic debris from surfaces, including the garden area, and disinfection of the environment as well as thorough bathing of the dog (first with a pet shampoo, taking care to remove all fecal material from the hair coat and perineum, followed by a quaternary ammonium compound, particularly soaking the perineum). Reinfection is the most likely explanation because the dog had close contact with other dogs and was allowed to run free in potentially contaminated areas.

It is important to realize that tests are available to detect fecally excreted *Giardia* antigen (coproantigen). These tests are specific for *Giardia* spp., but can yield positive results due to persistent antigen excretion for several weeks or even months after successful elimination of the parasite. Thus, these tests are not useful for monitoring the success of therapy. This, however, was not the reason for the continuously positive result in this dog, because zinc sulfate flotation was used.

2 How should the dog be treated? As the dog was apparently healthy, the best advice would be to stop treating and testing. This dog was neither tested nor treated further. The fecal consistency improved and became normal when the dog was 1 year old. A *Giardia* test at the age of 1.5 years was negative.

CASE 160

1 What are the most likely differential diagnoses for the problems of unilateral epistaxis and ipsilateral lymphadenopathy? Nasal neoplasia and aspergillosis should be highest on the differential diagnoses list, although occasionally dogs with lymphoplasmacytic rhinitis can present with epistaxis rather than nasal discharge; this can be unilateral, and can be associated with regional lymphadenopathy. Blepharospasm is suggestive of facial pain, which would be more likely with aspergillosis. Preservation of nasal airflow is more suggestive of aspergillosis or inflammatory rhinitis. While systemic causes of epistaxis such as coagulopathies can lead to unilateral bleeding, it would be unusual for a coagulopathy alone to result in lymphadenopathy.

2 If only one diagnostic test was allowed in this patient, what would you perform? Currently, the single most useful non-invasive diagnostic test in this patient is agar gel immunodiffusion for *Aspergillus* spp. serum antibodies. While a negative test does not rule out disease, a positive test makes it highly likely that sinonasal aspergillosis is the cause of the clinical signs. A lymph node aspirate would not be an incorrect diagnostic test; however, aspergillosis is usually not a systemic disease when nasal discharge is present and so fungal hyphae would not be expected on cytologic examination of a lymph node aspirate. A swab of nasal discharge or collection of a blind nasal sample for cytology or culture is unlikely to yield a diagnosis.

3 If the owner agreed to a full work-up, what would you recommend? Full work-up would entail a minimum database (CBC, chemistry profile, urinalysis) as well as lymph node aspirates, followed by anesthesia for CT and rhinoscopy. If rhinoscopy failed to identify fungal plaques, but CT showed evidence of an amorphous soft tissue density in the frontal sinus, trephination and sinusocopy should be performed.

CASE 161

1 What is your interpretation of the lymph node cytology? The nucleated cells consist of a heterogeneous population of lymphocytes in which small mature lymphocytes predominate and are admixed with an increased population of intermediate-sized lymphocytes and plasma cells. This is consistent with a reactive lymph node.
2 What is your interpretation of the CT images? There is marked turbinate destruction in the right nasal cavity with increased soft tissue opacity lining the nasal cavity caudally. There are irregular soft tissue densities within the right frontal sinus. There is no evidence of cribriform plate destruction, although thinner sections should be obtained through this region of interest because of the concerns about topical treatment in a dog with cribriform plate destruction. The dog was suspected to have sinonasal aspergillosis. A rhinoscopy was performed and biopsy samples were collected for histopathology and culture. This confirmed the diagnosis of sinonasal aspergillosis.

CASE 162

1 What are the main differential diagnoses? Tick bite hypersensitivity, bacterial pyoderma (post trauma or tick bite), or possibly a kerion (a dermatophyte infection that has led to localized furunculosis) are the main differential diagnoses. A histiocytoma is another possibility, although the lesion is atypical in that it is rather small and crusting, and erythema is normally only present in the end stages of a histiocytoma, whereas in this case it was present when the lesion first appeared.
2 What would you recommend as the minimal diagnostic approach for this case? The simplest approach would be to obtain an impression smear from the bottom of the removed crust or the underlying eroded epidermis and evaluate it for inflammatory cells and bacteria. If there are only eosinophils, the lesion can be due to a tick bite and topical anti-inflammatory therapy could be considered. If, however, there are neutrophils and cocci, topical antimicrobial therapy should be added to the treatment regimen. If many macrophages and neutrophils are seen without bacteria, a dermatophyte infection should be considered as a possible option and a dermatophyte culture could be considered.
3 What is the most complete diagnostic approach to this case? The most complete approach would be to collect a swab for bacterial culture and susceptibility, perform an impression smear, fungal culture, and surgically excise the lesion and submit it for histopathologic evaluation, freezing a portion for PCR if needed based on the histopathology findings. In addition to the above-mentioned diagnoses, neoplastic

skin disease would be identified using this approach, and special stains or PCR could identify unusual infectious organisms that might be present depending on the histopathologic changes. In this dog, impression smears showed neutrophils and cocci, and topical antimicrobial therapy as well as topical anti-inflammatory therapy was initiated, and the skin lesion improved within a week.

CASE 163

1 What differential diagnoses should be considered? Head tilt, circling and falling, and positional strabismus are suggestive of left-sided peripheral vestibular disease. Horner's syndrome and facial nerve paralysis suggest involvement of the middle and inner ear. Post-ganglionic sympathetic fibers are responsible for the autonomic innervation of the eye and these, along with cranial nerve VII, pass near the petrous temporal bone and tympanic bulla. A central vestibular disorder was less likely because neurologic examination revealed no abnormalities in mentation, placing reaction abnormalities, limb paresis/paralysis, or involvement of other cranial nerves. Based on the acute onset, the progressive nature of the clinical signs, and the dog's age, inflammatory/infectious causes seemed most likely, although neoplasia should also be considered.

2 What is your initial diagnostic plan? Initial investigations should include otoscopic examination of both ears to evaluate for otitis media, and imaging of the ear under general anesthesia. Otoscopy or video-otoscopy should be performed under deep sedation or general anesthesia and should involve thorough examination of the external ear canal and tympanic membrane (to assess for a ruptured, opaque, or bulging tympanic membrane). Open-mouth anterior–posterior radiographs of the skull can detect severe abnormalities of the bullae (such as lysis, thickening, and presence of fluid or tissue inside the bulla). However, CT is more sensitive for detection of otitis media and should be recommended in this case following otoscopy, should the owner's finances allow.

CASE 164

1 What is your diagnosis? The dog has chronic bilateral otitis externa and otitis media. The left ear is more severely affected and there is likely to be secondary otitis media, based on the clinical signs present.

2 What additional diagnostic tests might be useful to better understand the condition? Otitis media is frequently caused by extension of otitis externa. Otitis externa is the consequence of a primary skin disease promoting bacterial and yeast overgrowth. The most common underlying disease in dogs is allergic dermatitis, but foreign bodies, hypothyroidism, mite infestations, and cornification disorders (such as seborrhea in Cocker Spaniels) can also predispose to otitis externa.

Bacterial infections (such as those caused by *Staphylococcus pseudintermedius*, *Pseudomonas aeruginosa*) and yeast (*Malassezia*) infections are perpetuating factors, and the chronic inflammation produces progressive pathologic changes in the external ear, including the tympanic membrane. Therefore, the underlying cause of chronic or recurrent otitis externa should be investigated and treated if possible. Cytology and culture (ideally of material obtained from the middle ear) are useful to guide the choice of systemic antimicrobial drug therapy. Cytology of both external ear canals should be performed, at a minimum, to confirm the presence of bacteria and yeast together with neutrophils.

3 What treatment is indicated? Ear flushing under anesthesia should be recommended. A 3–4-day course of systemic glucocorticoids can reduce stenosis due to inflammation and make otoscopic evaluation without anesthesia, ear cleaning, and topical treatment possible. Owners should be educated regarding the complications of ear canal flushing (e.g. Horner's syndrome, facial nerve paralysis, vestibular signs, and deafness). Topical combination therapy with glucocorticoids, antibiotics, and antifungal drugs is then indicated to control infection, pain, pruritus, and inflammation. A variety of combination preparations are available and selection depends largely on clinician preference. In case of *Pseudomonas aeruginosa* infection, topical treatment with fluoroquinolones can be potentiated by combination therapy with topical Tris-EDTA or dexamethasone solutions. In severe cases, systemic glucocorticoids and antimicrobial drugs can be combined with topical therapy. When there are advanced pathologic changes of the ear canal (stenosis and calcification) and otitis media, total ear canal ablation and bulla osteotomy might be required. Addressing the underlying causes is also recommended when possible.

CASE 165

1 What is the most likely differential diagnosis? Aujeszky's disease (pseudorabies) is the most likely cause of this dog's signs, based on the history and physical examination findings. Aujeszky's disease was confirmed at necropsy in this dog. This disease is caused by a herpesvirus. Domestic pigs as well as wild boars serve as reservoirs of the virus. On rare occasions, dogs (and cats) can be infected and develop an acute or peracute disease with excessive salivation, lethargy or agitation, with rapid progression of neurologic signs due to encephalitis, leading to coma and death. In many dogs, intense pruritus, especially in the head and neck region, occurs. Affected dogs violently rub their heads against walls or the floor and scratch at their faces and ears. This leads to severe self-mutilation, with erythema, excoriation, and severe ulceration. Often the lesions are asymmetric. Neurologic signs due to brainstem involvement are also often unilateral, and include anisocoria, absent pupillary light reflexes, trismus, facial muscle paresis or paralysis, head tilt, and impaired swallowing.

2 What other differential diagnoses are there for the neurologic signs combined with fever? Other differential diagnoses for the neurologic signs should include rabies in endemic areas, because of the public health risk. Both rabies and pseudorabies are acute, fatal, can result in similar behavioral changes early in the course of illness (excitation or lethargy), and progress with other signs of encephalitis. Although rabies always follows a bite wound, many owners of rabid dogs are not aware that a bite wound has occurred, nor is it often visible by the time clinical signs occur, owing to the long incubation period. Pruritus is usually present in pseudorabies but rarely seen in rabies. Unprovoked aggression, typical of rabies, is rare in Aujeszky's disease. However, many rabid dogs show the so-called "paralytic form" of the disease without aggression. Another differential diagnosis for a dog with fever and neurologic signs is acute encephalitis due to canine distemper virus. However, distemper encephalitis has a slower progression, is usually accompanied or preceded by respiratory and/or gastrointestinal signs, and pruritus is absent.
3 What is the prognosis? Aujeszky's disease is rapidly fatal in dogs, therefore the prognosis is grave.

CASE 166

1 How is a diagnosis of Aujeszky's disease confirmed? Analysis of the CSF in dogs with pseudorabies can reveal elevated total nucleated cell counts and elevated total protein concentrations. However, this is not specific for pseudorabies. The disease progresses so rapidly that antibodies to the virus are hardly detectable. In addition, virus isolation from the saliva or oropharynx has a low sensitivity in dogs. Thus, the diagnosis is usually made at necropsy. Histopathology reveals eosinophilic, intranuclear inclusion bodies in the brain. Specific confirmation of infection can be performed by using immunostaining for viral antigen or by PCR on brain or tonsillar tissue.
2 What was the likely source of this infection in this case? Direct contact with infected pigs places dogs at risk for infection. Although the virus is quickly inactivated by drying and ultraviolet light, it can survive in carcasses over long periods (e.g. at 25°C for up to 40 days, longer at lower temperatures). Carnivores are almost invariably infected by consumption of raw tissues of domestic or wild pigs. The pigs can appear healthy, but have subclinical infection. Thus, in regions where Aujeszky's disease in pigs is still endemic, raw pork should not be fed to dogs. Aujeszky's disease has been eradicated from domestic pigs in many countries as a result of vaccination programs, but continues to circulate in wild boar and feral pigs. As was the case for this dog, contact with wild boar and their carcasses is a risk factor, and cases of Aujeszky's disease in hunting dogs have been described in many countries.

3 Can a dog with Aujeszky's disease infect other animals? The reservoir hosts for suid herpesvirus-1, the cause of Aujeszky's disease, are domestic and wild pigs, because only in pigs are subclinical infections possible. Many other mammalian species are also susceptible to infection and sporadically develop disease (including cattle, small ruminants, horses, and cats). In contrast to pigs, these species are considered as "end hosts" that acquire the infection from pigs and die before spreading it to other hosts. Direct transmission from dog to dog does not occur.
4 Is Aujeszky's disease a zoonosis? Humans are refractory to Aujeszky's disease, being an exception among mammals. There are anecdotal reports of suspected Aujeszky's disease in humans, based on development of pruritus around a wound after close contact with pigs, but the disease has never been confirmed in humans.

CASE 167

1 What are the differential diagnoses for nodular ulcerative skin lesions? Differential diagnoses include granulomas caused by foreign bodies, fungi, bacteria, protozoa, or helminth or arthropod parasites, or immune-mediated or neoplastic disorders.
2 What would be the diagnostic plan to evaluate the skin lesions? The initial diagnostic plan would be to obtain fine needle aspirates of the lesions followed by cytologic examination of stained specimens. Radiographs can be performed to determine whether there are any underlying bony lesions responsible for or associated with the nodules. Underlying osteomyelitis can either be a cause or a result of chronic ulcerative skin lesions. If the results of these diagnostic tests are uncertain, a CBC, biochemical profile, urinalysis, and biopsies of the lesions should be performed. Specimens should be obtained using aseptic technique and submitted for fungal and bacterial cultures. Specialized laboratories can perform antibody or PCR testing on blood or tissue specimens to help determine whether an organism is causing these lesions.

CASE 168

1 What are the treatment options for *Pythium insidiosum* infection? Surgical drainage and lesion removal with debridement can be attempted initially to reduce the tissue mass and to improve drainage and facilitate drug penetration. Treatment with itraconazole and terbinafine, in combination, has been recommended. However, the effectiveness of antifungal drug therapy has been limited with this infection. Presumably, the poor response is caused by an absence of chitin and ergosterol in the cell wall of these organisms.

Immunotherapy, consisting of a vaccine containing the isolated organism and an adjuvant, has been proposed to facilitate regression of the fungal infection. Although empirical and controversial, it has been used to treat one dog with

Pythium spp. infection with a positive outcome. The specific effect of the vaccine, however, was difficult to determine because the infection resolved over several months using a combination of surgical resection and drainage, antifungal chemotherapy, and the autogenous vaccine.

Spending time in lake water was likely a predisposing factor for exposure to and dermal entry of this infection. To prevent reinfection, recommendations should be made to restrict the dog from further unlimited access to the lake.

2 What other genera of bacteria or fungi can cause ulcerated (with or without drainage) nodular granulomatous or pyogranulomatous skin lesions in dogs? Other bacteria or fungi that can cause ulcerated nodular granulomatous or pyogranulomatous skin lesions with or without drainage in dogs include *Nocardia* spp., *Mycobacterium* spp., *Blastomyces* spp., *Histoplasma* spp., *Cryptococcus* spp., *Coccidioides* spp., and many other saprophytic fungi.

CASE 169

1 What coronaviruses are known to infect dogs, and what is their role as pathogenic agents? In dogs, two different coronaviruses, canine enteric coronavirus (CECoV) and canine respiratory coronavirus (CRCoV), have been recognized. In addition, a highly virulent CECoV strain (pantropic CCoV) was isolated a few years ago that was responsible for an outbreak of fatal systemic disease in puppies. CECoV was first isolated in 1971 in dogs with acute enteritis in a canine military unit in Germany, and experimental administration of the isolated strain to young dogs reproduced the gastrointestinal signs. Since then, several CECoV outbreaks have been reported worldwide, showing that CECoV can be an enteropathogen in dogs. However, the true importance of CECoV as a pathogen is unknown, because many clinically healthy dogs shed CECoV in their feces. Most likely, changes in virulence and tissue tropism leading to disease outbreaks occur through genetic variations in structural and/or non-structural proteins. Antibody and RNA prevalence studies have shown that CECoV is widespread in the dog population, primarily in kennels and shelters. It is unclear how often and why clinical signs appear, and differentiation of CECoV from other infectious causes of enteritis is difficult, because many healthy dogs shed CECoV. Therefore, detection of CECoV in dogs with diarrhea is not proof of causation. If it causes clinical signs, infection is usually restricted to the alimentary tract, with sudden onset of signs typical of gastrointestinal involvement including loss of appetite, vomiting, diarrhea, dehydration, and rarely death. Fatal disease can occur as a consequence of mixed infections (e.g. with canine parvovirus or canine distemper virus). CECoV can mutate to more virulent strains (pantropic CCoV). Outbreaks of severe disease with systemic spread of the virus and high mortality in puppies have been reported in the USA, England, Sweden, and Australia.

CRCoV was identified in 2003 in the respiratory tracts of dogs housed in a rehoming kennel in England with a history of endemic respiratory disease. CRCoV is closely related to a bovine coronavirus. Since its first description, CRCoV has been detected in many countries worldwide. CRCoV can be responsible for mild to moderate respiratory signs and is one of the etiological agents of canine infectious respiratory disease. In one study, CRCoV RNA was only detected in the respiratory tracts of dogs with respiratory signs, and not in healthy dogs. Replication of CRCoV in the respiratory epithelium can damage the mucociliary system, and this can lead to a more severe clinical course of infections caused by other respiratory pathogens.

2 Is it necessary to treat this dog for coronavirus infection? Treatment is not necessary in this dog because the dog is subclinically infected and apparently healthy dogs can shed coronaviruses without developing disease.

CASE 170

1 What are the main problems in this dog, and what are the most important differential diagnoses? The main problems are pancytopenia, likely caused by bone marrow disease, hyperglobulinemia, hypoalbuminemia, and proteinuria, which suggest a chronic persistent infection leading to glomerulonephritis associated with immune complex deposition. Two infectious agents that would cause such a combination are *Ehrlichia canis* and *Leishmania infantum*. Multiple myeloma can have a very similar presentation and should also be considered.

2 What diagnostic procedures should be performed next? Antibody tests or PCR assays can be used for diagnosis of both *E. canis* and *L. infantum* infections. To detect *E. canis*, PCR can be performed on blood as well as on lymph node or spleen aspirates or bone marrow. *L. infantum* PCR can be performed on blood (low sensitivity), lymph node aspirates, conjunctival swabs, or bone marrow aspirates (highest sensitivity). Osteolytic bone lesions, hypercalcemia, the identification of a monoclonal gammopathy, and Bence–Jones proteinuria can be indicative of multiple myeloma, although (rarely) *E. canis* infections are also associated with monoclonal gammopathies. The diagnosis of multiple myeloma can also be established by cytology of bone marrow aspirates. Clonality PCR can also be used to confirm the presence of neoplasia, as opposed to reactive plasmacytosis.

CASE 171

1 What are possible complications in this dog secondary to the abnormalities identified? Hyperproteinemia with very high concentrations of immunoglobulins can induce hyperviscosity syndrome leading to thrombocytopathy, hypervolemia, myocardial hypoxia, and increased cardiac workload. Thrombocytopenia and thrombocytopathy can lead to severe generalized hemorrhage (potentially including the brain and lungs) and cause blood loss anemia. Neutropenia can increase susceptibility to bacterial infections. Glomerulonephritis can gradually lead to secondary renal tubular failure.

2 **What treatment should be given and what is the prognosis?** The prognosis is guarded because the dog already has two major complications of both infections: bone marrow suppression and glomerular disease. Treatment of choice for the *Ehrlichia canis* infection is doxycycline (5 mg/kg PO q12h or 10 mg/kg PO q24h). In chronic ehrlichiosis, doxycycline treatment should be continued until the platelets are in the RI, which can take several months. Some dogs fail to respond to antimicrobial therapy. Leishmaniosis is treated with allopurinol (10 mg/kg PO q24h usually lifelong) in combination with meglumine antimonate (100 mg/kg SC q24h for 4 weeks) or miltefosine (2 mg/kg PO q24h for 4 weeks).

CASE 172

1 **How should the ELISA result be interpreted in this case?** The positive C6 ELISA indicates exposure to *Borrelia burgdorferi*. However, >90% of infected dogs in the USA show no clinical signs after infection and have antibodies that persist for months to years after exposure, so associating the positive test result with disease can be challenging. The C6 ELISA result is not affected by vaccination against *B. burgdorferi*.

2 **What other diagnostic tests should be considered?** A definitive diagnosis of Lyme disease can only be obtained by direct detection of the organism in conjunction with typical clinical signs. Blood PCR assay is insensitive for detection of *B. burgdorferi* infection because the spirochete is a connective tissue pathogen and is rarely present in the bloodstream. Synovial fluid can be considered for PCR testing in dogs with polyarthritis. Skin biopsies also can be used for PCR but are only confirmative if positive. Evaluation of the UPCR is recommended in this case to evaluate for evidence of glomerulonephritis. Diagnostic tests for other pathogens that can cause polyarthritis (such as *Anaplasma* spp., *Ehrlichia* spp., endemic fungi such as *Blastomyces*, *Bartonella* spp.) should also be considered (i.e. PCR and antibody testing). Non-infectious causes of polyarthritis should also be considered, including systemic lupus erythematosus and erosive and non-erosive immune-mediated polyarthritis.

3 **What treatment should be recommended?** Doxycycline (5 mg/kg PO q12h for 4 weeks) is recommended for dogs with clinical manifestations consistent with Lyme disease. Dogs with Lyme polyarthritis generally respond within 24–48 hours. Failure to respond within this time period suggests that an alternative disease is present. Dogs with Lyme glomerulonephritis require additional management of protein-losing nephropathy. This dog improved with doxycycline treatment. Therefore, Lyme disease (or another doxycycline-responsive infection) was suspected.

4 What is the prognosis? If treated with doxycycline, dogs with Lyme polyarthritis have a good prognosis. Lyme glomerulonephritis has a guarded to poor prognosis.

CASE 173

1 Considering that the dog did not show aggression, could this still be rabies? Rabies must be considered in a dog with a history of a bite exposure within last few months and sudden unexplained neurologic abnormalities that progress quickly, especially in this case when the dog lived close to the border of Ukraine, where rabies is still endemic in foxes. Classically, the clinical course of rabies in dogs has been divided into three phases, each lasting 1–3 days. In the prodromal stage, fever, anorexia, and behavioral changes are seen. During the furious phase, restlessness, irritability, vocalization, and aggressiveness predominate. Affected dogs bite humans, animals, or inanimate objects with no apparent reason. The last phase is the paralytic stage with cranial nerve deficits, salivation, seizures, limb paralysis, coma, and death. However, not all cases fit these categories, and many dogs show the "silent" form of rabies, in which the paralytic stage immediately follows the prodromal stage.

2 Could detection of antibodies have been helpful to confirm or rule out rabies in this dog? Antibody detection cannot be used for diagnosis of rabies. Although rabies virus is highly immunogenic, little antigen is presented to the immune system during the early stages of infection, and the virus is able to evade detection by the immune system by hiding in nerve cells. Thus, antibodies cannot protect against rabies, nor do they have diagnostic value. In contrast, antibody testing can be helpful to confirm immunity after vaccination.

3 How should dogs be protected from rabies? Rabies vaccines are very effective, safe, and inexpensive. Most commercial products induce immunity lasting up to 3 years in a very high percentage of vaccinated dogs. Thus, all dogs living in or travelling to endemic countries should be vaccinated against rabies, and in many countries vaccination is required by law.

CASE 174

1 What are the main differential diagnoses for the vomiting and diarrhea before the laboratory results are available? Before the blood test results become available, in a young dog that has never been vaccinated, canine parvovirus infection still is possible, despite a negative antigen test. As many as 50% of fecal antigen test results can be negative in dogs with parvovirus enteritis. Other causes of acute hemorrhagic diarrhea and vomiting include a gastrointestinal foreign body, acute pancreatitis, liver disease, hypoadrenocorticism, and toxicities such as non-steroidal anti-inflammatory drug toxicity. Idiopathic acute hemorrhagic diarrhea syndrome, which was called hemorrhagic gastroenteritis until recently, is another important differential diagnosis. The history makes drugs and toxins less likely. The pyrexia suggests an infection.

2 What are the main differential diagnoses after the laboratory results become available? The clinical and laboratory findings suggest the presence of acute liver cell destruction. Canine adenovirus-1 (CAV-1) infection has been associated with tonsillitis and hepatitis in dogs. CAV-1 causes an acute viremic disease (infectious canine hepatitis [ICH]) characterized by hepatitis, generalized vascular endothelium damage, nephritis, DIC, and later uveitis with corneal edema. Icterus is a rare event in ICH. Leptospirosis has also been associated with liver enzyme elevation, but this is usually accompanied by renal failure. Other infectious causes of acute liver disease include bacterial cholangiohepatitis, liver abscesses, and protozoal infections (e.g. toxoplasmosis, sarcocystosis). Severe acute pancreatitis can also be associated with gastrointestinal signs, fever, and liver enzyme elevation (but would usually also be accompanied by hyperbilirubinemia).

3 What other diagnostic tests should be performed? Abdominal ultrasound should be recommended to evaluate the liver and biliary tract. Given the presence of thrombocytopenia, coagulation testing should be considered to identify DIC and assess the safety of liver fine needle aspiration. Depending on the ultrasound results, testing for leptospirosis and CAV-1 infection should be considered. Antibody testing is widely used to diagnose leptospirosis. A 4-fold MAT titer increase (2 titer steps) over a 1–2-week period is considered diagnostic of leptospirosis in dogs with suggestive clinical signs. PCR can also be used to detect the DNA of leptospires in urine or blood. CAV-1 infection can be confirmed by antibody testing and demonstration of a 4-fold titer increase within 2 weeks. Alternatively, demonstration of viral DNA by PCR in blood in the early phase of disease is confirmative. During the acute stage of disease, viremia occurs and the virus is present in all body tissues and secretions, but 10–15 days post infection viremia is cleared and virus can only be isolated from the kidney or from urine, in which CAV-1 is excreted for as long as 6 months.

CASE 175

1 What is the pathogenesis of the ocular changes? Corneal clouding ("blue eye") occurs in about 20% of dogs with infectious canine hepatitis (ICH). It results from deposition of CAV-1 antigen–antibody complexes in the corneal endothelium. Endothelial cells are normally responsible for removal of fluid from the cornea into the anterior chamber. Thus, damage to the endothelium causes edema within the corneal stroma that is visible as corneal opacity. Corneal edema commonly appears during recovery from acute ICH, typically at least 7 days after the onset of clinical signs. Sometimes it can be the only sign of an otherwise subclinical CAV-1 infection. Typically, it is unilateral, but both eyes can be affected. Signs of ocular pain can occur at the onset of ocular lesions, but they subside once complete corneal opacity results. In the past, use of modified live CAV-1 vaccines resulted in blue eye in a low percentage of vaccinated animals. For this reason, vaccines against CAV-1 now contain attenuated CAV-2, which provides solid cross-protection against CAV-1 without the risk of corneal edema.

2 **What is the prognosis for this dog?** Corneal edema is usually self-limiting. In most cases, the endothelium regenerates and the edema resolves within about 2 weeks.

3 **How should the ocular disease be treated?** No treatment is needed for ICH-associated ocular disease if the dog shows no ocular discomfort. If pain is present, topical anti-inflammatory drugs can be indicated, with or without topical atropine, depending on the presence of concurrent uveitis.

4 **What could have been the source of CAV-1 infection in this dog?** Because of widespread vaccination with effective vaccines, ICH is nowadays a very rare disease worldwide. However, CAV-1 still circulates in wild carnivores belonging to the Canidae, Mustelidae, and Ursidae families. In European red foxes, CAV-1 infections have been recently demonstrated in the United Kingdom and Italy. Thus, considering the long-term shedding of the virus in urine and the high resistance to environmental inactivation of this agent, wild carnivores can still serve as a CAV-1 reservoir for dogs.

CASE 176

1 **What is your interpretation of the radiograph?** The thoracic radiograph shows normal cardiopulmonary structures.

2 **What differential diagnoses should you consider?** Given the age and breed of this patient, the top differential diagnoses are tracheal collapse and canine infectious respiratory disease complex (CIRD), although the course of illness is long for the latter condition. Occasionally, bordetellosis or mycoplasmosis can be associated with a chronic cough that lasts weeks to months, but this is unusual. The owners should be questioned about whether the onset of cough followed intubation for the spay operation and should be asked about exposure to other dogs that are coughing.

3 **What additional diagnostic tests should be performed?** A CBC could be considered, although it is unlikely to be abnormal if the patient has only local (i.e. tracheal) inflammation. Fluoroscopy would be valuable to investigate the possibility of airway collapse. Given the long duration of the history, the owners should be encouraged to pursue bronchoscopy and bronchoalveolar lavage. A short course of doxycycline could be considered for treatment of bordetellosis or mycoplasmosis.

CASE 177

1 **With what disease process are the bronchoscopic image and the histopathology most consistent?** The nodular lesions in the carina and the findings on biopsy are consistent with *Oslerus osleri* infection.

2 Is there an additional diagnostic test that could have provided the diagnosis prior to bronchoscopy? Fecal Baermann analysis can be used to detect larval stages of airway parasites such as *O. osleri*. The larvae are coughed up into the mouth, ingested, and passed in the feces. Tests can be falsely negative owing to intermittent appearance of parasites in the feces.

CASE 178

1 What influenza viruses can infect dogs? Influenza in dogs can be caused by several influenza A viruses. Influenza A viruses belong to the Orthomyxoviridae family and are negative single-stranded, segmented RNA viruses. The various influenza A virus subtypes are named according to an H number (for the type of hemagglutinin) and an N number (for the type of neuraminidase). There are 18 different known H antigens (H1 to H18) and 11 different known N antigens (N1 to N11). Strains of all subtypes of influenza A virus can be isolated from wild birds, but birds usually do not develop disease. Some variants also cause disease in humans or other mammals, including dogs and cats.

Most reported influenza outbreaks in dogs have been with subtype H3N8, which originated from horses. Canine H3N8 influenza virus was first detected in 2004 as a cause of a respiratory disease outbreak in racing Greyhounds in Florida, USA. Exposure occurred at horse race tracks that were also used for dog racing. Since then, outbreaks have been described in different states in the USA as well as in Europe. In some areas in the USA, such as New York, southern Florida, and northern Colorado/southern Wyoming, H3N8 is meanwhile considered endemic in the dog population.

A second dog-adapted subtype, H3N2, was identified in 2006 in South Korea and southern China. Outbreaks in the USA were first reported in the Chicago area in early 2015, and in several other USA states during the spring and summer of 2015.

Influenza A virus subtypes that infect humans have been very rarely found in dogs. H5N1 ("avian influenza") was the cause of death in one dog in Thailand, following ingestion of an infected duck.

2 Are dogs with influenza virus infection a zoonotic risk? There is no evidence that H3N8, the most common subtype infecting dogs, can be transmitted to people, cats, or other species. For subtype H3N2, no infections in people have been detected. If dogs are infected with H5N1 (which occurs only extremely rarely), they theoretically could pose a risk to humans. Thus, most cases of canine influenza do not represent a risk of transmission to humans.

3 What is the risk of the husband transmitting infection to the dog? Most of the influenza subtypes that cause "flu" in humans are not infectious to dogs, but routine hygienic measures, such as hand disinfection, should generally be taken with every sick human being or dog.

CASE 179

1 What other differential diagnoses should have been considered in this dog before the results of cytology were available? Other differential diagnoses that should have been considered were infiltrative neoplastic processes, such as lymphoma or mast cell tumor, as well as other infectious agents that can infiltrate the intestinal tract, especially *Cryptococcus neoformans*, *Prototheca* spp., and *Pythium insidiosum*.
2 What is the normal geographic distribution of *Histoplasma capsulatum*? *Histoplasma capsulatum* is especially found in the Ohio and Mississippi river valleys of the USA and in Latin America, but foci of endemicity also occur in northern and southern California. Infections have been reported sporadically in other parts of the world, such as Brazil, Italy, Australia, and Japan. *H. capsulatum* can be found in the intestinal tract and guano of bats, which constitute the primary reservoir of the organism and serve to disseminate it geographically.
3 What are the anatomic sites of predilection of *Histoplasma capsulatum* in dogs? After inhalation, *Histoplasma* yeasts migrate to local lymph nodes (such as the hilar lymph node) and other tissues that contain mononuclear cells, such as the liver and spleen. In addition to lymph nodes, liver, and spleen, other common sites of dissemination in dogs include the bone marrow, small and/or large intestinal tract, the skin, bones, CNS, and eye. Dogs with histoplasmosis in the USA appear to be particularly susceptible to intestinal involvement.
4 How could the success of antifungal drug therapy be monitored in this dog? The success of antifungal drug therapy in dogs with histoplasmosis could be monitored through serial abdominal ultrasound examinations or by monitoring urine *Histoplasma* spp. antigen titers. Unfortunately, in this particular case, the baseline urine *Histoplasma* spp. antigen test was negative, which underscores the potential for false-negative urinary antigen test results.

CASE 180

1 What are the main differential diagnoses for this dog's neurologic abnormalities based on the physical and neurologic examination findings? The presence of multifocal areas of spinal pain is most suggestive of inflammatory disease, such as meningitis or discospondylitis. Other inflammatory diseases that cause pain on manipulation of the spine or palpation of the paraspinal musculature are polyarthritis or osteoarthritis of the articular facets, polymyositis, or spinal empyema. Non-inflammatory diseases only rarely lead to multifocal areas of spinal pain (e.g. multiple sites of intervertebral disc protrusion, extensive syringomyelia).

2 How would you interpret the radiographs? The radiographs of the cervical and thoracolumbar spine show several abnormal intervertebral disc spaces with an irregular contour and lytic appearance of the adjacent vertebral endplates, which is most suggestive of vertebral endplate lysis. Additional findings are ventral and lateral spondylosis and endplate sclerosis of the vertebral endplates. Based on these findings, the radiographic diagnosis is discospondylitis at the C5–C6, T13–L1, and possibly also at the T11–T12 and L1–L2 intervertebral disc space. It is possible that even more sites are involved, based on the multifocal pain on palpation, because radiographic findings can lag behind physical examination findings by 4–6 weeks. Only CT or MRI can identify evidence of discospondylitis within the first few weeks.

3 What are the next diagnostic steps? Discospondylitis is the result of bacterial infection or filamentous fungal infections. Hematogenous spread and slowing of blood flow in the vertebral endplates are considered responsible for the seeding of bacteria or fungi in most cases of discospondylitis. In rare cases, migration of an aspirated grass awn, extension from bite wounds, or infection of a surgical site can be the cause. The source of infection can be the skin, the genitourinary tract, endocarditis, an abscess, or oral or respiratory infections. Thus, these sites should be evaluated carefully. However, the original site of infection often remains obscure despite intensive investigations.

Culture of blood and urine should be performed in order to identify the infecting agent in any case of suspected discospondylitis. For this purpose, ideally 10 ml of blood is collected with a syringe under strict aseptic conditions from three separate venipuncture sites and transferred to a blood culture bottle. Urine for culture should be obtained by cystocentesis. Blood culture bottles are stored at room temperature until they are submitted to the laboratory. It is commonly recommended to collect the three blood samples at different times during the day (8 hours apart) to enhance the diagnostic yield. Blood should ideally be cultured aerobically and anaerobically. An alternative diagnostic approach is bacterial and fungal culture of a fine needle aspirate of the affected disc space under fluoroscopic or CT guidance under anaesthesia. This procedure should be considered for severely affected cases or dogs with a suspected fungal infection (e.g. dogs that are refractory to antibiotic therapy). The sensitivity of this approach has varied between 30 and 70% in different studies. Discospondylitis can also be diagnosed by culture of surgical biopsies when severely affected dogs undergo decompressive surgery.

Testing for *Brucella canis* should be performed in all dogs with discospondylitis and in any dog with a history of traveling to countries where *B. canis* is still endemic. *B. canis* is a gram-negative aerobic bacterium, which is sexually or vertically transmitted. It is frequently associated with discospondylitis as well as orchitis, epididymitis, and prostatitis. Other clinical signs include abdominal lymphadenopathy and hepatosplenomegaly, or signs of dermatitis, uveitis, endocarditis, and, rarely, meningoencephalitis. Among fungi, mainly *Aspergillus* spp. are associated with discospondylitis, especially in predisposed dog breeds (e.g. German Shepherd Dog, Rhodesian Ridgeback). An *Aspergillus* spp. antigen test can be performed on serum or urine for diagnosis of *Aspergillus* discospondylitis. In this dog, *B. canis* was grown from blood cultures.

4 What treatment would you recommend? Treatment of discospondylitis generally requires a minimum of 6–8 weeks of antibiotics, but treatment might have to be continued for many months up to 1 year (until all lytic lesions have resolved). Providing adequate analgesia and restriction of movement is an important part of the treatment protocol for discospondylitis.

Antibiotics that can be used to treat brucellosis include doxycycline in combination with either a short course of an aminoglycoside antibiotic (e.g. streptomycin), rifampin, or combined treatment with doxycycline and enrofloxacin for 2–3 months. The owner should be informed about the (low) zoonotic potential of *B. canis*, which can be relevant to immunocompromised individuals.

CASE 181

1 What are the main differential diagnoses for the skin changes in this dog? Diseases that cause alopecia, scaling, and crusting that should be considered in an immunosuppressed dog from this region would be dermatophytosis, mange (demodicosis or scabies), bacterial pyoderma, and leishmaniosis.

2 What diagnostic tests should be performed? Dermatophytosis is investigated by performance of a trichogram, Wood's lamp test, and fungal culture of scales and hair. Diagnosis of demodicosis is based on multiple deep skin scrapings. Cytology of crusts is helpful to evaluate the number and shape of intra- and extracellular bacteria. *Leishmania* spp. antibody testing should also be performed.

CASE 182

1 What are the therapeutic options? Dermatophytosis can be self-limiting in a few weeks or months in immunocompetent dogs. However, treatment should be recommended because of zoonotic concerns. Puppies, immunosuppressed dogs (as in this case), and Yorkshire and Jack Russell Terriers can be more likely to develop generalized disease. In this case, systemic treatment is required; the most commonly used systemic drugs are azoles (itraconazole, fluconazole) and terbinafine. Itraconazole is the drug of choice. Oral therapy should continued until two consecutive cultures at a 2–4 week interval are negative, and usually must be continued for several months.

2 What should be done to reduce contamination of the environment? Decontamination of the dog's hair is important, and shampoo therapy with a miconazole–chlorhexidine shampoo should be started while culture is pending (growth can require several weeks incubation). Lime sulfur shampoos are more effective than miconazole–chlorhexidine shampoos if they are available, and should be applied twice weekly. Long-haired dogs should be clipped, preferably with scissors to avoid skin trauma and further dissemination on the healthy skin. Infected dogs should be handled with disposable gloves, cap, and gown. Hospitalization should be avoided but, if necessary, affected dogs should be housed in the isolation ward. Decontamination of the environment can be extremely difficult. Contaminated objects in the home environment should be discarded if possible. Thorough vacuuming and steam cleaning of the household is recommended to reduce the spore burden in the environment. Disinfection of hard surfaces should be performed with 1:10 to 1:100 bleach solution, 0.2% enilconazole solution, or (where available) an enilconazole fogger. Vehicles and carriers used to transport animals must also be appropriately cleaned. Concentrated (1:16) accelerated hydrogen peroxide solutions can also inactivate dermatophytes and reduce environmental contamination.

CASE 183

1 What are the most important findings of the necropsy and histopathology of the heart? Several areas of hemorrhage in the epicardium, myocardium, and endocardium are seen (**183a**, between white arrows). Fibrin deposition is seen on the epicardium (**183b**, white arrow). Histopathology indicates mononuclear cell infiltration (**183c**, white arrow), myocardial hemorrhage (**183c**, black arrows), and necrosis, consistent with myocarditis.

2 What are the differential diagnoses for these abnormalities in this case? Myocarditis can have numerous causes, such as infectious agents, nutritional deficiencies (taurine, carnitine), vascular disorders (coronary arterial embolus, vasculitis), drugs, and toxins. Infectious agents are most likely in this case based on the history, presentation, and laboratory abnormalities. Infectious causes of myocarditis in dogs include parvovirus (before or in the first weeks after birth), West Nile virus (rare), *Bartonella* spp., *Rickettsia rickettsii*, *Ehrlichia canis*, *Trypanosoma cruzi*, *Toxoplasma gondii* and *Neospora caninum*, *Babesia rossi* infection (South Africa), *Leishmania* spp. infection, and bacteremia/sepsis. In this case, infection with *E. canis* was suspected as the cause of the myocarditis on the basis of severe pancytopenia, a positive PCR result for *E. canis* on whole blood, and negative test results for other vector-borne pathogens.

CASE 184

1 How would you treat the dog? A registered adulticidal spot-on containing selamectin or moxidectin every 2 weeks for three treatments will usually resolve clinical signs of scabies very quickly. Other effective miticidal products are available and might be indicated in individual cases, but can be associated with more severe adverse effects or a higher rate of adverse effects. As it is not uncommon for dogs to develop an increase in pruritus for several days after miticidal treatment is initiated, 3–5 days of anti-pruritic therapy with glucocorticoids or oclacitinib can be beneficial in such cases.

2 How would you treat the owner? Although owners of dogs infected with *Sarcoptes scabiei* var. *canis* often develop pruritus, the mites do not reproduce on humans, and treatment of the dog usually leads to resolution of signs in the owner. In some cases, where dogs have a high number of mites, owners can be affected for up to 2 weeks after miticidal therapy has been administered to the dog.

3 How would you treat the environment? As *Sarcoptes* mites cannot survive away from the host for a long period, environmental treatment for these mites is not required, as long as all in-contact animals entering or living in the household are treated for at least 4–6 weeks.

CASE 185

1 What are your differential diagnoses for the skin lesions? The most likely differential diagnoses are leishmaniosis, vasculitis, fly strike, and, less likely, dermatomyositis (predominantly seen in younger Collies and Shelties). Leishmaniosis is an important differential diagnosis because the dog has come from Spain and shows scaling and alopecia, two of the most common clinical signs of leishmaniosis. Vasculitis is often the cause of scaling and alopecia of ear tips in the dog, but is more often seen in special breeds, such as the Jack Russell Terrier, and often during winter. Fly strike is more often seen in outdoor dogs and in summer.

2 What tests are indicated in this dog? A good history could provide diagnostic clues for either vasculitis, fly strike (possibly flies observed by the owner and head shaking without otitis externa), or leishmaniosis. Dogs with leishmaniosis might have a history of other systemic signs such as weight loss or lameness. On physical examination, lymphadenopathy is present in many dogs with leishmaniosis and lymph node aspirates can reveal *Leishmania* organisms. Mild footpad hyperkeratosis can escape the owners' attention but might be detected on physical examination. A serum biochemistry panel and urinalysis could identify hyperglobulinemia and/or findings consistent with a protein-losing nephropathy in dogs with leishmaniosis. A *Leishmania* spp. antibody titer is the most commonly used diagnostic test for leishmaniosis and is high in most dogs with clinical disease. Alternatively, or in addition, PCR of bone marrow aspirates (most sensitive), lymph node aspirates, conjunctival scrapings, or blood (least sensitive) can be performed. Cytologic evaluation of impression smears of the pinnal lesion might reveal eosinophilic dermatitis in dogs with fly strike, or macrophages with intracytoplasmic *Leishmania* spp. amastigotes. If vasculitis or dermatomyositis is higher on the list based on the history and other findings, biopsy of the pinna with histopathology is recommended for diagnosis.

3 What is the prognosis for each of the major differential diagnoses? For leishmaniosis, the presence of hypoalbuminemia, proteinuria, and lymphopenia is associated with a significantly shorter survival time. With fly strike, keeping the dog indoors and using fly screens on windows and doors can lead to resolution of lesions. If the dog is kept outdoors, the prognosis for remission during the warm season is guarded, although use of fly repellents can be helpful. Dogs with severe dermatomyositis typically have progressive disease with a poor prognosis. Prognostic factors for vasculitis are not known.

A high *Leishmania* spp. antibody titer was detected in this dog, so the dog was diagnosed with leishmaniosis.

CASE 186

1 What would be an adequate analgesia protocol for painful oral ulceration? An adequate analgesia protocol would include fentanyl as a continuous rate infusion (2–5 μg/kg/min) or methadone (0.2 mg/kg q4h). Opioids (μ-agonists) provide adequate analgesia in the mouth and also in the kidneys. However, they can cause decreased intestinal motility, nausea, and vomiting. Buprenorphine might not provide sufficient analgesia in this case. Non-steroidal anti-inflammatory drugs are contraindicated because they can lead to further kidney injury.

Adequate mouth hygiene (e.g. flushing with chlorhexidine q8h) can help to reduce the bacterial load in the mouth and bacteria-induced inflammation. Some clinicians also recommend oral rinses with lidocaine-containing solutions. This can have an effect for up to 2 hours. However, some lidocaine will be swallowed and could result in systemic adverse effects, such as seizures and bradycardia.

2 What would be appropriate routes for food administration in this dog? Nutrition should be provided as soon as possible via the enteral route, for example by using a nasoesophageal feeding tube or esophagostomy tube. Nasoesophageal tubes can be easily placed, but should be used with caution if thrombocytopenia or other coagulation disorders are present. The small tube diameter also limits the amount of food that can be administered. To place an esophagostomy tube, general anesthesia with intubation is required, which could potentially result in further insult to this dog's kidneys. Esophagostomy tube placement should be avoided if hemostatic disorders are present. However, the larger diameter would allow administration of larger amounts of food. Parenteral nutrition could also be used to provide nutrition to this patient but should be reduced to a minimum, because of higher risks associated with parenteral nutrition and greater benefits of enteral nutrition to gastrointestinal health.

CASE 187

1 What are the main differential diagnoses for the genital lesion? Proliferative lesions on the penile mucosa can have an inflammatory or neoplastic origin. Papillomatosis, squamous cell carcinoma, fibrosarcoma, lymphoma, or vascular tumors are infrequently detected. Transmissible venereal tumor (TVT) can affect sexually active dogs in enzootic tropical and subtropical areas. The genital tract is also frequently involved in *Leishmania infantum* infections and is responsible for the venereal transmission of the disease. Nodular or ulcerative mucosal lesions are described in dogs with leishmaniosis.

2 What diagnostic tests should be performed? Cytology of impression smears and fine needle aspiration of the lesion, as well as fine needle aspiration of the enlarged lymph nodes, should be performed at a minimum. Cytology of impression smears of the lesion revealed the presence of *L. infantum*.

CASE 188

1 How should the dog be treated? In contrast to anaphylactic shock, local anaphylactic reactions (angioedema and urticaria) are in many cases self-limiting. Antihistamines (e.g. diphenhydramine [1–2 mg/kg IV] and prednisolone [1 mg/kg PO q12–24h]) are indicated until the signs resolve. During the first few hours after the onset of the clinical signs, the patient should be monitored for laryngeal edema and signs of shock.

2 Is this dog at higher risk for allergic reactions after future vaccinations? Although each exposure to allergen is unique and the consequences of future vaccinations are unpredictable, the risk of adverse reactions with subsequent vaccinations is higher in animals that have a history of allergic reactions than in those that do not. In most cases, these reactions seem to be induced not by antigens of infectious agents in the vaccine, but by fetal calf serum derived from the culture media used for vaccine production or by stabilizer proteins. As these components are present in many vaccines, use of any product subsequently that may contain these components can represent a risk to this dog.

3 How should this dog be vaccinated in the future? Unnecessary vaccination should be avoided in this dog. Many vaccines induce immunity lasting for 3 years or more. For some pathogens, such as canine distemper virus, canine adenovirus, and canine parvovirus measurement of antibodies could be considered to determine whether booster vaccination is needed after a 3-year interval. If vaccination is deemed necessary, diphenhydramine (1 mg/kg IV) can be given 10 minutes before vaccination. If possible, adjuvanted vaccines should be replaced by non-adjuvanted ones, because adjuvants could induce allergic reactions. The dog should be closely observed for an hour after vaccination in the clinic. In addition, the owner should watch the dog closely for several hours at home for development of any abnormal signs.

CASE 189

1 What is the ocular diagnosis based on the clinical presentation and ocular examination? The ocular diagnosis is corneal edema and scleritis in the right eye. The intraocular pressure was low and although the anterior chamber could not be examined in detail, the presence of anterior uveitis was suspected. There was mild corneal edema in the left eye.

2 Which underlying disease would you suspect based on the clinical findings and history? The travel history of this dog together with the skin and ocular lesions are strongly suggestive of an infection with *Leishmania* spp. Clinically, the condition is suspected based on chronic weight loss, facial and pinnal dermatitis, and a history of regular visits to an endemic area. Leishmaniosis is endemic in many southern European countries (including Greece, Spain, Italy, Portugal, and Turkey). Dogs are primary reservoirs and transmission occurs through the bites of infected sandflies (*Phlebotomus* spp.). The incubation period is between a few months and many years. Ocular manifestations occur in up to 80% of dogs with leishmaniosis. They include blepharitis, simple or granulomatous conjunctivitis, scleritis, superficial or deep keratitis, anterior uveitis, keratoconjunctivitis sicca, and secondary glaucoma. Signs are typically bilateral.

3 What further diagnostic tests do you suggest? Diagnosis of leishmaniosis is made by finding the organism (amastigotes, which are round to oval and 2.5–5.0 µm by 1.5–2.0 µm in size) in bone marrow aspirates, lymph node aspirates, or skin impression smears. Other diagnostic tests include antibody tests or PCR performed on bone marrow, lymph node aspirates, blood, or conjunctival scrapings. Conjunctival scraping PCR was positive for *Leishmania* spp. in this dog.

4 What is your ocular and systemic treatment plan for this dog? Ocular treatment includes anti-inflammatory treatment with a topical glucocorticoid (e.g. dexamethasone or prednisolone acetate, q6–8h). Uveitis treatment also includes topical 1% atropine q12–24h, which releases painful ciliary muscle spasm, stabilizes the blood–aqueous barrier, and dilates the pupil, thereby preventing formation of posterior synechiae. The intraocular pressure should be carefully monitored.

Systemic treatment for leishmaniosis includes lifelong allopurinol (to avoid xanthine stone development, strict adherence to a specific low purine diet is recommended). Adjuvant treatment can include domperidone to increase the T-helper cell (Th1) response. In periods when clinical signs appear, meglumine antimoniate or miltefonsine should be given in addition to allopurinol for 4 weeks.

CASE 190

1 What are the differential diagnoses for the main problem in this dog? Icterus is the most specific problem in this case, and can be prehepatic, hepatic or posthepatic. Common prehepatic causes of icterus include immune-mediated hemolytic anemia (primary or secondary) and hemolysis due to infection, toxins (e.g. zinc), or transfusion. Hepatic causes include infectious diseases (such as leptospirosis, infectious canine hepatitis), chronic hepatitis, toxins, or neoplasia. Posthepatic causes include gallbladder disease, pancreatitis, and peritonitis. Based on the presence of fever, splenomegaly, and abdominal pain, an inflammatory or infectious cause is suspected.

2 What are the next diagnostic steps? A work-up for icterus should include a CBC, serum biochemical panel, urinalysis, and abdominal ultrasound. Subsequent diagnostic tests would depend on whether the problem appears to be prehepatic, hepatic, or posthepatic on the basis of those initial diagnostic tests.

3 Does this patient represent a risk for transmission of infection to other dogs and to humans? The combination of icterus and fever in a dog from Brazil should result in suspicion of leptospirosis, and so this dog should be handled with appropriate precautions until an alternative diagnosis is made. Isolation is not required, because dogs with acute leptospirosis require critical care, but personal protective equipment, including gloves, disposable gowns, and eyewear or face shields, should be worn at least until appropriate antimicrobial drugs have been administered for 48 hours. Warning signs should be posted, and movement around the hospital should be minimized. Pregnant women should not work with dogs that are suspected to have leptospirosis. Most disinfectants are appropriate for hospital decontamination. Indwelling urinary catheters are recommended for monitoring urine output in oliguric/anuric animals and to facilitate the containment of potentially contaminated urine. The dog should be treated with an antibiotic that reduces *Leptospira* spp. shedding (e.g. penicillin derivative).

CASE 191

1 What are the abnormalities seen on the blood smear? *Babesia* spp. are seen within red blood cells, and based on the morphology of the parasite and the geographic region, this is suggestive of *Babesia vogeli* infection. However, *Babesia* spp. cannot be speciated solely on the basis of morphology. PCR confirmed *Babesia vogeli* infection in this case. Interestingly, North American strains of *B. vogeli* rarely cause severe anemia in immunocompetent dogs, so it is possible that strain differences exist internationally. Alternatively, unidentified co-infections in this dog may have contributed to the severity of disease.

2 How did this dog become infected with these organisms? Most species of *Babesia* are transmitted by ticks. *Babesia gibsoni* can also be directly transmitted by bites, mainly within fighting breeds, or perinatally.

3 How should this disease be treated? *B. vogeli* is effectively treated with two doses of imidocarb diproprionate (6 mg/kg SC) 14 days apart. Dogs treated with imidocarb diproprionate should be premedicated with atropine (0.5 mg/kg SC) 30 minutes before injection to avoid parasympathetic adverse effects, such as salivation, vomiting, and occasionally diarrhea.

4 What is the prognosis? With treatment, the prognosis for dogs with *B. vogeli* infection is good.

CASE 192

1 What is Lyme disease, and how is it transmitted? Lyme disease is a tick-borne spirochetosis caused by *Borrelia burgdorferi* sensu lato, which is divided into several species affecting people and dogs worldwide. *Borrelia* spp. are small, corkscrew-shaped, motile, microaerophilic bacteria. *B. burgdorferi* sensu stricto predominates in people and dogs in the USA. It is also found in Europe but only in about 10% of the isolates. *Borrelia garinii* and *Borrelia afzelii* are the main species infecting people and dogs in Europe. The presence of disease and its clinical features are dependent on the isolate in a given geographic region.

Borrelia spp. do not survive freely in the environment. They are host associated, being transmitted between vertebrate reservoir hosts and hematophagous arthropod vectors. The principal vectors of *Borrelia* spp. are various species of hard ticks of the *Ixodes* complex. These small (<3 mm) ticks generally feed on more than one host during their life cycle. Infected nymphs overwinter, and in the spring they transmit infection to reservoir hosts, which in turn infect feeding larvae. Larvae and nymphs feed primarily on rodents and small mammals or reptiles, whereas adult ticks feed on deer or larger mammals. People and companion animals are usually infected by nymphs or adult ticks. Other ticks and insect vectors have been found to harbor *Borrelia* spp. but do not seem to maintain infection or be important in transmission. Direct transmission of *Borrelia* spp. between reservoir hosts is unlikely, as is transovarial transmission in ticks. In a natural infection model, control dogs in direct contact with infected dogs for up to 1 year did not develop antibodies, and organisms could not be isolated from the urine of infected dogs. There is also no evidence of *in-utero* spread in dogs.

2 How common are clinical signs in dogs? Most infected dogs never develop clinical signs. *B. burgdorferi* sensu stricto seems to be more pathogenic in dogs than the *Borrelia* spp. mainly found in Europe. About 5–10% of dogs with antibodies in endemic areas in the USA are thought to develop clinical signs within 2–5 months after infection; the percentage of dogs that develop clinical manifestations appears to be much lower in Europe. The number of infected ticks, immunosuppression of the animal, and co-infections with other pathogens could influence the development of clinical manifestations.

3 Is it possible that the infection was transmitted from the dog to the owner? There is no evidence that infected pet dogs pose a direct risk to humans except by introducing unfed tick stages into a household. The ticks do not survive long indoors and, if fed, tick stages do not reattach without molting. However, partially fed ticks can re-feed and can pose a risk of infection. No correlation has been observed between antibody prevalence in hunters when compared with their dogs. Dogs and people are incidental hosts for a sylvan cycle that exists in nature, and Lyme disease in humans is usually associated with outdoor activities, such as hunting, that result in exposure to tick vectors.

4 How could you quickly rule out a diagnosis of Lyme disease in this dog? The SNAP 4Dx Plus test (IDEXX Laboratories) is a rapid in-house test, a component of which detects (among other infectious agents) antibodies to the C6 peptide of *Borrelia* spp. There is a long incubation period for Lyme disease in dogs (i.e. there is adequate time to show an antibody response before clinical signs are present). Thus, if this test is negative, it makes active *Borrelia* spp. infection and Lyme disease extremely unlikely. The SNAP 4Dx Plus test was negative in this dog. Other assays are available that also detect antibodies to *Borrelia* antigens, such as the Antech Accuplex assay.

CASE 193

1 What treatment is indicated for leptospirosis? It is important to start antimicrobial therapy as early as possible, and this is usually based on suspicion before the diagnosis can be confirmed. Penicillin or an aminopenicillin (e.g. ampicillin 20 mg/kg IV q6–8h) is usually recommended for initial therapy if vomiting is present. As soon as oral drug administration is possible, a change to doxycycline (5 mg/kg PO q12h for 2 weeks) is recommended, because this antibiotic is most effective in eliminating bacteria from the kidneys. Dehydration should be treated aggressively with IV fluid therapy. Hydration status and urine output should be monitored carefully to ensure that overhydration, oliguria, or anuria does not develop. In dogs with inadequate urine output that are developing volume overload, hemodialysis is required. Early referral to a center that has dialysis capabilities is recommended whenever possible to improve outcome.

2 Are other dogs in this household at risk of infection? Following bacteremia, which lasts 7–10 days, bacteria are shed in the urine. In incidental hosts, this shedding is usually brief and of low magnitude, but when reservoir hosts are infected, shedding can continue for weeks. Direct transmission to other animals can occur through contact with contaminated urine and, less commonly, by venereal or placental transfer or ingestion of infected tissue. Most infections occur as a result of contact with urine-contaminated water sources or moist soil. Depending on environmental conditions, the organism can survive in these sources for hours to several weeks and can infect other animals and humans through contamination of skin wounds or intact mucous membranes. Although the other dogs in the household have the potential to be infected as a result of contact with urine from the affected dog, it is more likely that they would be exposed from the same environmental source of infection. Many dogs that are exposed are subclinically infected and recover without illness.

3 Could handling this dog represent a risk for humans? Leptospirosis is an important zoonosis worldwide, especially in countries with a warm climate. Urinary shedding by subclinically infected or sick dogs can represent a risk to humans. Therefore, precautions should be taken, especially avoidance of contact with urine, if handling a dog suspected of infection. As is the case for other dogs in the household, humans are, however, more frequently infected through exposure to contaminated water sources. Heavy rainfall and flooding are risk factors for leptospirosis in humans and dogs.

CASE 194

1 Based on the ophthalmic findings in the left eye, what is your ocular diagnosis? The ocular findings in the left eye are suggestive of anterior uveitis and possibly retinitis or chorioretinitis. The mainstay finding of uveitis is a low intraocular pressure and flare (positive Tyndall effect) in the anterior chamber. Aqueous flare is caused by the breakdown of the blood–aqueous barrier (tight junctions between non-pigmented ciliary body epithelial cells, and tight junctions and gap junctions in the iris vascular endothelium and non-fenestrated impermeable capillaries in the iris). The pupil is usually miotic owing to increased activity of inflammatory mediators (mainly the effect of prostaglandins). Uveitis is always initiated by tissue injury, which can be caused by trauma, bacteria, fungi, parasites, viruses, immune-mediated disease, or neoplastic disease (mainly lymphoma).

2 What ocular treatment would you suggest? Treatment of uveitis should include a topical glucocorticoid (e.g. dexamethasone, prednisolone acetate) or non-steroidal anti-inflammatories (e.g. ocufen, ketorolac). The anti-inflammatory medications will help to re-establish and stabilize the blood–aqueous barrier. The second most important medication is a parasympatholytic drug (atropine), which is important to relieve painful ciliary muscle spasm and induces pupillary dilation, which decreases the risk of posterior synechiae formation and secondary glaucoma.

3 What further diagnostic tests would you perform to identify the underlying etiology? The next diagnostic steps should consist of a CBC, biochemistry panel, urinalysis, and assays for infectious diseases including (depending on the geographic location) toxoplasmosis, neosporosis, tick-borne diseases, systemic fungal infections, leishmaniosis, and leptospirosis. In the present case, testing for *Toxoplasma gondii* revealed a moderately high IgM titer and a high IgG titer and repeat testing 2 weeks later supported the diagnosis with 4-fold rise in the IgM titer. Oral clindamycin was started at 25 mg/kg q12h for 30 days. The dog recovered completely.

CASE 195

1 What is the most likely underlying cause for the pyoderma? In young dogs, allergic dermatitis is the most common cause of pyoderma. If this is the first time this dog has developed the lesions, treatment with an antibacterial shampoo should be the only recommendation. If the pyoderma is recurrent, sequential trial therapy to identify likely underlying diseases is indicated. Retrievers in most countries are predisposed to allergic skin disease. Fleabite hypersensitivity should be considered first, especially because flea preventives have not been used. The type of flea control used (spot-ons, tablets, sprays, collars, environmental treatment) depends on the owner's preferences and the dog's environment, but in general the more animals there are in the household and the warmer the climate, the more aggressive flea control needs to be. If flea control for 2–3 months does not prevent recurrence of pyoderma, hypersensitivities to food or airborne allergens should be considered, and an elimination diet trial is indicated. A diet should be selected that consists of a protein and a carbohydrate source never fed before.

2 How would you treat this dog? In most situations, epidermal collarettes are the only lesions and these can be treated successfully with an antibacterial shampoo containing chlorhexidine or benzoyl peroxide. The shampoo should be applied 2–3 times weekly for 2–3 weeks. Shampoos that contain benzoyl peroxide are drying, and should be followed by a moisturizing lotion or rinse for a dog with dry or normal skin. However, to optimize treatment outcome, the shampoo should be left on the skin for at least 10 minutes and then rinsed off.

3 Does the treatment have consequences for any tests used to identify underlying disease? If the flea control used for this patient is a spot-on treatment, then frequent shampooing will remove active ingredients and so the spot-on will need to be applied more frequently than normally recommended. The frequency of application required depends on: (1) the shampoo, because benzoyl peroxide more efficiently removes oils on the skin surface that contain the active ingredients of most flea products; (2) the shampooing technique, because the more vigorously and longer the dog is shampooed, the more active ingredients will be removed; and (3) the flea product itself, because some products are only present on the surface of the skin and thus will be affected more by shampooing, whereas other products are absorbed to a degree and distributed via the circulation and sebaceous glands. Typically, twice-monthly applications are recommended but in some situations even weekly application should be considered.

CASE 196

1 What would be your assessment of the vaccination history of this dog? The dog had received a full primary vaccination series, with the third vaccine administered at week 16. At this time, it is unlikely that maternal antibodies would have interfered with the vaccination. She also had received a booster at 1 year. Such a vaccination protocol is considered to give good and long-lasting protection against infection with canine parvovirus, potentially lifelong. This dog, however, is receiving chronic immunosuppressive drug therapy, which might influence immunity.

2 Could vaccination against parvovirus infection present an increased risk of adverse effects for this dog? Dogs with immune-mediated thrombocytopenia should not be vaccinated (if avoidable), as the antigenic stimulation might predispose to relapse of disease.

3 What would you recommend as an alternative to vaccination? The best recommendation for this dog would be to test for parvovirus antibodies, which, if present, are an excellent predictor of immunity. This dog had a moderate parvovirus antibody titer and vaccination was not considered necessary.

CASE 197

1 What is the significance of finding *Aspergillus terreus* in this dog's urine? *Aspergillus terreus* is an important cause of disseminated aspergillosis in dogs. German Shepherd Dogs are predisposed to this infection, and female German Shepherd Dogs are overrepresented. The other major *Aspergillus* spp. that causes canine disseminated aspergillosis is *Aspergillus deflectus*. In contrast, *Aspergillus fumigatus* complex organisms, which cause sinonasal aspergillosis in dogs, do not cause disseminated disease. Because *A. terreus* has not been associated with isolated lower urinary tract infections in dogs, its presence in the urine strongly suggests that this dog had disseminated aspergillosis. Many dogs with disseminated aspergillosis have infections of the renal pelvis; this can result in the formation of large balls of mold within the pelvis, which can be visualized grossly at necropsy or on abdominal ultrasound. However, not all dogs with disseminated aspergillosis have positive urine cultures for *Aspergillus* spp.

2 What is the likely cause of the pelvic limb paresis? *A. terreus* frequently infects the intervertebral discs; thus, the most likely cause of the pelvic limb paresis in this dog is *Aspergillus* spp. discospondylitis. This could be confirmed using spinal radiographs.
3 Had the urine culture been negative, what additional test could have been performed to make a diagnosis? The diagnosis of disseminated aspergillosis in this dog could also have been confirmed by performing an *Aspergillus* spp. galactomannan antigen ELISA. Although the cut-off for a positive test result in dogs is >1.5, most dogs with disseminated aspergillosis have titers >5. Owing to cross-reactivity, a positive antigen test can also occur in dogs with other fungal infections, and especially other disseminated mold infections (such as paecilomycosis), so positive results do not confirm disseminated aspergillosis. Strongly positive test results can also occur in dogs receiving Plasmalyte®.
4 What treatment would be recommended, and what is the prognosis? Treatment that can be effective in obtaining remission is amphotericin B, with or without concurrent azole therapy (e.g. itraconazole). Although isolates of *A. terreus* are often resistant to amphotericin B *in vitro*, clinical responses have been documented using this combination. Fluconazole is not active against *Aspergillus* spp. and other molds. In human patients, the treatment of choice for disseminated aspergillosis is voriconazole. Posaconazole appears to have had efficacy in some cases, but both voriconazole and posaconazole can be prohibitively expensive for some owners. When effective, treatment usually results in temporary remission rather than cure, so lifelong treatment is recommended.

CASE 198

1 What is the diagnosis? The blood smear shows large *Babesia* spp. trophozoites within an erythrocyte. Thus, the dog has an infection with a large *Babesia* spp. There are three major large Babesia species in dogs: *B. vogeli*, *B. canis*, and *B. rossi*. *B. rossi* is the most pathogenic species, but mainly occurs in southern Africa, and *B. vogeli* is the least pathogenic species and typically only causes severe disease in very young puppies or splenectomized dogs. Other large *Babesia* spp. have been reported to infect dogs in the UK and the USA.

In Southern Europe, *B. vogeli* is endemic and transmitted by *Rhipicehalus sanguineus*. In Eastern Europe, *B. canis* is endemic and transmitted by *Dermacentor reticulatus*. The fact that the dog was so severely anemic and had recently travelled to Croatia makes *B. canis* infection more likely.
2 What is the prognosis? With early treatment, the prognosis is usually good for dogs with babesiosis. Immediate supportive and specific antiparasitic treatment is indicated to address the severe anemia.

3 How should the dog be treated? Supportive care includes supplemental oxygen and blood transfusions to improve tissue oxygenation. Specific anti-babesial therapy consists of imidocarb dipropionate (6 mg/kg SC) twice at a 14-day interval. Pre-treatment with atropine (0.5 mg/kg SC 30 minutes before the imidocarb dipropionate injection) can be administered to avoid anticholinesterase effects.

CASE 199

1 What are the clinically relevant findings from the ophthalmic examination? The white membrane seen through the dilated pupil is a detached retina showing focal areas of intraretinal hemorrhage. The iris shows rubeosis iridis, which in association with low IOP and scleral injection suggests uveitis.

2 What are the most likely diseases causing these problems? Uveitis and retinal detachment can have intraocular or extraocular causes. Bilateral uveitis with other systemic signs suggests extraocular causes, such as neoplastic, immune-mediated, or infectious (bacterial, fungal, protozoal or viral causes) diseases. The heavy tick infestation in this case should lead to suspicion of infection with one or more of the vector-borne pathogens that cause uveitis, such as *Ehrlichia* spp. or *Rickettsia* spp. Because the dog was a stray with unknown travel history, pathogens such as *Brucella canis*, *Leptospira* spp., and *Leishmania* spp. should also be considered. Fungal pathogens, such as *Histoplasma* spp., *Cryptococcus* spp., and *Coccidioides* spp. are also possible.

This dog tested positive for *Ehrlichia canis* by PCR despite a lack of morulae on blood smears, which are insensitive for diagnosis. An IFA antibody titer to *E. canis* was also high at 1:12,800. Ehrlichiosis predisposes to uveitis and retinal detachment by causing vasculitis, intraocular hemorrhages, and hyperviscosity syndrome secondary to hyperglobulinemia.

3 What is the prognosis for this dog? Permanent blindness is a frequent consequence of total retinal detachment. Given the severe ocular changes and the very high antibody titer, chronic ehrlichiosis is likely, which has guarded prognosis despite appropriate antibiotic therapy. The possibility of co-infections with other vector-borne pathogens or other concurrent diseases causing the ocular signs should also be considered in this dog, because this can influence prognosis.

CASE 200

1 Given that this puppy has never been vaccinated before, could the vaccine be the cause of anaphylactic shock? Anaphylaxis (type I hypersensitivity) is a systemic reaction caused by rapid, IgE-mediated release of histamine and other mediators from mast cells and basophils. It can occur when there is re-exposure to the same

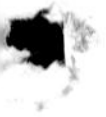

antigen following previous sensitization. Such a reaction can be induced by vaccine antigens or other vaccine components, such as fetal calf serum (FCS). Therefore, FCS in any vaccine can induce anaphylaxis in a dog that has been vaccinated previously against another disease. Occasionally, anaphylactic reactions have been observed even following the first vaccination in puppies up to 3 months of age. Food sensitization to beef allergens is suspected in these cases.

2 How common is postvaccinal anaphylaxis in dogs? Anaphylactic shock is a rare complication of vaccination. In a recent large-scale study in Japan, the incidence of anaphylactic shock was 7.2 cases per 10,000 vaccinated dogs. Small breed dogs (<10 kg) are more likely to show severe adverse reactions to vaccination, such as anaphylaxis. Local type I hypersensitivity reactions, such as angioedema or urticaria, are more common than systemic anaphylaxis.

3 How would you treat this dog? Rapid administration of epinephrine to control hypotension is the most important aspect of the treatment of anaphylactic shock. Epinephrine is diluted to 0.1 mg/ml (1:10,000) and administered intravenously at a dose of 0.05–0.1 ml/kg (maximum dose 2 ml). If intravenous administration is impossible, twice the dose can be administered into the trachea. Isotonic fluids (50–150 ml/kg IV) should also be administered over 1–2 hours to maintain blood pressure. Also, to maintain blood pressure, dobutamine (2–5 μg/kg/min IV) should be considered. Bradycardia can be treated with atropine (0.02–0.04 mg/kg IV). Animals that develop pulmonary complications might require treatment with supplemental oxygen and bronchodilators. Short-acting IV glucocorticoids are commonly administered, but evidence to support their use is lacking. Antihistamines are useful in the treatment of local anaphylaxis (angioedema, urticaria, pruritis) but are less effective in treatment of shock owing to slower onset of action and minimal effect on blood pressure. The animal should be hospitalized and closely monitored for 24 hours, because clinical signs can recrudesce during this period.

CASE 201

1 What is tick-borne encephalitis? Tick-borne encephalitis is a viral disease (caused by a flavivirus) of the CNS transmitted by bites of various *Ixodes* ticks. Tick-borne encephalitis virus is transmitted immediately after the tick bite; thus, early removal of ticks does not prevent transmission. The range of tick-borne encephalitis virus spans an area from France and Scandinavia, across Europe (Central European tick-borne encephalitis), to far eastern Russia (Russian spring–summer encephalitis). Dogs become readily infected with tick-borne encephalitis virus but they are considered end-stage hosts. The disease occurs relatively frequently in non-vaccinated people. In contrast, most dogs develop antibodies without clinical signs after infection, but only rarely develop clinical disease. However, if dogs do become ill, the course of disease is usually severe and commonly fatal.

2 What are the typical clinical signs? The incubation period in dogs is up to 2 weeks. Dogs that develop the disease can present with fever, behavior changes, vestibular signs, optic neuritis, ataxia, or tetraparesis, reflecting multifocal lesions in the cerebrum and the brainstem. Most dogs progress to development of motor failure with reduced proprioception and hyporeflexia in the thoracic and/or pelvic limbs.

3 What is the prognosis? The prognosis is very poor. Many dogs will die regardless of medical intervention. The few dogs that survive typically need intensive supportive treatment and a period of 6–12 months for resolution of clinical signs.

Conversion factors

To convert from SI units to Old/conventional units, multiply by the conversion factor.

	SI units	Conversion factor	Old/conventional units
Haematology			
Hematocrit	l/l	100	%
Hemoglobin	mmol/l	1.6113	g/dl
RBCs/erythrocytes	$\times 10^{12}$/l	1	$\times 10^{6}$/µl
Reticulocytes	$\times 10^{9}$/l	n/a	% of RBCs
Platelets	$\times 10^{9}$/l	1,000	/µl
WBCs/leukocytes	$\times 10^{9}$/l	1,000	/µl
Neutrophils	$\times 10^{9}$/l	1,000	/µl
Band neutrophils	$\times 10^{9}$/l	1,000	/µl
Lymphocytes	$\times 10^{9}$/l	1,000	/µl
Basophils	$\times 10^{9}$/l	1,000	/µl
Monocytes	$\times 10^{9}$/l	1,000	/µl
MCV	fl	n/a	fl
MCH	pg	n/a	pg
MCHC	g/l	0.1	g/dl
Biochemistry			
ALP	U/l	1	IU/l
ALT	U/l	1	U/l
Albumin	g/l	0.1	g/dl
Bilirubin	µmol/l	0.058	mg/dl
Calcium	mmol/l	4.008	mg/dl
Chloride	mmol/l	1	mEq/l
Cholesterol	mmol/l	38.67	mg/dl
Creatine kinase (CK)	U/l	1	U/l
Creatinine	µmol/l	0.011	mg/dl
Globulin	g/l	0.1	g/dl
Glucose	mmol/l	18.0	mg/dl
Phosphorus	mmol/l	3.007	mg/dl
Potassium	mmol/l	1	mEq/l
Protein, total	g/l	0.1	g/dl
Sodium	mmol/l	1	mEq/l
Thyroxine (T4)	nmol/l	0.0777	µg/dl
Urea nitrogen	mmol/l	2.8	mg/dl

Index

Note: References are to case numbers, not page numbers.